THE ULTIMATE WOMEN'S GUIDE TO BEATING DISEASE

AND LIVING A HAPPY, ACTIVE LIFE

2025

FROM THE EDITORS OF BOTTOM LINE

Belvoir

**The Ultimate Women's Guide to Beating Disease
and Living a Happy, Active Life**

Bottom Line Books® is an imprint of Belvoir Media Group, LLC.

Belvoir

© 2024 Belvoir Media Group, LLC.

10 9 8 7 6 5 4 3 2 1

All rights reserved. No part of this publication may be reproduced, scanned, distributed or transmitted in any form, by any means, electronic or mechanical, without permission in writing from the publisher. For more information, write to Permissions, Belvoir Media Group, 535 Connecticut Avenue, Norwalk, CT 06854-1713.

ISBN 978-0-88723-032-5

Bottom Line Books® publishes the advice of expert authorities in many fields. These opinions may at times conflict as there are often different approaches to solving problems. The use of this material is no substitute for health, legal, accounting or other professional services. Consult competent professionals for answers to your specific questions.

Telephone numbers, addresses, prices, offers and websites listed in this book are accurate at the time of publication, but they are subject to frequent change.

Bottom Line Books® is a registered trademark of Belvoir Media Group, LLC.
535 Connecticut Avenue, Norwalk, CT 06854-1713

Belvoir.com || BottomLineInc.com

Bottom Line Books® is an imprint of Belvoir Media Group, LLC, publisher of print and digital periodicals, books and online training programs. We are dedicated to bringing you the best information from the most knowledgeable sources in the world. Our goal is to help you gain greater wealth, better health, more wisdom, extra time and increased happiness.

Printed in the United States of America

CONTENTS

Preface xi

1 • AGE WELL: STAYING YOUNGER LONGER

The Longevity Diet: How to Eat for
  a Long, Healthy Life 1
Obesity Worsens Menopause Symptoms 3
Anti-Aging Serums—Worth the Hype? 3
New Drug for Hot Flashes 4
Pursue a Positive Purpose for a Longer Life 4
Longevity Strategies from a
  102-Year-Old Doctor 5
Depression Hastens Aging 6
Stress Can Help You Live Longer 7
Learning Multiple New Skills Can Improve
  Cognition in Older Adults 8
Show Your Hands Some TLC 9
Could Your Hand Stiffness
  Be Dupuytren's? 10
The Four Fitness Tests That Matter 11
Resources for Older Drivers 12
Bursts of Activity Help You Live Longer 13
Addressing Droopy Eyelids 13
Medications That May Cause
  Eyelid Drooping 14
Options to Treat Age-Related Macular
  Degeneration 14
Foods to Boost Eyesight 15
Preventing Major Eye Diseases 17
ARMD vs. Cataracts 17
Nearsightedness and Dry Eye Are
  Linked to Screen Time 18
Stuck Stem Cells Responsible for Gray Hair ... 18
That Bump on the Head May Be a Bigger
  Problem Than You Think 18
Eye Drops for AMD 19
How to Protect Yourself from
  Noise Pollution 21
Braces Are for Grown-Ups, Too 23
Now Don't Hear This 23
Self-Directed Ageism Causes Real Harm 24
Finding a Caregiver 24
Confused by Medigap? What You
  Need to Know 24
Don't Take Metformin to Boost Longevity 25
We Do Mellow with Age 26
Medicare Advantage Ads May
  Be Misleading 26
Free University Tuition for Older Students ... 27
Exposure to Microplastics May Lead
  to Behavioral Changes in Older Adults 27
Older Drivers with ADHD Have
  More Accidents 27
Seniors: Be Careful with Cannabis Products ... 28
Our Body Temperature Changes 28
Digestive Health and Loneliness 29
Babies and Pets Help the Aging Brain 29

2 • BRAIN HEALTH

Exciting Developments in
  Alzheimer's Research 31

Contents

Hormone-Replacement Therapy: The Earlier the Better to Protect Against Alzheimer's ... 33
Does COVID Increase Alzheimer's Risk? 33
Can You Reduce Your Risk of AD? 34
For Cognitive Benefit, Dancing Beats the Treadmill 34
Take Steps to Avoid Dementia 34
Warning Signs to Discuss with Your Doctor 36
New Risk Factors for Early Dementia 36
Belly Fat Link to Alzheimer's Disease 36
Certain Vaccines Lower Alzheimer's Risk 37
Heart Health = Brain Health 37
Multivitamin Reduces Age-Related Memory Decline 38
Proceed with Caution with the Direct-to-Consumer Alzheimer's Disease Blood Test ... 39
Should You Get a Cognition Test? 39
Alzheimer's Spotted During Eye Exam 40
Scents May Boost Memory 40
What Is Frontotemporal Dementia? 40
Who's at Risk? 42
Coping with a Dementia Diagnosis 42
Where Can Families Find Help? 43
Don't Forgo Laxatives for Fear of Dementia 44
Brain Health in a Bottle? 44
Proven Ways to Protect Cognition 45
Saunas May Help Head Off Alzheimer's 46
Another Promising Alzheimer's Drug 46
Positive Thinking May Reverse Mild Cognitive Impairment 46
Traumatic Brain Injury May Become a Chronic Condition 46
How Diet Affects Your Brain 47
Freezing Up: What Does It Mean? 47
Don't Delay, Call 911 48
Mediterranean Diet May Improve Memory in People with MS 49
Traffic Noise Increases Risk of Tinnitus 50
Turn Down the Volume on Tinnitus 50
Can CBD Help Tinnitus? 51
Ultrasound May Treat Parkinson's Symptoms 52
Parkinson's Disease Linked to Mitochondria 52
Head Pain When Bending Down 53
Brain-Computer Interface Translates Brain Signals to Speech 53
Bad Air Affects Brain Health 53
Internet Use Is Linked to Lower Dementia Risk 54
Controlling Light Exposure May Help Sundowning 54

3 • CANCER BREAKTHROUGHS

How to Catch Cancer Early 55
The Next Generation in Screening: Multi-Cancer Early Detection Tests 57
Air Pollution Increases Breast Cancer Risk 58
Artificial Intelligence Can Predict Breast Cancer Chemotherapy Outcomes 59
A False-Positive Is a Cancer Warning 59
Which Women Benefit from Medication for Breast Cancer Prevention 60
Why Breast Cancer Survival Has Improved ... 61
Artificial Sweetener May Increase Cancer Risk 62
Get a Second Opinion for Cancer Diagnosis 63
Does Eating Organic Foods Protect You from Cancer? 63
Red Meat and Dairy Appear Protective Against Cancer 63
Weight-Loss Surgery in Women Reduces Blood Cancer Risk 63
How to Survive the No. 2 Cause of Death in America 65
Liquid Biopsy for Lung Cancer 65
Mortality Risk from Lung Cancer May Be Cut in Half 66
Skin Cancer—Not a Deadly Diagnosis Anymore 67
Nail-Gel Dryers Boost Cancer Risk 67
The ABCs of Melanomas 68
Ultra-Processed Foods Linked to Higher Cancer Risks 69
Food Wrappers Contain Dangerous Chemicals 70
Cancer Treatment Gets Personal 70
Common Biomarkers 71
The Thymus Is Important After All 72
Alternatives to Colonoscopy 72
Colorectal Cancer Is Skewing Younger 73
New Diabetes Drugs Can Reduce Risk of Colon Cancer 73
For Treating Some Cancers, Less May Be More 74
Don't Trust ChatGPT for Cancer Information 74

4 • DIABETES BREAKTHROUGHS AND BLOOD SUGAR CONTROL

How to Reverse Prediabetes............................. 75
Testing for Prediabetes 76
The Cause of Prediabetes 77
Red, Purple, Blue Foods Reduce
  Risk of Diabetes 78
Easy, Delicious Low-Carb,
  Low-Sugar Recipes 78
High Doses of Vitamin D Slash
  Diabetes Risk... 80
Phthalate Exposure Is Associated with
  Diabetes, Endocrine Disorders.................... 80
Women Who Are "Night Owls" Are at
  Higher Risk for Diabetes 80
Just a Little Sleep Loss Affects Diabetes
  Risk in Women 81
The Skinny on Sugar 82
More Evidence of Sugar's Harm..................... 84
Non-Sugar Sweeteners Won't Help
  You Lose Weight.. 84
Are Sugar Alcohols Safe for Diabetics?........... 84
What You Drink Has a Major
  Health Impact.. 85
Type 2 Diabetes Can Directly Cause
  Lung Complications 85
Bariatric Surgery Improves Neuropathy......... 85
Afternoon Exercise Is Better for
  Blood Sugar... 85
COVID Still Increases Diabetes Risk 86
Older Diabetes Patients Face
  Growing Cancer Risk................................. 86
Plastic Chemicals Are Linked to
  Diabetes Risk... 86
Diabetes and Frozen Shoulder 86
Stress Link to Metabolic Syndrome................ 87
Can Foot-Warming Socks Relieve
  Foot Neuropathy? 87
Your Voice May Indicate Diabetes 88

5 • EMOTIONAL RESCUE

A Better Marriage Means Better Health 89
Oh, Brother (or Sister)................................... 91
Gardening Lifts the Spirits 92
Drug Add-on Boosts
  Antidepressant Effects 93
Seven Habits to Fight Depression 94
Nondrug DIY Treatments for
  Depression All Backed by Research 94
Can Probiotics Help Depression? 96
The Rising Risk of Suicide............................. 96
Watch for Your Loved Ones........................... 97
Finding the Mental Health Help You
  Need…When You Need It......................... 99
New Therapy for Depression—ADepT 100
Depression Doesn't Affect All
  Aspects of Life... 101
The Disease of Loneliness 101
When Your Fear Is Actually a Phobia…
  and What to Do About It 102
To Combat Your Mind's Negative Chatter.... 104
Success Secrets from a 78-Year-Old
  Ironman World Champion....................... 104
To-Do Items Can Be Threats for
  People with Task Paralysis 106
Breath Work Improves Mood and
  Reduces Anxiety...................................... 106
How to Beat Medical-Test Anxiety................ 106
Crying Is Good for You 106
Recovering Your Mental Health After
  a Medical Emergency 107
What Not to Do When You're
  Stressed Out 107
Reminiscence Therapy Benefits
  Older Adults 108
Hyperbaric Oxygen for Opioid Addiction.... 109
Cannabis-Use Disorder Is Linked to
  Schizophrenia Risk 109
Forgotten Courtesies We All Need
  to Practice 109
Stress Really Does Make Your Hair Gray 109
How to Benefit from Pet Therapy................. 110
Food and Mood 111
Colorful Environments Boost Mood 112

6 • FOOD, DIET, AND FITNESS

Finding the Best Weight-Loss Program
  for You 113
10 Tips for MediterAsian Eating 115
Dieters Beware... 115
5 Percent Weight Loss Improves Health 116
To Maintain Weight Loss, Sleep Matters....... 116
Artificial Sweeteners Are Fattening 117
The USDA's MyPlate Should Not Be
  Your Plate 117
Secret Superfoods 118
Foods You Should Refrigerate 120
Low-Calorie Sugar Substitute Danger 120
Skip the Banana to Boost Flavanols 120
Almonds Keep Your Gut Healthy 121
Fiber Makes You Fuller, Especially
  This One 121

Contents

Kidney Beans Caution 121
Most Eco-Friendly Straws Contain
  Toxic Chemicals 122
Revisiting Dairy.................................... 122
Common Beverages Contain Toxic Metals ... 123
Dairy Is Not for Everyone...................... 123
Should You Go Gluten-Free? 124
Most Healthful Deli Meat Options 125
Truffles Are Worth a Try 126
The Health Benefits of Eating Insects 126
Easy Egg Substitutes 126
Should Your Oil Be Cold-Pressed
  or Refined?................................... 126
Don't Throw Out Overripe Avocados........... 127
Choose Your Chocolate Carefully 127
The World's Most Nutritious Vegetable......... 127
The Best Rx: Take a Walk 128
When You Exercise Affects Weight Loss 130
Water Workout.................................... 130
Simple Exercises for Strength and
  Energy…In Just 6 Minutes 133
11 Minutes of Activity to Lower
  Disease Risk 135
8,000 Is the New 10,000…Steps, That Is...... 136
Exercises to Improve Your Balance 136
Get the Most from a Standing Desk............ 138
Offset Sitting with Just a Little Exercise 138
Women Need Less Exercise Than Men 139
Difficulty Walking Predicts Higher
  Fracture Risk 140
Running Doesn't Harm Your Knees—
  It Protects Them 140

7 • GET THE BEST MEDICAL CARE

Depersonalized Health Care 141
Shop Around for Care........................... 142
Medical Gaslighting: Don't Let Your
  Doctor Dismiss Your Symptoms 142
When to Go to the Emergency Room........... 144
Don't Drive Yourself to the ER.................. 146
Beware These Risks When You're
  in the Hospital................................ 146
Take Care at Urgent Care Centers 147
Private Equity Increases Adverse Events 149
Understand What Your Medical
  Specialist Does 149
Micro Hospitals—A Growing Trend 149
Home Medical Essentials 150
Limitations of the Apple Watch..................152
Beware of Oxygen Machines Sold Online 152
Health Screening Tests...........................152

Take Your Temperature with Your Phone.... 153
Genetic Testing and Medication.................. 153
Genetic Testing and Your Current Drug
  Intake 155
Is Your Medicine in Short Supply? 155
The New Obesity Drugs: Is One Right
  for You?.. 157
Compounded Obesity Drug Is a Bad Idea ... 159
Unsafe Supplements............................. 159
Antibiotic Overuse Can Be Harmful............ 160
The Dangers of Polypharmacy.................. 161
If You're Taking a Drug, Don't Take
  This Herb...................................... 162
Some of Your Meds May Cause
  Hearing Loss.................................. 163
What Triggers a Drug-Drug Interaction? 163
New Safety Warnings on Opioid Pain
  Medicines..................................... 164
High-Intensity Interval Training (HIIT)
  Before Surgery Can Speed Recovery 164
For Hip Replacement, Pay Attention to
  the Surgeon's Level of Experience 165
You Could Be Rejected by a Hospital
  or Surgeon 165
Doctor Dilemmas 165
Were Your Medical Records Stolen?............ 166
Watch Out for Medical Billing Scams 166
Beware Special Financing for Health Care... 166
Less Expensive Medical Care from Costco... 166
10 Drugs Medicare Will Negotiate 167
Watch Out for the Sun If You Take
  These Drugs 167
Are Steroid Drugs Safe? 167
Did You Take Zantac? What You
  Need to Know 167
Lifestyle Changes for Heartburn 168
How Safe Are Proton Pump Inhibitors? 168
Time to Talk to Your Doctor 169
How to Create Your Family
  Medical History 170
What Is Palliative Care? 171

8 • HEART AND STROKE HEALTH

Understanding and Preventing
  Heart Attacks................................. 173
Certain Heart Attacks Affect Women
  More Than Men............................. 175
When Your Heart Skips a Beat 175
Stress and Insomnia Could Increase A-Fib
  Risk After Menopause...................... 175
Atrial Fibrillation and PVCs 176

Early Cardiac Arrest Warning Signs 177
A Keto Diet Could Hurt Your Heart 177
Should You Treat High Triglycerides? 177
Nearly One-Quarter of Coronary
    Stents Are Unnecessary 179
500 Steps Lowers Heart Disease Risk 179
Climb Stairs for Your Heart 179
Couples' Guide to Keeping Your
    Heart Healthy 179
Plant-Based Diet for a Healthy Heart 180
Heart Shape Predicts Risk 181
Beyond Pacemakers 181
You Can Save a Life 183
How Cardiac Arrest Is Treated 184
Hypertension in Women Linked
    to Insomnia 184
Keep Your Blood Pressure Under Control ... 185
What Makes Your Blood Pressure Rise 186
Don't Put a Saltshaker on Your Table 188
Is It Safe to Take Glucosamine If You
    Also Take a Diuretic? 188
Cut Salt, Cut Blood Pressure 188
High Blood Pressure When Lying Down 188
Fluctuations in Cholesterol
    Increase Dementia Risk 189
Another Statin Alternative
    Proves Effective 189
Weight-Loss Drug Improves Cardio
    Outcomes 189
Shingles and Your Heart 189
What Is Shingles? 190
Other Risks from Shingles 191
Biologic Therapy for Psoriasis
    May Reduce Heart Disease 191
The Cardiovascular Risks of Psoriasis 191
Cardiac Stents Work for Stable Angina 193
Cognitive Decline Is Common
    After Bypass Surgery 194
Ablation Protects the Brain 194
Essential Activities for Post-Stroke
    Recovery 194
Your Gut and Sleep Patterns
    Affect Stroke Risk 195
Get the Care You Need 196
Radon Exposure May Increase Stroke
    Risk in Women 196
A-Fib Affects Your Cognitive Health Even
    Without a Stroke 197
What You Can Do to Reduce Risk
    of Heart Disease 197

9 • INFECTIOUS DISEASE

Pneumonia: Prevention Is Your
    Top Priority 199
Painkillers Can Make Infections
    Last Longer 201
Shingles Vaccine Reduces
    Dementia Risk 201
COVID-Negative Long Haulers 202
Healthy Lifestyle May Protect Against
    Long COVID 203
Sleep Well to Stop Long COVID 203
Patient Beware: Hospital Acquired
    Infections 204
Fungal Infections on the Rise 205
Natural Medicine and Respiratory
    Syncytial Virus 207
RSV Vaccine Is Available 207
More Severe Strep Throat 208
When Are You No Longer Contagious? 208
Travel Health: How to Keep It in Check 209
First-Aid Basics for Travel 210
Managing Motion Sickness 211
Infections May Worsen Cognition 211
Best Foods to Eat After a Stomach Virus 211
Lesser-Known Tickborne Illnesses
    Are Spreading Fast 212
Why You're a Mosquito Magnet 212
Mosquitos Like Red! 212
Beware Malaria 212

10 • KIDNEY, BLADDER, AND LIVER HEALTH

Your Kidneys Are Fragile 213
Added Salt Linked to CKD 215
Is Your Chicken Dinner Causing
    Your UTI? 215
First New Antibiotic for Urinary
    Tract Infections 216
Keep Your Gallbladder Healthy 217
GLP1 Agonists May Be Good for the Liver... 219

11 • NATURAL REMEDIES AND SUPPLEMENTS

The Power of Prebiotics 221
Disease-Busting Prebiotics 223
Ginger Stimulates the Immune System 224
The Pet Prescription 224
Preparing for a Pet 225
Supplements: An Inflation-Friendly
    Nutrition Strategy 226
Be Selective About Supplements 228

Contents

The Sunshine Vitamin: Vitamin D Is Even
  More Important Than You Think 228
Best Ways to Get Your Vitamin D 229
Benefits from Specific Kinds of Massage 231
You Need More Procyanidins....................... 231
Herbs for Stress 231
Should You Drink More Red Wine? 232
The Good Medicine of Onions...................... 234
Does Melatonin Really Help You Sleep?....... 235
Inhaling Fragrances During Sleep
  Boosts Memory 236
Look to Bees to Boost Your Health 236

12 • PAIN RELIEF AND AUTOIMMUNE DISEASE

The Pain Gap: Women Experience
  More Pain Than Men 237
New Nasal Spray for Migraine Approved
  by the FDA 239
New Ways to Fight Migraine Pain 239
Pain on the Brain 239
You Don't Have to Live with Chronic Pain ... 241
To Treat Sunburn Pain… 242
Breakthrough Therapies for Chronic Pain..... 244
Halt Lower Back Pain with Exercise 244
Spinal Cord Stimulation Does Not
  Provide Long-Term Relief 245
5 Strategies to Protect Your Back 245
When Is the Right Time for Back Surgery? .. 247
Causes of Back Pain 247
Tummy Troubles 249
Could Your Stomach Pain Be a
  Heart Attack? 250
When Is Constipation Pain Serious? 251
Food Dye Can Trigger IBS............................ 251
Exercise Eases Arthritis Pain 251
Ginger Fights Autoimmune Symptoms 252
Music Soothes Pain 253
Is It Gout…or Pseudogout?.......................... 253
Give Foot Pain the Boot 253
Knee Arthritis: Questioning the
  Standard of Care 256

13 • PHYSICAL INJURY AND BONE HEALTH

Getting a Grip on Carpal Tunnel
  Syndrome 257
Walking a Leashed Dog
  Can Be Dangerous 258
Are You Getting the Right Bone
  Density Test? 259
Preventing Carpal Tunnel Pain 259
Osteoporosis Is Underdiagnosed 260
Yes…Yoga Can Make Your Bones Strong 261
12 Bone-Centric Yoga Poses......................... 262
Beyond Calcium: Minerals That
  Protect Bone Density 264
7 Things You Are Doing Wrong
  When Exercising 264
Prep Your Joints for Chilly Weather 267
When to Get Guidance for Injuries 267
Keep Yourself Safe: Top 10 Winter
  Hazards… 268
Replace Old Fire Extinguishers—
  Even If Unused 268
SUV, Pickup Truck Blind Spots Put
  Pedestrians at Risk 269
Choose the Best Footwear to Protect
  Against Winter Falls 270
TLC for Chronic Wounds 270
The Healing Power of Hyperbaric
  Oxygen Therapy 271

14 • RESPIRATORY HEALTH AND ALLERGIES

COPD Deaths Are Rising in Women 273
Misdiagnosis of COPD in Women 274
A New Breathing Device Improves
  COPD Breathlessness 275
Beetroot Juice Beneficial for
  People with COPD 275
Halt a Lingering Cough 275
New Strategy for Severe Asthma 276
Poor Sleep May Increase the
  Risk of Asthma 277
CPAP Mask Comparison 277
Persistent Asthma May Increase
  Stroke Risk 277
Airway Mechanics 278
Mouth Exercises That Reduce Snoring 278
Bet You Know Someone Who
  Still Smokes 279
Cannabis Concerns...................................... 280
The Reward for Quitting............................... 281
DIY Ways to Quit Vaping 281
Stuffy Air Can Give You Brain Fog 282
You Probably Have "Screen Apnea" 282
How to Prepare for Allergy Season 282
Don't Sleep with a Fan If You
  Have Allergies 284
Natural Ways to Beat Sinusitis 284

Double Check on a Penicillin Allergy 285
Plants Improve Indoor Air Quality 286

15 • SLEEP AND RESTORATIVE HEALTH

Countdown to Your Best Night's Sleep 287
What Is the Ideal Sleeping Temperature? 288
Best Cooling Pillows 288
Some Like It Hot, Some Like It Cold 289
Proven! You Can Think Your Way
  to Better Health 291
The Strangest Sleep Disorder:
  Sleep Paralysis 293
Yes...You Can Fix Your Genes 294
Go to the Beach for Your Health 296
Living in Harmony with the Seasons 297
The Time of Your Life 299
SCN: The Master Clock 300
App to Find Rainbows! 301
Secrets to Slowing Down the Clock 301
The Best Times...to Exercise...Nap...
  Take Medication...and More 303
Are You Sleepy...or Tired? 305
Cannabis Might Not Improve Sleep 306

16 • VERY PERSONAL

Breast Reduction Surgery Helps More
  Than Appearance 307
For Many Women, Pain During Sex
  Is Treatable 308
Even Older Adults Can Get STIs 308
Cannabis Might Improve Sex 309
How to Discuss STI Testing with
  a New Partner 309
Reading Erotica Can Rekindle Romance 310
Sex Before Bed Works as Well as
  Sleeping Pills 310
Intimacy and Relationship Status 310
Skin Lightening Products Can
  Be Dangerous 310
Battling Bloat 311
FODMAPs to Avoid 312
A Vibrating Capsule Can Treat
  Constipation Without Drugs 312
Natural Ways to Treat Irritable
  Bowel Syndrome 312
Laxative Shortage Tied to Hybrid Work 314
When Varicose Veins Cause Pain 314
Index 315

PREFACE

We are proud to bring to you *The Ultimate Women's Guide to Beating Disease and Living a Happy, Active Life 2025*. This essential volume features trustworthy and actionable life-saving information from the best health experts in the world—information that will help women beat the most deadly conditions. In the following chapters, you'll find the latest discoveries, best treatments, and scientifically proven remedies to keep you living a long, happy, and active life.

Whether it's heart care, the latest on breast cancer prevention and treatment, breakthrough treatments for hot flashes or cutting-edge nutritional advice, the editors at Bottom Line Books talk to the experts—from top women's health doctors to research scientists to leading alternative care practitioners—who are creating the true innovations in health care.

Over the past four decades, we have built a network of literally thousands of leading physicians in both alternative and conventional medicine. They are affiliated with the premier medical and research institutions throughout the world. We read the important medical journals and follow the latest research that is reported at medical conferences. And we regularly talk to our advisors in major teaching hospitals, private practices and government health agencies for their insider perspective.

In this 2025 edition, we've gone beyond diseases and have included additional chapters of life-enhancing information on fitness, nutrition, mental health, sleep habits, quality medical care, pain relief, and aging...all of which are essential to living a happy, active life. And it's all backed by breaking studies and top health experts.

The Ultimate Women's Guide to Beating Disease and Living a Happy, Active Life 2025 is a result of our ongoing research and connection with these experts, and is a distillation of their latest findings and advice. We trust that you will glean new, helpful, and affordable information about the health topics that concern you most...and find vital topics of interest to family and friends as well.

As a reader of a Bottom Line book, be assured that you are receiving well-researched information from a trusted source. But please use prudence in health matters. Always speak to your physician before taking vitamins, supplements, or over-the-counter medication...stopping a medication...changing your diet...or beginning an exercise program. If you experience side effects from any regimen, contact your doctor immediately.

Be well,
The Editors, Bottom Line Books
BottomLineInc.com

Chapter 1

AGE WELL: STAYING YOUNGER LONGER

The Longevity Diet: How to Eat for a Long, Healthy Life

Want to extend your life for a few more years? Then consider eating what the longest-lived populations on the planet eat! Scattered around the globe are a handful of "Blue Zones," regions where life spans are impressively long—Ikaria, Greece...Nicoya, Costa Rica...Okinawa, Japan...Sardinia, Italy...and the Seventh Day Adventist community in Loma Linda, California. There are more 100-year-olds in these areas than anywhere else, and their rates of heart disease, dementia, and diabetes are a fraction of those in the overall U.S. Genetics alone do not explain this longevity. People living in these communities consume diets that help them live long lives.

Recent research suggests that the rest of us might be able to live significantly longer, too, if we ate the way they do—potentially 10.7 years longer for women (13 years longer for men), according to a team at Norway's University of Bergen. Substantial longevity gains appear feasible even for people who have consumed a typical Western diet for many decades—up to perhaps 8.8 extra years for those who make these eating changes at age 60...or 3.5 years at age 80.

How do you get started? *Here are key Blue Zone dietary guidelines, based on an analysis of more than 150 surveys...*

• **Eat more plants and less meat.** Blue Zone dining does not require you to become a vegetarian, but it does mean eating a lot less meat than the average American does. The diets of people in these long-lived communities are at least 90 percent plant based, and they consume meat only five times per month or less. By comparison, people in the U.S. consume meat five times a week, on average.

Despite what many meat fans fear, switching to a plant-focused diet does not doom you to disappointing dining. Americans often are less than thrilled when they first attempt to cook without meat. But that's not

---

Dan Buettner, founder of Blue Zones, an organization that works with governments, employers and health insurance companies to promote longer, healthier, happier lives. He is a National Geographic Fellow and author of several books, including *The Blue Zones American Kitchen: 100 Recipes to Live to 100*. DanBuettner.com

because plant-based dishes can't be tasty. It's because people who have been eating mostly meat-based meals their whole lives often lack experience preparing plant-based dishes. Keep at it for a few months and experiment with a wide range of recipes from around the world, and you will discover plant-based dishes that you love.

Another meat-eater fear—that a plant-based diet won't provide enough protein—also is inaccurate. Plenty of plants are excellent sources of protein, including broccoli, spinach, and beans.

Helpful: Meat fans who think they dislike tofu might try cooking with extra-firm tofu, which is popular in Okinawa, Japan. It replicates meat's texture better than other, softer tofu varieties.

Also: Cooking in a healthful fat can make plant-based dishes more satisfying. Olive oil, popular in Ikaria, is among the healthiest fats—drizzle it over vegetables… and/or use it to sauté ingredients at temperatures no higher than 350°F.

• **Limit fish consumption.** Surprisingly, the longest-lived populations tend to consume no more than three servings of fish per week—even though most of them are located near coasts. This might come as a surprise, since seafood is considered a healthy alternative to meat. When Blue Zone communities do consume fish, it tends to be relatively small fish from the middle of the ocean food chain, such as sardines and anchovies. Ocean predators such as swordfish can contain troublingly high levels of mercury, among other dangers.

• **Reduce dairy and egg consumption.** In the U.S., milk and eggs often are presented as ultra-healthy protein sources, but that's largely because these products have extensive lobbying and marketing campaigns. In fact, no Blue Zone community consumes much cow's milk. Goat and sheep milk do have a place in Sardinian and Ikarian diets, but largely in the form of cheese and yogurt. It is not common in these cultures to drink a glass of any type of milk.

Eggs play only a modest role in Blue Zone diets—people in these places eat eggs only two to four times per week, on average, and the eggs they consume are inevitably from free-range chickens.

• **Drink water, coffee, red wine, and/or tea.** People in Blue Zones drink little or no soda. But they do consume a rich range of beverages—in addition to water, many of them enjoy coffee, red wine and tea (typically green or herbal) virtually every day. Nutritionists have been debating the healthfulness of coffee and red wine for years, but the fact that the people who live the longest drink lots of these seems like compelling evidence that, on balance, they must not be too bad for us.

• **Eat beans.** Blue Zone populations often eat a cup of beans per day. Beans have more nutrients per gram than any food group…are wonderful sources of protein and complex carbohydrates…and are so fiber-rich and satisfying that they reduce the temptation to overeat. Experiment with a range of beans—in Nicoya they often use black beans…in Okinawa, it's soybeans… and in Ikaria and Sardinia, favorites include garbanzos, white beans, and lentils.

Helpful: Add beans to your diet slowly to reduce the odds of digestive distress. Seasoning bean-based dishes with turmeric, ginger, and/or fennel also helps control this problem.

• **Make nuts a go-to snack.** Any diet plan that requires you not to snack is likely to fail. Instead, replace life-shortening snacks with one that extends lives—eat two to four ounces of nuts each day. Nut consumption is common in Blue Zones—almonds are favored in Ikaria and Sardinia, and pistachios in Nicoya. A study of nearly 100,000 members of the Seventh Day Adventist Church by researchers at Loma Linda University concluded that nut eaters outlived people who don't eat nuts in that community by an average of two to three years.

• **Eat naturally sweet foods…skip sugar-added foods.** Blue Zone populations don't avoid sweet foods—they just choose naturally sweet fruit rather than sugar-added snack products. Based on the eating habits of these long-lived populations, it seems that we can treat ourselves to more or less all the fruit we want without shortening our lives.

Blue Zone diets tend to include no more than seven teaspoons of added sugar per day, one-fifth of what the average American consumes. Much of the added sugar consumed in these regions is stirred into coffee or tea. Blue Zone groups eat virtually no processed snack foods.

•**Choose either sourdough or whole-grain bread.** Most bread sold in the U.S. is made from bleached white flour, which the body metabolizes into sugar. It has been linked to higher risk for life-shortening health issues including obesity and diabetes. People in Blue Zones favor sourdough or whole-grain bread. Several studies, including one by researchers at Canada's University of Guelph, have found that sourdough has a low glycemic index, meaning that it helps keep blood sugar levels in check. Whole-grain breads, such as whole wheat, are high in healthful fiber.

Warning: Many breads marketed as "sourdough" are not baked using the lactobacilli that sets true sourdough bread apart...and some breads marketed as "whole grain" or "whole wheat" are not really 100 percent whole grain. Either bake these breads yourself—Breadtopia.com is a good place to find recipes—or buy from a highly regarded local bakery, and ask for confirmation that it's a true sourdough or 100% whole-grain bread.

•**Eat foods that look like what they looked like on the farm.** The majority of the food consumed in Blue Zones enters people's kitchens looking more or less like a part of a plant—or, less often, a part of an animal—straight from a farm.

Obesity Worsens Menopause Symptoms

Menopause.

Women with obesity experience more menopausal symptoms and get less relief from hormone therapy than women without obesity, according to a small, retrospective study. Women with obesity were more likely to report vasomotor symptoms, genitourinary/vulvovaginal symptoms, mood disturbances, and decreased libido. They were much less likely to see a satisfying reduction in their menopausal symptoms with the use of hormone therapy. Among the 20 women receiving systemic hormone therapy in the study, only one of the 12 with obesity reported improvement in symptoms, compared with seven of eight women without obesity. Among 33 women using localized hormone therapy, 46 percent of the 24 women with obesity vs. 89 percent of the nine women without obesity experienced symptom improvement.

Anti-Aging Serums— Worth the Hype?

Angela J. Lamb, MD, board-certified dermatologist and associate professor of dermatology at Icahn School of Medicine at Mount Sinai in New York City. Icahn.MSSM.edu

Sales of anti-aging serums are expected to triple in the next 10 years to $150 million. There already are thousands of over-the-counter products making promises of fewer lines and wrinkles. How do you decide which one to try? *Start by looking for these key ingredients in the formula, says dermatologist Angela J. Lamb, MD...*

•**Retinol.** This is a mild retinoid derived from vitamin A. Retinoids can brighten skin and ease the appearance of fine lines. The topical retinoid with the best anti-aging properties is tretinoin (Retin-A), available by prescription. It has been proven to increase cell turnover and stimulate collagen to refresh the skin.

I like: Philosophy Ultimate Miracle Worker Fix Face Serum Roller Uplift & Firm, which also contains hyaluronic acid and glycolic acid.

For sensitive skin: An alternative is bakuchiol, made from the seeds of the babchi plant.

I like: Bakuchiol Retinol Alternative Smoothing Serum from Herbivore Botanicals.

• **Hyaluronic acid.** This substance, found naturally in the body, can plump skin from the outside, easing lines and wrinkles and creating a dewy look.

I like: Hyaluronic Acid Intensifier from SkinCeuticals.

• **Ferulic acid.** This powerful antioxidant protects skin from free radicals in the environment and, when included in formulas with vitamins C and E, can intensify anti-aging effects.

I like: C E Ferulic from SkinCeuticals.

• **Copper peptides.** Copper has anti-inflammatory properties to help skin heal, and it can boost collagen, make skin more supple and soften wrinkles.

I like: Bioevolve Serum with a copper peptide complex and various botanicals from Veracity.

• **Glycolic acid.** One of the milder alpha-hydroxy acids, it helps exfoliate dead skin cells and boosts skin tone along with texture.

I like: Regenerating Infusion with 8% glycolic acid, niacinamide (vitamin B-3) and benthi plant peptides (another retinol alternative) from Veracity.

Get the Most from Your Serum

• **Aim for consistency.** You won't see a dramatic improvement after just one week, but over time, you'll notice better texture, tone and light reflection.

• **Cost contributes to effectiveness.** Higher prices often reflect active ingredients with a higher potency or better-quality antioxidants than less expensive brands.

When You Need More Than Serum

If topicals just aren't enough, ask your dermatologist about treatments. Lasers are great for natural-looking rejuvenation—they help your skin rebuild collagen and stimulate regrowth. Next in line are muscle-relaxing injections, such as Botox, and fillers, such as Restylane, that bolster collagen.

New Drug for Hot Flashes

Chrisandra Shufelt, MD, associate director of Women's Health Research Center and chair of the general internal medicine division at Mayo Clinic, Jacksonville, Florida. MayoClinic.org

The FDA has approved *fezolinetant* (Veozah), the first non-hormonal medication for menopausal hot flashes and night sweats. The drug, which blocks brain receptors involved in regulating body temperature, is an option for women who can't or choose not to use menopausal hormone therapy (HT).

Pursue a Positive Purpose for a Longer Life

Cynthia Covey Haller, oldest daughter of Stephen R. Covey. She is coauthor of *Live Life in Crescendo*. FranklinCovey.com

A study involving more than 43,000 elderly Japanese people found that those who practiced *ikigai*—a philosophy of developing positive purpose and a sense of satisfaction—were significantly less likely to die during the following seven years than those who did not. Other researchers have found links between being motivated to achieve a purpose and reduced rates of depression…and between believing one's life has meaning and lower rates of cancer and heart disease.

Yes, it's true that caring deeply about something also can bring stress (for more on how stress can help you, see page 7)—but despite what many people believe, stress is not a killer. One study by Stanford University researchers that tracked participants for more than eight decades—from childhood until death—concluded that carefree people tend to die sooner than those who push themselves to reach goals. The moderate stress that might come from pushing oneself to do something meaningful is more likely to extend your life than shorten it.

Longevity Strategies from a 102-Year-Old Doctor

Gladys McGarey, MD, cofounder and past president of the organization now known as the Academy of Integrative Health and Medicine and author of *The Well-Lived Life: A 102-Year-Old Doctor's Six Secrets to Health and Happiness at Every Age*. GladysMcGarey.com

Gladys McGarey, MD, has a very busy professional life. A pioneer in the holistic medicine movement, she offers life consultations…is working to launch a "village for living medicine"…and recently authored a book. What might surprise you is that she is…102 years old! *We asked Dr. McGarey to share her strategies for living a long, healthy and productive life…*

•**Walk even when walking isn't easy…move even when you sit.** The mobility challenges that come with age are not a valid excuse for becoming sedentary. These days, I get my daily 3,800 steps with the help of a walker…and I ride an adult tricycle rather than a bicycle. I'm often in motion even when I'm not going anywhere—wiggling around in a chair is better for the body than total stillness. Analysis of data from the large-scale UK Women's Cohort Study found that habitually sitting for more than seven hours a day significantly increases overall mortality risk…except among people who frequently fidget.

•**Eat a diet that leaves you feeling healthy—but don't deprive yourself of foods you love.** Most days I eat a high-fiber breakfast of raisin bran and prune juice, salad for lunch and soup for dinner. I don't do this because studies say eating light is a path to longevity—I do it because I feel my best when I eat this way. There is no secret ingredient or vitamin supplement that unlocks a long healthy life—the key is to pay close attention to how you feel when you're eating in a particular way, then settle on foods, portion sizes, and other eating habits that make your body feel its best.

Of course, eating isn't only about giving the body what it needs—I eat cake and chocolate sometimes, too, and I drink a cup of coffee every morning. These are things I enjoy, and in moderation they don't make my body feel noticeably worse.

•**Get in touch with other people…literally.** I hug loved ones as often as I can. Physical touch is comforting and good for our health. A study by researchers at Carnegie Mellon University found that hugging reduces the odds of contracting respiratory infections, perhaps because physical contact reduces stress and stress can reduce the effectiveness of the immune system. If daily hugs with loved ones aren't an option, get a pet…or if you can't care for a pet, get a houseplant. Researchers at Korea's Chungnam National University found that simply repotting a houseplant reduces stress and lowers blood pressure.

I get a full-body massage every week, too. Massage doesn't just feel good. It stimulates the lymphatic system, which plays an important role in keeping the body healthy. A study by researchers at Cedars-Sinai Medical Center found that even a single massage session measurably improves lymphatic system function.

• **Pay attention to your body's aches and pains.** When something hurts, it's tempting to take a painkiller to make the discomfort go away. When muscles feel weak, it's tempting to take it easy on them. But pain and muscle fatigue are messages from the body. When we take painkillers or ease up on weak muscles without first considering what that message is trying to tell us, we fail to solve our body's underlying problem…and often end up feeling even worse.

Example: My bedroom is at the top of a staircase. When I'm tired, walking up those stairs can be difficult. But I've learned that when I skip the stairs and rest downstairs, it's even more difficult to climb those stairs the next day. My body is sending me a message—I have to climb stairs regularly, or I may lose my ability to do so at all.

• **Have a 10-year plan at any age.** Having a long-term plan means having a purpose—and having a purpose is among the keys to remaining mentally and physically healthy as we age. A recent study by researchers at University of Michigan confirmed that having a strong life purpose is associated with lower mortality rates among people over age 50. My current 10-year plan is to create a "village for living medicine," featuring a birthing center and a research facility.

It can be tempting to choose shorter, more easily achieved plans, but those soon will be completed, leaving us feeling purposeless once again. Also, it's usually the ambitious plans that seem most meaningful to other people, drawing compatriots to the cause. Fostering a network of relationships is an important part of having a long, healthy life as well.

Related: If your occupation is a core component of your identity, don't ever fully retire. I've thought of myself as a physician for a century—when I was a young child, my dolls were my patients—so I continued offering life consultations even after I retired from my full-time practice.

• **Dwell in gratitude.** Researchers at University of California, San Diego, have found that gratitude is good for the heart—literally. Patients who are thankful for the good things in their lives have lower levels of inflammatory biomarkers related to cardiac health problems. They sleep better, too, which also is healthful. I focus on what I still have and what I've gained. I am surrounded by wonders—we didn't have a phone when I was young, but now I can connect with people around the world. I don't take that for granted—the modern world is an incredible place, and every day I'm grateful to be in it.

Whatever it is that I've lost along the way hasn't been anything I couldn't live without. Declining eyesight has cost me my ability to read, but the world has given me audio books—and unlike printed books, I can enjoy those and still have my hands free for knitting.

Depression Hastens Aging

University of Connecticut.

Older adults with depression age faster than their peers, new research from the University of Connecticut suggests. As cells age, they function less efficiently and often produce proteins that promote inflammation and illness. Investigators found elevated levels of these proteins in 426 people with late-life depression. They also found that people with higher levels of these aging-associated proteins were more likely to have high blood pressure, high cholesterol, multiple medical problems, and worse performance on tests of brain health, such as working memory and other cognitive skills.

Stress Can Help You Live Longer

Elissa Epel, PhD, professor and vice chair in the department of psychiatry at University of California, San Francisco, and director of UCSF's Aging, Metabolism, and Emotions Center. She is author of *The Stress Prescription: Seven Days to More Joy and Ease.* AMECenter.UCSF.edu

Stress gets a bad rap. We're often warned that stress is a killer, increasing our risk for heart disease, obesity, type 2 diabetes, depression, dementia, and more. And stress feels terrible, tying us up in knots of anxiety. But while chronic stress is indeed toxic, there's increasing evidence that short, concentrated bursts of stress actually can be extremely good for us...and even life-extending. We asked Elissa Epel, PhD, a longevity expert and author of *The Stress Prescription*, how your stress can help you live longer.

Short bursts of stress, also known as hormetic stress, trigger the body's stress response just as chronic stress does—but because hormetic stress is over in just seconds or minutes, the stress response is quickly followed by the body's stress shut-off process, called the vagal rebound. This rebound not only feels good, it triggers autophagy, a process of cellular cleanup that is strongly linked to longevity.

Example: In a study by researchers at Sanford Burnham Prebys Medical Discovery Institute, worms that were subjected to brief bursts of high temperatures to induce stress and autophagy lived longer than worms that were not subjected to elevated temperatures—even though the temperatures were high enough that they would have killed the worms with longer exposure.

Additional studies, including one conducted by Firdaus Dhabhar, PhD, from University of Miami, have shown that short-term stress enhances the immune response in humans. That makes it very different from chronic stress, which can interfere with immune response. Research suggests that repeated exposure to short-term stress also might boost cognitive and physical performance...and it likely enhances our resilience during larger stresses in the future. So not only can living through frequent brief stresses make us more psychologically resilient, it can improve the body's overall stress response.

Even better: We can put this "positive hormetic stress" to use in our own lives in just a few minutes per week.

We asked Dr. Epel to share the "stress fitness" exercises that trigger longevity-promoting hormetic stress. Try doing one or more of the following a few times or more each week...

•**Get quick bursts of physical exercise.** Vigorous physical activity triggers the body's positive hormetic stress process—and you don't need an extended workout to benefit.

Strategy: Do an aerobic exercise for 30 seconds...take a 10-second break...then repeat the exercise/rest cycle for a total of seven minutes. What exercise you do during this high-intensity interval training is up to you—pushups, jumping jacks, jumping rope, or quick sprints are among the many options. What's important is that the exercise increases your heart rate and breathing rate. Even just walking briskly could be sufficient if you're out of shape. But those exercises should be done with enough intensity that you feel mild-to-moderate discomfort. That discomfort indicates that your body is under stress, which is precisely what's required to reap the longevity benefits of short-term stress.

Bonus: There's strong evidence that high-intensity interval training also is a mood booster. One recent study by Harvard University researchers found that just 15 minutes per day of high-intensity exercise significantly reduces the odds of depression.

•**Take cold showers.** Researchers at Washington University School of Medicine in St. Louis found that daily immersion in cold water increases the life spans of lab rats—the jolt the body experiences when hit by a blast of icy water triggers positive hormetic stress. Fortunately, you don't have to immerse yourself in cold water to take advantage—you don't even have to give up your hot showers.

Strategy: Shower at whatever temperature you find comfortable...but before stepping out of the shower, turn the temperature to cold for at least 15 to 30 seconds. If this doesn't cause you discomfort, spend more time under the cold water or lower the water temperature further—if there's no discomfort, there probably isn't any positive hormetic stress.

Bonus: Showering and/or immersion in cold water have been shown to decrease inflammation and improve circulation.

Added benefit: A study conducted at Virginia Commonwealth University School of Medicine found that cold showers reduced symptoms of depression.

• **Take saunas.** Exposing the body to a cold shower's icy water triggers positive hormetic stress...and exposing it to heat can do so as well. Saunas can help accomplish this. Researchers at University of Eastern Finland found that middle-aged men who took four to seven saunas per week were 40 percent less likely to die during a 20-year period than were men who took saunas less frequently.

Strategy: Take periodic 30-minute saunas. Both steam and infrared saunas appear to be effective. The sauna temperature should be high enough—and your time in the sauna long enough—that you experience a measure of discomfort.

Caution: If you have heart issues, first confirm with your doctor that sauna use is safe for you.

Bonus: Sauna use improves cardiovascular function...and it's been shown to be a helpful treatment for depression, according to researchers at University of Arizona, Tucson.

• **Try hypoxic breathing techniques.** Researchers at University of Amsterdam have confirmed that hypoxic breathing techniques—which combine quick inhales, slow exhales and breath-holding—trigger positive hormetic stress. One easy protocol for hypoxic breathing was developed by the Dutch extreme athlete Wim Hof, who helped popularize it—he also is a pioneer in harnessing the health benefits of cold-water immersion.

Strategy: Inhale quickly, deeply and vigorously...exhale slowly but powerfully and not all the way...repeat this inhale/exhale technique 30 to 50 times...take one more quick, deep inhale...exhale part way...then hold your breath for as long as you can without feeling faint or dizzy. This breath-holding should last long enough that it becomes uncomfortable. After a short break, repeat this entire process two more times. Hypoxic breathing shifts blood oxygen levels and causes other bodily responses that trigger hormetic stress.

Related: Modifying the pace at which you breathe also can help you calm down when you're agitated...or pep you up when you need an energy boost.

When you want to be calmer: Consciously slow your breathing to around six breaths per minute for at least three to five minutes.

When you're feeling tired and need to reinvigorate yourself: Try stimulating breath practice—while seated, inhale and exhale rapidly through your nose with your mouth closed for around 10 seconds...breathe normally for 15 to 30 seconds...then repeat this process at least several more times.

Learning Multiple New Skills Can Improve Cognition in Older Adults

Rachel Wu, PhD, associate professor of psychology at UC Riverside, California.

In a new study, adults ages 55 and older spent 15 hours per week for three months learning at least three new skills, such as Spanish, using an iPad, and photography. At three months, six months, and one year after the intervention, their cognitive scores, which measured attention, inhibition, and short-term memory, were significantly higher than before the intervention.

"Our finding of continuous cognitive growth in older adulthood is unique because most studies show only maintenance of cognitive abilities or cognitive decline over time," Dr. Wu said.

Along with Dr. Wu's previous research, this study suggests that key factors to enhancing cognition include learning multiple things at once, believing that effort will improve results, and approaching learning without a fear of criticism.

Show Your Hands Some TLC

Taylor Pendergast, MS, OTR/L, CHT, advanced clinician at the Hand and Upper Extremity Therapy Center of the Hospital for Special Surgery and HSS Hudson Yards Rehabilitation in New York City. HSS.edu/specialty-hand-therapy.asp

Many of us have trouble opening stubborn jars—that can happen at any age. But as you get older, specific issues with your hands—weakness, pain, joint stiffness, swelling, decreased dexterity—may affect your ability to perform normal daily activities. These symptoms often stem from degenerative changes caused by osteoarthritis, osteoporosis, rheumatoid arthritis, and other conditions—they are called intrinsic factors.

Extrinsic factors also can play a part. External influences that add to inflammation and wearing down of cartilage include placing unnecessary stress on the small joints of the hands through overuse or repetitive motions. For instance, rather than stopping an activity when our hands are getting tired, we switch hand positions to keep going. Even diet can have a negative impact—too much salt and fatty foods, not getting enough fluids, and not eating enough fruits and vegetables. All too often, we take our hands for granted. Here's how to show them the TLC they deserve.

Give Your Hands a Break

Use these strategies to make everyday activities easier on your hands...

•**Use your larger and stronger joints rather than your hands and wrists to do heavy lifting.**

Examples: Use your arm to push open doors rather than your fingers. When carrying a bag with a strap, sling it over your shoulder or place it in the crook of your elbow. If you must use your hands, use your palms, not your fingertips.

•**Conserve energy.** Take intermittent breaks during activities that last longer than 30 minutes, such as gaming or knitting.

•**Try adaptive tools to reduce the workload on your hands.**

Examples: To open jars and containers, use a nonslip rubber jar opener or an opener with long levers. Or consider a multi-function kitchen tool—a six-in-one or five-in-one container opener that works for jars, bottles, wine bottles, cans, and more. No single adaptive device is right for everyone, so it may take some trial and error to find what's best for you.

•**Avoid using your fingers when you don't have to.** Hold your phone with a grip band or a knob.

Examples: The PopSocket, available on Amazon for about $10, adheres to the back of your phone, allowing you to hold it between your index and middle fingers. Rest a book (or Kindle) on your lap or a table rather than holding it in your hands.

•**Increase the diameter of objects you must hold to reduce the stress on your hands.**

Examples: Use a pen grip or an ergonomic pen, such as the PenAgain (available on Amazon.com), when writing. Add a grip enhancer to your toothbrush and kitchen utensils—you can find foam tubing made for this exact purpose online.

Soothing Treatments

•**Fingerless compression gloves,** available online or at drugstores, provide light thermal heat and compression to reduce swelling and pain.

Caution: The gloves should feel like a light hug on your hands. Seams should be on the outside to prevent impressions in your skin.

•**Ice or heat modalities, including ice packs and heating pads.** Heat helps with blood circulation, joint mobility, and pain. A heating pad placed over your hands often does the trick.

Caution: If your fingertips have decreased sensation, be careful with any hot or cold approach.

Could Your Hand Stiffness Be Dupuytren's?

Dupuytren's contracture is believed to be a hereditary condition that primarily affects the hands, although it also can affect the feet (known as Ledderhose disease). The first signs are small palpable nodules and cords in the palm of the hand. For some people, this may be the only symptom that occurs throughout their lifetime. But for others, it can progress into fixed bent positions of the fingers, otherwise known as flexion contractures. It can affect one or multiple fingers in one or both hands, and the progression can be aggressive or slow in nature.

Best: Avoid aggressively stretching or massaging the hand. Once the contracture begins interfering with your daily activities, see a hand surgeon. There's no cure for Dupuytren's contracture, but there are treatments that can break up the cords that are restricting movement.

—Taylor Pentergast, MS

When to see a hand therapist: Consider seeing a therapist as soon as you notice changes, such as weakness, pain, or numbness in your hands.

To find a certified hand therapist (CHT): Go to HTCC.org. A CHT can be a physical or occupational therapist who specializes in treating the hand. He/she will provide information based on each person's individualized needs, analyze how you perform various activities, and offer modifications that will get you back to doing the things you love. He also can tailor an individualized home exercise program based on your needs and provide splinting options, if necessary. At most comprehensive clinics, you can test-drive assistive devices, so you'll know exactly which ones work for you. One session with a hand therapist is enough for many people.

Exercises for Better Hand Mobility

The following exercises are safe for everyone, whether you have mobility issues or simply want to help prevent these issues from developing.

Gentle movements can help with range of motion and weakness in your hands. Here's a simple program you can follow daily, up to three times throughout the day. Repeat each exercise three to five times with each hand.

Important: Exercises should never cause pain. If these do, stop and contact a hand expert.

•**Tendon Gliding Exercises.** Start with fingers straight, palm open. Begin slowly transitioning to a table top position by bending the fingers at the knuckles while keeping the other two joints straight. Move to a half fist by bending the middle joints and keeping the top joints straight. Next move into a full fist by curling the top joint into the palm. End by rolling up into a hook fist—keep the top and middle joints bent while extending the knuckles.

Age Well: Staying Younger Longer

- **Thumb Opposition with Finger Slide.** Touch the tip of the thumb to the tip of each finger, starting with the index and working one finger at a time to the pinky. When performing this exercise, try to focus on making an "O" with the thumb and each finger. Next work on sliding your thumb down the length of each finger to where it meets the palm.

- **Webspace Massage.** Massage the webbed area between your thumb and index finger with lotion to loosen up the muscles.

Caution: Don't be too aggressive.

- **Thumb C Isometric.** Wrap your hand around a small stress ball, making a C shape with your index finger and thumb. Be sure the ball is placed in the palm of your hand—don't force it into the webspace. Gently squeeze the ball to create a muscle contraction. The goal is to not squeeze hard, but rather to produce enough force for a muscle contraction only. Stress balls are available on Amazon.com for about $10.

- **Index Abduction.** Place your hand flat on a table. Move your index finger out to the side and then back next to the middle finger.

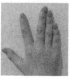

- **Wrist Isometrics.** Protect your fingers by also protecting your wrists. For each of these exercises, use only moderate resistance to counter the pressure from your other hand.

Wrist extension: Place your wrist in a slight extension (pressed back toward the forearm), and use your other hand to apply a downward pressure.

Wrist flexion: Place your wrist in slight flexion (lowered away from the forearm), and use your other hand to apply a downward pressure.

Ulnar deviation: Make a fist with your right hand, and use your left hand to apply an upward pressure on the pinkie side of your wrist. Press down with your wrist to resist the pressure.

Radial deviation: Make a fist with your right hand, and use your left hand to apply downward pressure on the thumb side of your wrist. Press up with your wrist to resist the pressure.

The Four Fitness Tests That Matter

Greg Hartley, DPT, PT, vice president and immediate past president of APTA Geriatrics, an academy of the American Physical Therapy Association. He is associate professor of clinical physical therapy at University of Miami Miller School of Medicine. Med.Miami.edu

How are you really holding up? There's a strong correlation between how well aging people do on the following four physical tests and whether they're likely to experience major health problems, dangerous falls and/or end up in nursing homes in the near future.

Good news: A poor score on these tests doesn't mean undesirable health outcomes are inevitable. It means that it's time to get fit—so put on your comfy shoes and give them a try.

If you struggle with these tests: You can improve your results, and thus your health, by getting at least 150 minutes per week of moderate-to-vigorous aerobic activity...plus two low-impact strength-training sessions per week.

- **Walking-pace test.** Time yourself as you walk at your natural pace over a measured distance—ideally 20 feet—indoors on a flat path. Then calculate your walking speed in feet per second.

Example: If your path is 20 feet, divide 20 by your time. Don't rush—what

> ### Resources for Older Drivers
>
> CarFit (Car-Fit.org) checkups are a free program from AAA, AARP and the American Occupational Therapy Association. An occupational therapist suggests adjustments and helps optimize your vehicle's ergonomic features to make you more comfortable in the driver's seat, particularly if you've gotten smaller with age. Refresher course—online and classroom courses with driving instructors can bring you up to date on new laws, driving techniques and technology. Check out AAA's RoadWise Driver, online course (from $16 for members, $25 for nonmembers) and AARP Smart Driver online course (AARP.org, about $30). If you are concerned about changes in your driving, ask your doctor for a referral for a formal driving assessment—in which an occupational therapist and a driving instructor ride along with you while you drive and make recommendations to improve your performance. Cost is about $600 or more, not covered by insurance. Driver rehabilitation—for people with conditions such as neuropathy or Parkinson's disease or who had a stroke or other injury, a certified driving rehabilitation specialist can teach you how to make adaptations, use adaptive equipment, practice difficult on-the-road scenarios, and develop safe habits. Cost is $100 per hour, not covered by insurance.
>
> *Harvard Health Letter. Health.Harvard.edu*

matters is your normal walking speed, not the top speed you can achieve—and don't chat during this walk. Slow natural walking speeds often suggest that serious health issues might be looming. One study by researchers at the University of Sydney in Australia found that for men age 70 and older, walking speeds slower than about 2.7 feet per second—around 1.8 miles per hour—are correlated with dramatically increased risk for death in the coming year. None of the men in that study who walked faster than 4.5 feet per second—around three miles per hour—died during the ensuing year.

- **Sit-to-stand test.** Sit on a stable, straight-backed, armless chair—one where the seat is about 17 inches from the floor—with your arms crossed over your chest. The back of the chair should be against a wall so it won't move. See how many times you can stand up and sit back down in 30 seconds without using your arms. A woman in her 60s should be able to do at least 11…10 in her 70s…eight in her 80s…and four in her early 90s, according to the Centers for Disease Control and Prevention (CDC). (A man…12 in his 60s…11 in his 70s…eight in his 80s…and seven in his early 90s.) Lower scores are correlated with falls and higher levels of dependence on others for care and are predictive of a move into assisted living.

- **Timed up-and-go test.** Place a piece of colored masking tape on the floor 10 feet in front of a stable, nonmovable chair. Ask someone to time how long it takes you to rise from the chair once he/she says "go," walk past the tape at your normal walking pace, turn, and return to sit in the chair. He should stop the timer as soon as your backside hits the seat. You may use any walking aid (cane, walker) you would normally use. Times above 12 seconds are predictive of significant fall risk, according to research in *Journal of Geriatric Physical Therapy*.

- **Four-stage balance test.** Stand near enough to a kitchen counter that it could support you if you had to grab it. Place your feet side by side, so close that they touch, then hold this position for 10 seconds. Next, move one foot slightly forward so that its instep is in contact with the other foot's big toe, and hold this stance for 10 seconds. Third, position one foot directly in front of the other—heel touching toe—and hold that for 10 seconds. Finally, stand on one foot for 10 seconds. Being unable to maintain any of these positions for at least 10 seconds is correlated with increased risk for falls, according to the CDC.

Bursts of Activity Help You Live Longer

Emmanuel Stamatakis, PhD, professor of physical activity, lifestyle, and population health at The University of Sydney's Charles Perkins Centre and the Faculty of Medicine and Health in Australia. He chaired WHO's Physical Activity Guidelines Development Group in 2020 and is senior adviser to the *British Journal of Sports Medicine* and lead author of the study cited above. Sydney.edu.au

People who don't exercise can reap tremendous benefits by briefly increasing their exertion level during everyday activities. A recent study by Australia's University of Sydney used data from more than 25,000 users of wearable fitness trackers to compare those who never engage in vigorous activity and those who occasionally get their heart rates up for a minute or so.

Result: Non-exercisers who exert themselves now and then tend to outlive those who don't ever exert themselves.

Especially notable: Engaging in several short bursts of vigorous activity totaling just three to four minutes per day is associated with a 49 percent reduction in death from cardiovascular disease and up to a 40 percent reduction in "all-cause" and cancer-related mortality. Feeling slightly out of breath is a clue that your heart rate is elevated. For most adults, walking at a pace of 120 to 130 steps per minute or above for at least 30 to 40 seconds will do the trick. A pace as modest as 110 steps per minute might be sufficient for people who are unfit or older.

"Vigorous activity" options: Walking at a more modest pace but up hills or stairs… tackling household chores with more gusto than usual.

What to do: Find opportunities for short bursts of vigorous activity each day. You might push your pace for several 30-to-60-second segments of an otherwise leisurely stroll, for example.

The most dramatic longevity gains are achieved by shifting from no vigorous activity to three to four minutes of vigorous activity per day divided into several short bursts. Getting even more bursts of activity is better—11 brief activity bursts a day is associated with a 65 percent reduction in cardio death risk compared with people who engage in no vigorous activity.

Addressing Droopy Eyelids

Mithra Gonzalez, MD, associate professor in the department of ophthalmology at the University of Rochester School of Medicine and Dentistry, New York.

If you've noticed that your eyelids are looking a little droopy as you age, you're not alone. Two different conditions can cause this common sign of aging—which can be merely cosmetic or interfere with your vision—and both are treatable.

•**Ptosis.** Ptosis (toh-sis) refers to a falling or dropping. When it applies to the eyelid, it is called blepharoptosis (blef-a-rop-toh-sis) drooping. Bleph means eyelid. It is caused by an issue with one or both of the muscles that lift the eyelid. Some people are born with it, while others develop it with age or as the result of trauma. The most common form is involutional blepharoptosis. This is primarily age-related and occurs due to the stretching, weakening, or separation of the muscles responsible for lifting the eyelid.

Less often, ptosis may be the result of a structural abnormality (such as a cyst), a neuromuscular disorder, or trauma from accidents, surgeries, preferentially sleeping on one side, sleeping in contact lenses, or repeated eye injections.

Several medications have been reported to potentially cause or contribute to ptosis as well. (See sidebar on next page.)

•**Dermatochalasis.** Another cause of droopy eyelids is excess skin or fat (dermatochalasis [derm-ay-toe-kuh-lay-sis]) on the lid.

Treatment

These conditions can occur together or separately, but they have different treatment options.

If you need muscular repair, you would see an oculofacial plastic surgeon—an ophthalmologist who has also trained in plastic surgery. If you have excess skin, an oculofacial plastic surgeon, ophthalmologist, or general plastic surgeon could perform a procedure called blepharoplasty to remove it. If you have both conditions, the oculofacial plastic surgeon can address both in a single surgery. The risks of surgery are scarring, asymmetry, dry eye, and in rare cases, a bleed that can cause vision loss.

Eye Drops for Droopiness

There is also a prescription eye drop, oxymetazoline hydrochloride ophthalmic solution 0.1% (Upneeq), that temporarily improves droopy eyelids for people with acquired blepharoptosis. Oxymetazoline hydrochloride is the same primary ingredient in decongestant nasal spray, such as Afrin. In nasal spray, it causes blood vessels to contract. In Upneeq, it causes an involuntary eyelid muscle to contract.

In clinical studies, the drop lifted the eyelid by an average of 1 millimeter for about six hours. Side effects may include eye inflammation or irritation, redness, dry eye, blurred vision, headache, inflammation of the cornea, and eye pain. Upneeq may affect blood pressure and may interfere with some prescription medications, including antihypertensive medications, beta-blockers, cardiac glycosides, and monoamine oxidase inhibitors.

Both conditions are normally considered to be cosmetic, so insurance doesn't cover care unless the eyelid is so droopy that it impairs vision and affects activities such as driving or reading.

Medications That May Cause Eyelid Drooping

- **Muscle relaxants.** Medications such as *baclofen*, used to treat muscle spasms and spasticity, can occasionally cause ptosis as a side effect.
- **Antihypertensive drugs.** Some blood pressure medications, particularly alpha-adrenergic blockers like *clonidine* or *methyldopa*, have been reported to cause ptosis in rare cases.
- **Antidepressants.** Certain antidepressant medications, including tricyclic antidepressants like *amitriptyline* or selective serotonin reuptake inhibitors (SSRIs) like *fluoxetine*, have been associated with ptosis as a potential side effect.
- **Antipsychotic medications.** Some antipsychotic drugs, such as *chlorpromazine* or *haloperidol*, have been linked to the development of ptosis.
- **Anti-Parkinson's medications.** Certain drugs used in the treatment of Parkinson's disease, like *levodopa* or dopamine agonists (e.g., *pramipexole, ropinirole*), have been reported to cause ptosis in some individuals.
- **Ophthalmic medications.** Certain eye drops or ophthalmic medications, particularly those containing beta-blockers (e.g., *timolol*) or prostaglandin analogs (e.g., *bimatoprost*), can occasionally lead to ptosis as a local side effect.

Options to Treat Age-Related Macular Degeneration

Mark H. Nelson, MD, MBA, an assistant professor of ophthalmology, Atrium Health Wake Forest Baptist, in Winston-Salem, North Carolina. He is a leading authority on imaging biomarkers and combination treatments utilizing anti-VEGF drugs and PDT laser in exudative ARMD.

Macular degeneration, also known as age-related macular degeneration

(ARMD), is a degenerative disease of the macula, a part of the retina. Vision loss begins with central vision, which mainly affects reading, but it can later spread into peripheral vision, and can lead to profound visual disability if not treated.

There are two types of ARMD: dry (nonexudative) and wet (exudative). The term wet refers to leakage of fluid and blood from abnormal vessels below the retina (neovascularization). Vision loss can occur from both nonexudative and exudative ARMD; however, the latter is rapidly progressive and largely treatable.

Signs and Symptoms

Though ARMD has often been attributed to aging, many patients develop changes as soon as the fifth decade, especially if there is a family history. While early ARMD has no symptoms, more advanced ARMD has patterns of blind spots called *scotomas,* distortion called metamorphopsia, and varying degrees of vision loss. Very often, these changes affect the quality of vision, most commonly reading vision, and is often manifested as missing words or words jumping.

An eye-care professional will see drusen, or yellow spots under the retina, and/or areas of retinal damage in nonexudative ARMD, or leakage of fluid or blood in exudative ARMD. He or she will then commonly refer the person to a retinal physician.

The retinal specialist might then use advanced imaging techniques, such as fluorescein angiography or indocyanine green imaging, in which dyes are injected into the vein for visualization of damage, and/or optical coherent tomography (OCT) angiography, a new technique that allows for visualization of damage without the dye injection. The presence of early or intermediate ARMD can be monitored for progress. This process can take years and then abruptly cause severe vision loss if unrecognized. To paraphrase Ernest Hemingway, vision loss from ARMD occurs, "in two ways...gradually and then suddenly."

Foods to Boost Eyesight

Goji Berries for Better Vision

Age-related macular degeneration (AMD) is the leading cause of vision loss in older adults. Risk can be assessed by measuring macular pigment optical density (MPOD).

Recent finding: People who ate about one ounce of dried goji berries five times a week for 90 days had increased density of protective pigments in their eyes. People who consumed a commercial eye-health supplement that included lutein and zeaxanthin, antioxidants known to benefit eye health, did not show any increase. Because of the small study size, further research is needed. Dried goji berries taste somewhat like raisins and can be added to other foods or eaten as a snack.

Study by researchers at Department of Ophthalmology and Vision Sciences, University of California, Davis, published in *Nutrients*.

Grapes Are Good for Aging Eyes

In a 16-week study, people who consumed the equivalent of one-and-a-half cups of grapes per day had improvements in several indicators of eye health compared with people who consumed a placebo. Grapes improved levels of macular pigment optical density (MPOD) and plasma antioxidant capacity—two biomarkers of eye health. Those who consumed the placebo experienced increases in vision-damaging advanced glycation end products.

Study by researchers at National University of Singapore, published in *Food & Function*.

Treatment Options

The process that causes nonexudative ARMD to become exudative ARMD is unclear, but large clinical trials strongly suggest that taking a collection of over-the-counter vitamins called AREDS and AREDS2 can slow this progression. These contain slightly different combinations of vitamins, and your eye-care professional will suggest which version is better for you.

The treatment of moderate to severe nonexudative ARMD has been elusive, but recent FDA approvals of two new drugs are encouraging. They include *pegcetacoplan* (Syfovre) and *avacincaptad pegol intravitreal solution* (Izervay).

Anti-VEGF Injections

The treatment of exudative ARMD comes from groundbreaking research to suppress abnormal vessel growth in solid cancers. In exudative ARMD, neovascularization grows in the tissue below the retina (the choroid) in response to an unknown injury or stimulus. This process is mediated by a chemical called a cytokine, specifically vascular endothelial growth factor (VEGF). While VEGF naturally repairs damaged blood vessels in patients with a heart attack or stroke, it promotes abnormal neovascularization in exudative ARMD.

Injecting drugs that block the production of VEGF by the diseased choroid has been found to lead to visual improvement and/or stability in a large majority of patients.

There are four anti-VEGF drugs that are the standard of care…

- *Ranibizumab* (Lucentis) and *aflibercept* (Eylea) have been used for more than 10 years and are FDA approved.
- *Bevacizumab* (Avastin) is not FDA approved for ophthalmic use (it is for cancer), but it is widely used due to its affordability.
- A new entry, *faricimab* (Vabysmo) is now FDA approved and is becoming more commonly used due to its longevity and the need for fewer injections.

Originally, patients were given anti-VEGF injections monthly, but research has shown that some patients can be treated with fewer injections. We now know that every patient, and every eye, has different requirements for treatment. The goal is to reduce the number of treatments and have the best clinical effect. The use of anti-VEGF drug therapy is an ongoing process that may continue for years. The treating ophthalmologist must monitor the response to treatment by testing visual acuity and OCT imaging. Treatment that is not working has to be modified, either by increasing the frequency of injections or by changing the drug. Faricimab (Vabysmo) represents a new class of drugs as it suppresses two specific cytokines simultaneously.

Another treatment option is photodynamic therapy (PDT), which was largely abandoned after the start of the anti-VEGF era but is again being investigated in combination with anti-VEGF agents.

Ongoing Challenge

Even though patients can progress from nonexudative to exudative stages, the nonexudative changes continue in a slowly progressive manner. Despite successful resolution of neovascularization and leakage with anti-VEGF drugs, vision loss may still ensue over time. The next challenge for treatment will be integrating intraocular injections for both nonexudative and exudative ARMD together in a successful protocol.

Treating exudative ARMD with anti-VEGF drugs can help most people maintain or improve vision. The challenges in the future involve the mitigation of treatment burden,

Family History

Patients with family histories of ARMD may display imaging biomarkers, or measurable findings on imaging techniques, that may predict future progression. It is also clear that genetic predisposition increases the risk of developing ARMD and can predict future progression into the exudative form. Genetic tests are commercially available but not entirely definitive on their own. Patients with a strong family history should be followed by eye care professionals and have OCTs done routinely as early as age 40 or 50.

improved treatment response, and the successful treatment of nonexudative ARMD.

Anticoagulant Warning

The vision loss from ARMD is largely limited to the inability to read or drive, but the risk of severe vision loss is increased by the use of an anticoagulant drug. Despite this risk, it is imperative that a patient consult their primary care or specialist doctor on the discontinuance of anticoagulation, as this could cause serious consequences such as heart attack or stroke.

> **ARMD vs. Cataracts**
>
> Cataracts, or the clouding of a normal clear ocular lens, is a common cause of vision loss in the aging eye. It is essential to differentiate between the cataracts and ARMD because they have different treatments. Cataracts generally cause blurred vision, especially at night, and are easily removed with surgery. ARMD, on the other hand, causes changes in the quality of vision, with scotomas and metamorphopsia.

Preventing Major Eye Diseases

Marc Grossman, OD, LAc, doctor of optometry and licensed acupuncturist in New Paltz, New York. He is coauthor of *Natural Eye Care: Your Guide to Healthy Vision & Healing.* NaturalEyeCare.com

Many age-related eye diseases that cause vision loss in adults 60 and older have no early symptoms. Here's how to reduce your risk...

Glaucoma typically is caused by pressure in the eye that damages the optic nerve. But it can occur even with normal eye pressure—possibly from a sensitive optic nerve that receives limited blood flow. Over time, glaucoma causes loss of peripheral (side) vision. Diabetes, high blood pressure, thyroid disorders, and a family history increase risk. Treatments include prescription eyedrops, lasers and surgery.

Recent findings: Exercise may help to reduce eye pressure, slowing the progression and reducing risk, according to a study by researchers at University of Malaya Medical Centre in Malaysia. And researchers at Harvard Medical School are looking into gene therapy to reverse vision loss from glaucoma.

Cataracts, the leading cause of vision loss in the U.S., are a normal part of aging. Approximately half of all Americans will have cataracts by age 75. They cause clouding of the eye's lens, resulting in blurry, hazy vision and oversensitivity to light. Every year, doctors perform about 3.7 million surgeries to remove cataracts and replace the natural lenses with artificial lenses. Alternatives to surgery include homeopathic eyedrops, vitamins, and supplements (including a combination of the vitamins A and C and antioxidants).

Also: Walking, bicycling, and other types of exercise for an hour a day can reduce risk, according to researchers at Lawrence Berkeley National Laboratory in California.

Diabetic retinopathy results when the retina's blood vessels are damaged by uncontrolled high blood sugar. Symptoms include floaters and blurred vision. About half of people with type 1 or 2 diabetes will develop this condition, which can cause blindness. Eat properly, stay active, and manage your blood sugar levels. Women who had gestational diabetes may experience a rapid onset of diabetic retinopathy.

Also: Supplementing with antioxidants, amino acids, vitamins, enzymes, and fish oil may help preserve your vision, in particular, lutein, zeaxanthin, vitamins C, D, and E, zinc, copper, alpha-lipoic acid, n-acetylcysteine, and complexes of B-1, B-2, B-6, L-methylfolate, and methyl B-12.

Age Well: Staying Younger Longer

Nearsightedness and Dry Eye Are Linked to Screen Time

Rana Taji, OD, MSc, FAAO, owner and medical director, Toronto Medical Eye Associates, North York, Ontario, Canada, quoted in CBC News. TorontoMedicalEyeAssociates.ca

The more hours you spend looking at your computer or smartphone, the greater your risk for irreversible myopia (nearsightedness) or dry eye disease. Myopia can result from changes to the shape of the eye caused by screen time. Dry eye can develop because we blink significantly less often when looking at screens, damaging the glands that keep eyes moist.

Self-defense: Reduce screen time...every 20 minutes, take a 20-second break to blink 20 times...use preservative-free lubrication drops.

Stuck Stem Cells Responsible for Gray Hair

NYU Langone Health/NYU Grossman School of Medicine.

Stem cells that move between growth compartments in hair follicles, known as melanocyte stem cells, have been found to get stuck as people age, resulting in the loss of their ability to maintain hair color. Researchers suggest that this finding presents a potential pathway for reversing or preventing the graying of human hair by helping jammed cells to move again between developing hair follicle compartments.

That Bump on the Head May Be a Bigger Problem Than You Think

Christine Greiss, DO, double board-certified in physiatry and brain injury medicine, director of the Concussion Program at JFK Johnson Rehabilitation Institute, and clinical assistant professor in the department of physical medicine and rehabilitation at Hackensack Meridian School of Medicine and Robert Wood Johnson Medical School in New Jersey. HMSOM.org

Odds are it has happened to you. You wake in the middle of the night and have to use the bathroom. It is dark, difficult to see and...bam...you trip and clunk your head. After you get your wits about you, you figure you must be okay and head on to the bathroom and back to bed.

But maybe you're not okay—maybe you've just sustained a concussion and don't know it.

Most of the headlines about concussion involve well-known athletes, but Senator Mitch McConnell's fall and concussion in March 2023 brought to light the significant differences when an older person experiences a head injury. Concussions are classified as a mild form of traumatic brain injury (TBI), but in older adults, they may be anything but mild...and while we've learned a lot about how to help young people and athletes after concussion, the needs of the older brain aren't as well understood.

Why is there a difference? When an athlete suffers a concussion on the field, his/her brain is in a very specific and, in fact, optimal chemical state—primed for competition with the endorphins, or feel-good hormones, flowing. He/she is not only young but also likely to be in good physical condition. Age is on his side, and with the proper treatment and time, his healing potential is phenomenal.

An older person, on the other hand, may already be managing chronic conditions, such as high blood pressure, high cholesterol, or diabetes—factors that can impact the healing process. And in many situations, such as when an older person falls in the middle of the night, the brain is in a fatigued state, another factor that can make recovery more difficult.

Concussions in Seniors: A Silent Epidemic

About 12 percent of all hospitalizations nationwide are due to brain injuries such as TBIs, and the majority of those hospitalizations are adults 75 years and older who experienced a fall. That's more than the number of people of all ages whose TBIs stemmed from two other common causes—motor vehicle accidents and violent assaults. This silent epidemic is a major public health concern that needs a targeted, age-appropriate approach for care and, in particular, more research to overcome the challenges that older people face.

Following a concussion, older adults are at higher risk for severe complications, including a brain bleed.

Reason: Normal anatomical age-related changes in the brain cause it to shrink over time, leaving more room for it to shake and rattle during a head injury. More space between the brain and the inner wall of the skull gives even a slight bleed from a TBI space to grow or bleed more. Being on a blood thinner, as many older adults are, also increases bleeding risk.

Challenge to Diagnose

Identifying a concussion can be difficult even for health-care providers. The Glasgow Coma Scale (GCS) is a common assessment tool used to measure concussion effects, but it's very vague when it comes to the fine points. Example: The GCS considers whether you can move your arms and legs and open your eyes. If you can, you'll score pretty well...even if you have a concussion. In fact, older adults with a completely normal GCS score can show acute brain trauma on a CT scan.

Even brain scans have their limitations—they can't tell how severe a concussion is or how well you'll recover. There also are instances in which a CT scan looks normal at the time of the concussion, but the patient starts to experience symptoms in the days or weeks to come. In that situation, an MRI might be needed to identify problems.

When to Get Medical Attention

Senator McConnell was actually lucky to have fallen in public because people around him got him immediate attention. Many people who fall at home assume they're okay if they can get back up. But even if you think you're fine, a head trauma that shakes your brain causes chemical changes—the brain's normal workings may be impacted—so it is always best to get checked out when your head is shaken or rattled from a fall, a motor vehicle accident or even a low-impact event. And certainly get checked out if you feel that your functioning and/or thinking is off.

Keep an eye out for these three categories of concussion symptoms...

•**Physical symptoms.** Fatigue, dizziness, headaches, sensitivity to light and sound, nausea and/or vomiting, and problems with sleep.

Note: People used to be discouraged from going to sleep in the hours after a suspected

Eye Drops for AMD

A new compound could offer an alternative to injections to treat wet age-related macular degeneration (AMD). The drug, which can be delivered as an eye drop, can reverse damage from AMD and promote regenerative and healing processes. The compound targets a protein called end binding-3 in endothelial cells, which line the inside of blood vessels. In animal models, twice-daily treatment reduced eye damage within two to three weeks.

University of Illinois Chicago.

concussion. That's no longer the case, but needing too much sleep or not being able to get restorative sleep are concerns.

• **Cognitive symptoms.** Confusion, mental fog, and difficulty concentrating or remembering.

• **Emotional symptoms.** Anxiety, irritability, and worsening of existing mental health issues such as depression.

If any of these occur immediately after you have a head injury, call 911 or get to an emergency room for a neurological evaluation.

Problem: You might not feel symptoms right away. They can occur one, two, or even six months after a single fall, and people often fail to connect them to a head injury that occurred so much earlier. Signs that may occur later on include becoming fatigued faster than usual…needing to take daytime naps…yawning or feeling your eyes tiring after reading just three or four sentences…or feeling as though you're tripping over your own feet when you used to be able to run down stairs without a problem.

After a Concussion

As time passes, you may feel some of the following symptoms—all are signs to see your doctor or a neurologist for a neurological evaluation and possible treatment…

• **From two weeks to three months after a concussion or any head trauma.** You may feel depressed. That's because certain brain chemicals are at an all-time low—the brain depletes them while healing, and that may cause depression or even aggressive behavior. You might have trouble finding the right words, have difficulty with tasks that used to be automatic such as how to turn on your car, or forget recipes you've been preparing for years.

• **Between three months and two years.** Post-concussion syndrome can set in with post-traumatic headaches, vertigo and/or ringing in the ears and/or dizziness. After this long, most people have forgotten about hitting their head, so their doctor might order all sorts of tests unrelated to concussion without rooting out the true cause. What's needed is an evaluation by a neurologist of your balance and cognition and how you're processing information.

Recovery Road Map

There's no one-size-fits-all time frame for concussion recovery. It depends on your overall health, your lifestyle habits and, of course, the extent of your injury. It's not your age but the health of your brain that influences the healing process.

Example: If you experienced brain injuries in your youth or you've already had one or more concussions as an adult, your brain will be slower to heal from any new trauma. Depending on the extent of the injury, you may need a hospital stay, possibly followed by inpatient rehabilitation at a special facility, as did Senator McConnell. Rehab programs are tailored to each person's unique needs but typically focus on physical and mental therapies to help with movement and cognition and include a plan to gradually return to your everyday activities so that your brain has time to heal.

For a first-time concussion: Expect to feel extremely fatigued or wired for two to three weeks because of the chemical changes that took place in your brain. Your brain will use more than 300 calories a day to heal—that's why you may feel drained or excessively hungry, so boost your diet with healthy foods.

Other important steps: Get enough sleep…make sure you're getting needed vitamins…control any chronic conditions such as high blood pressure…and enlist loved ones to watch over you, drive you to follow-up appointments, help you prepare meals, and take medications as directed…and monitor pills and bills because the chances of making cognitive errors are high while you're healing from concussion.

How to Protect Yourself from Noise Pollution

Mathias Basner, MD, PhD, at the University of Pennsylvania Perelman School of Medicine, where he is professor in the department of psychiatry and director, unit for experimental psychiatry, division of sleep and chronobiology. He is president of the International Commission of Biological Effects of Noise (ICBEN).

You hear a lot about the health dangers of air pollution, but there's another type of pollution (a type you may not even realize is pollution) that can cause a host of health problems: noise pollution. The World Health Organization says noise pollution—formally defined as "unwanted and/or harmful sounds"—is the second-largest environmental cause of health problems, right after air pollution. And the U.S. Environmental Protection Agency says noise pollution can have "countless health effects." (Unfortunately, the EPA closed its Office of Noise Abatement and Control after it was defunded during the Reagan administration, leaving the U.S. population to fend for itself against the adverse effects of noise.)

The Damage Noise Can Do

The most common health problem created by loud noise—a one-time exposure such as a gunshot or long-term exposure such as working in a noisy factory—is noise-induced hearing loss, which affects 28 percent of American adults. Tinnitus—ringing in the ears—is also caused by both acute and chronic loud noise. But there are many other noise-related health problems—including the biggest killer of all, cardiovascular disease.

•**Cardiovascular disease (CVD).** Long-term exposure to environmental noise is bad for your circulatory system and heart. It raises blood pressure, heart rate, blood fats, blood sugar, and increases the thickness of the blood—increasing your risk for atherosclerosis, heart attack, and stroke. Every increase of 10 decibels increases the risk of CVD by 7 to 17 percent, according to a study in *The Lancet* on the effects of noise on health. (A decibel is a measurement of sound—a car in city traffic generates about 70 decibels, while a truck generates 80, a hairdryer 90, and a helicopter 100.)

•**Disturbed sleep.** Noise disturbs sleep in every way possible, making it harder to fall asleep, waking you up early in the morning, reducing deep sleep (slow-wave sleep) and dream sleep (rapid eye movement sleep), and generally increasing the time you are awake or in more superficial sleep stages. Deep, restful sleep is a must for health, with disturbed sleep linked to heart attack, stroke, kidney disease, diabetes, obesity, and depression—not to mention daytime fatigue, poor productivity, accidents and injuries, and lower quality of life. The people most at risk for disturbed sleep from noise are seniors, children, shift-workers, and people with a sleep disorder like sleep apnea.

•**Cognitive decline in adults.** A study from Germany involving more than 4,000 people showed that elevated levels of traffic noise were linked to lower cognitive scores. In a five-year study that was part of the Chicago Health and Aging Project, every 10-decibel increase in noise exposure increased the risk of cognitive impairment, up to 36 percent.

It affects kids, too. More than 20 studies show that children's ability to learn is harmed by noise because of communication difficulties, impaired attention, frustration, annoyance, and sleep disturbance. For example, a study showed that a 5-decibel increase in noise delayed reading age in children by two months.

•**Stress.** Loud noise causes stress, which lowers quality of life and can cause or complicate nearly every health condition and disease. Noises as low as 60 decibels can cause stress if they're unwanted and intrusive.

Reducing Noise...

There are several ways you can reduce noise in your environment and protect your health.

•**Protect your ears.** If you're exposed to loud noise—like when using a leaf blower, traveling by airplane, or attending a loud concert—always wear noise-reducing earmuffs. Earmuffs and earplugs are even better. Also consider using earplugs at night if noise is disturbing your sleep.

•**Use a decibel app to test your environment, and leave if it's too noisy.** An app like SoundPrint measures the decibels in your immediate environment so you can leave if the level of noise is damaging to health. It also provides a database of quiet restaurants and other quiet public venues based on other users' decibel measurements.

•**Buy quieter equipment.** Before buying a piece of conventionally noisy household equipment—for example, lawn and garden equipment, or appliances like dishwashers and blenders—check out which brands are quietest.

•**Don't be a noisy neighbor.** It's important to respect your neighbor's need for quiet, so do your best to maintain a quiet environment in your home or apartment. Follow this variation of the golden rule: Do unto your neighbor's ears as you would have them do unto your ears.

•**Be an activist for a noise-free world.** Many organizations are enlisting people in the fight against unwanted noise, and you can join. They include Quiet Communities (QuietCommunities.org), Quiet Parks International (QuietParks.org), and Right to Quiet (Quiet.org).

Home, Sweet Home...

There are many things you can do to reduce noise levels in your own home, according to Steve Haas, CEO and principal consultant for SH Acoustics, in Stamford, Connecticut, a firm that designs residential (and commercial) spaces that have quiet and controlled acoustics, to achieve what he calls "residential acoustical wellness."

•**First, understand your problem.** There are many factors that can affect the overall quality of sound in a home, including the size of the room, the furnishings, the adjacency to other rooms, the walls and windows, the noise-generating systems of the home, like plumbing, and heating and air conditioning, and exterior noises like vehicles, aircraft, and emergency sirens. There is also the fact that most homes are not designed and built to account for the control and quality of sound. Short of major renovations on your home by a designer and builder, here are some practical solutions to your sound problems and to achieving quieter and controlled acoustics:

•**Use carpets or area rugs with pads underneath them.** This gets rid of quite a bit of "footfall" noise, which can be very annoying in the room below the footfalls if you're trying to relax or sleep.

•**Insulate walls and ceilings.** Add another layer of sheet rock or drywall to each side of a wall or on a ceiling to reduce sounds from an adjoining room. Also add thermal insulation, when possible.

•**Consider acoustical panels.** These sound-absorbing panels can help reduce the noise in an echoey or reverberant room so you can hear a conversation during a party with a dozen friends. Make sure the panels are thick enough to make a difference (at least 1 inch) and that they blend in with the room rather than making it look like a sound studio.

•**Close the gaps.** Gaps or openings in a wall, like at the baseboard or where a pipe penetrates, allows sound to travel. Use caulk or other materials to seal them. An often overlooked gap is the areas around electrical boxes, outlets, and light switches.

•**Pay attention to doors.** They are the weak link in containing sound because they're of a much lighter weight than walls. To seal a door, use a professional-level gas-

Age Well: Staying Younger Longer

ket around all four sides of the door, not just at the bottom.

•**And windows, too.** Upgrading your windows is not inexpensive, but it can make a big difference in keeping out sound. Short of new windows, consider interior storm sashes, which fit on the inside of typical double-hung residential windows and make a noticeable difference in reducing sound.

•**Watch out for misinformation.** There is a lot of misinformation online when it comes to reducing sound in your home. Watch out for hyperbole. If a manufacturer claims their product will "solve all noise problems," or that a thin layer will "block all sound," stay away.

Braces Are for Grown-Ups, Too

Sercan Akyalcin, DDS, PhD, head of orthodontics, Harvard School of Dental Medicine, Cambridge, Massachusetts. HSDM.Harvard.edu

Changes to the mouth can make braces necessary even in middle age and older.

Not just cosmetic: A misaligned bite can lead to malnutrition. Crooked teeth are harder to clean, which can lead to gum disease. Bacteria can leak into the bloodstream and cause infection in heart valves. Gum disease bacteria also can lead to high blood pressure, diabetes, rheumatoid arthritis, osteoporosis, pneumonia, and even Alzheimer's disease.

Good news: Today's metal brackets are not painful the way braces were years ago…and clear aligners worn for 22 hours per day may be an option.

Cost: Depending on the complexity of the treatment and area of the country, braces cost between $5,000 and $12,000 and are not covered by Medicare and only partially paid for under some insurance policies.

Now Don't Hear This

There are many ways to protect your ears from loud and damaging noise, says Amy Sarow, AuD, the lead audiologist at Soundly (Soundly.com), a hearing-health education site.

•**Noise-canceling headphones.** These help keep volume in a safer range because you don't have to increase the volume over the sound of the background noise.

Two good products: AirPods Pro 2 and Bose QuietComfort Earbuds.

•**White noise.** White noise masks noise in the environment because it contains equal energy from all frequencies, high (bird song, sirens) or low (thunder, bass). Turn the volume up just to the level necessary to mask the bothersome sound.

Good products: the LectroFan EVO and Hatch Restore.

•**Earplugs.** There are many types. Look for a variety that fits you ear canal and effectively reduces noise. Silicone putty earplugs are a good option, particularly for hard-to-fit ear canals or people with sensitive ears.

Two good products: Mack's and Eargasm Squishies.

Also recommended: Loop earplugs are stylish, which encourages people to wear them. The Etymotic Research ER20XS is a high-fidelity earplug with a three-flange design that fits most ear canals.

•**Use headphones safely.** Keeping volume at 60 to 70 percent is generally a safe listening level.

A good rule of thumb: You should be able to hear a person speaking at an arm's length while listening with your headphones. If you can't, the volume is too loud.

Amy Sarow, AuD, lead audiologist at Soundly, a hearing-health education site. Soundly.com

Self-Directed Ageism Causes Real Harm

Julie Henry, PhD, professor, school of psychology, University of Queensland, Australia.

As people age, they're increasingly likely to believe negative stereotypes about seniors, which can lead to self-doubt ("I'm too old to learn this new technology") negative perceptions of one's own aging ("I'm so much worse at this than I used to be") and worries about being judged according to age-based stereotypes ("If I forget to do this, they're going to think it's because I'm old"). This internalized ageism has been linked to a shorter life span, a lower likelihood of trying new things, poorer physical and mental health, slower recovery from disability, and cognitive decline.

Finding a Caregiver

Charles B. Inlander is a consumer advocate and health-care consultant based in Fogelsville, Pennsylvania. He was the founding president of the nonprofit People's Medical Society.

Here are some tips to help you find competent and affordable caregiving services in your community.

•**Assess the need.** Be realistic in scoping out your or your loved one's caregiving needs. Speak with your doctor about what the short-term and long-term prognosis is in terms of the patient being able to regain function or how quickly further deterioration may occur. Many hospitals and home health-care agencies have home-care assessment teams that will come to your home to determine what equipment might be needed, such as lift chairs, hospital beds, walkers, ramps, and bathing or shower assisting chairs. If ordered by a physician, this type of equipment is often covered in total or in part by your medical insurance.

•**Finding reputable caregivers.** Most areas have a number of agencies that provide in-home caregivers. Start your search by contacting your county's Area Agency on Aging. These federally funded offices are administered by your state and are a great source of information. Ask for a listing of caregiver agencies in your community. Also search online for caregiving providers in your area. Speak to several providers. Ask for references and check them out with your state's department of health. Check as well to see if there are any complaints with the Better Business Bureau.

•**Help from family and friends.** Ask other family or friends if they have any caregivers or caregiver agencies whom they might recommend. Your church or synagogue can often recommend caregivers from their own congregations or organizations with whom they have an affiliation.

•**Is home care realistic?** If the family member's medical or lifestyle needs are significant, home caregiving may be inadequate or even dangerous. People in those situations may be better served by an assisted living or nursing home facility on either a short- or long-term basis. Making such decisions is extremely difficult but is usually in the best interest of the patient.

Confused by Medigap? What You Need to Know

Lauren Bigham, licensed insurance agent specializing in Medicare products at Boomer Benefits, a Fort Worth–based insurance agency. She previously served as Boomer Benefits' Client Service Team manager. BoomerBenefits.com

Medigap is an unfamiliar and confusing topic for many of us who are approaching retirement age—but the Medigap decisions we make now could dramatically affect our health-care costs for the rest of our lives.

What is Medigap exactly? Medicare does not cover all health-care costs. Enrollees face co-pays, co-insurance, deductibles, and a host of other out-of-pocket costs. Enrolling in a Medigap plan, in addition to Original Medicare, can fill many of those coverage gaps, greatly reducing out-of-pocket health-care costs in exchange for a monthly premium.

Unlike Medicare Advantage plans, which replace Original Medicare and have HMO-like provider networks, Medigap plans are used in conjunction with Original Medicare—in fact, they're sometimes called Medicare Supplement plans. You cannot enroll in both a Medigap plan and a Medicare Advantage plan.

Problem: There are a number of Medigap policies available, and the rules and benefits for each can cause confusion. Here's what you need to know before you make a choice...

• **If you choose Medigap, you'll probably choose Plan G or N.** There's an overwhelming alphabet soup of Medigap plans available—in most states, there are Plans A, B, D, G, K, L, M, and N...and that doesn't even include Plans C and F, which are available only to people who became Medicare eligible on or before January 1, 2020.

Reality: If you don't want to evaluate every one of those plans, you can focus on just two of them. Virtually everyone who decides to sign up for Medigap opts for either Plan G or Plan N.

Plan G covers the most Medicare out-of-pocket costs among the Medigap plans still available. If you want the most comprehensive coverage and you're willing to pay a potentially significant premium to obtain it, Plan G is likely for you. Plan G premiums average around $120 to $180/month.

Plan N provides much of the coverage of Plan G but at a lower cost. Plan N premiums can be as low as $80 to $100/month.

Main difference between Plans G and N: Plan N has co-pays for certain services—up to $20 for some office visits and up to $50 for some emergency room visits—and it doesn't cover the "excess charges" imposed by a small percentage of health-care providers. Plan G has no co-pays.

• **You don't have to sign up for the same Medigap plan as your spouse**—but you might save some money if you do. Medicare and Medigap policies cover individuals, not couples or families—one spouse's premiums, deductibles and out-of-pocket maximums are completely separate from those of the other spouse. There's usually no need for one spouse to consider the other's health-care needs when choosing a Medigap plan.

But there is one potential exception—companies that issue Medigap plans sometimes offer household discounts of as much as 10 to 15 percent when two or more people living at the same address sign up. That can be a significant incentive for a married couple—or any other Medicare-eligible individuals who share an address—to obtain Medigap plans from the same company.

Don't Take Metformin to Boost Longevity

The diabetes drug *metformin* has been used by nondiabetic "biohackers" trying to extend their lifespans, after mouse studies and observational studies in humans had suggested a benefit. But more research shows that not only does metformin not increase lifespan in people without diabetes, it blunts the benefits of exercise and lowers testosterone.

Better: Pursue longevity through diet, exercise, and sleep.

Brad Stanfield, MD, primary care physician in private practice in Auckland, New Zealand. DrStanfield.com

We Do Mellow with Age

Study of 3,000 American adults ages 22 to 77 led by researchers at Penn State University, University Park, Pennsylvania, published in *Developmental Psychology*.

Based on interviews over several eight-day periods between 1996 and 2017, it appears that stress diminishes as we get older. When younger, interviewees experienced more stress and anxiety and had fewer psychological resources to help them cope. By the time they reached their 40s and 50s, they faced less stress and had more settled emotional lives.

Medicare Advantage Ads May Be Misleading

David A. Lipschutz, JD, associate director of Center for Medicare Advocacy, a national nonprofit law organization that works to advance access to Medicare coverage, Washington, DC. MedicareAdvocacy.org

Beware: The federal government has deemed many claims in Medicare Advantage (MA) insurance ads "fraudulent" and "misleading." Some ads imply that the Centers for Medicare & Medicaid Services endorses or prefers a specific plan...others promise more cost savings than you really get. And if you choose the wrong plan, your doctor may not be a member of that plan's network...or you may end up paying out-of-pocket for medically necessary care.

In September 2023, the U.S. Department of Health and Human Services began cracking down on these ads, but you still need to practice self-defense...

•**Stay focused on what's most important to you in a plan.** Does it cover the doctors you like and facilities you normally go to? Are all of your prescription medications on the drug plan's formulary? Are you eligible for all the benefits you hear about in the ad for the plan? MA plans are organized around networks of providers in defined geographic areas, so a particular plan may not offer certain features in your town.

•**Reach out to your local State Health Insurance Program (SHIP) at SHIPHelp.org or call 877-839-2675.** These nonprofit agencies are funded by the federal government through the Administration for Community Living, a branch of Health and Human Services. They are available in every state to help you navigate Medicare's complexities by providing unbiased one-on-one counseling and assistance to individuals, their families, and caregivers.

•**Investigate free vision, hearing, and dental benefits.** MA plans often include such benefits, unlike traditional Medicare, but the ads may exaggerate the advantages.

Examples: A plan that offers free dental coverage may cover only cleanings and x-rays. Extensive procedures such as root canals or caps may not be covered...or the plan may limit the dollar amount it pays.

•**Be realistic about claims that there are no monthly premiums.** Even if it's true, you are responsible for your original Medicare costs including your Part B premium and deductibles and copays for covered services. Moreover, you may have to pay more out-of-pocket if you see a doctor outside the network.

Also: If the plan is an HMO, it generally doesn't cover non-emergency care out-of-network, so an individual may be responsible for full costs. A PPO, on the other hand, allows people to go out of network, but they generally have to pay more to do so.

•**Report misleading claims** to the Senior Medicare Patrol Resource Center at SMPResource.org/you-can-help/report-fraud or by calling 800-447-8477.

Free University Tuition for Older Students

BestColleges.com

Earn a college degree while paying for only textbooks, fees, and some other costs. University of Alaska gives free tuition to state residents over age 65 on a space-available basis. University of Arkansas has a similar program for Arkansas residents over age 60, as does Clemson University for South Carolina residents at least 60 years old. University of Connecticut waives tuition for state residents who are at least 62. University of Delaware has a similar arrangement for Delaware residents age 60 or older. Georgia Institute of Technology has a space-available graduate-studies program for state residents who are at least 62. Other universities may allow older students to audit classes for free, without working toward a degree.

Exposure to Microplastics May Lead to Behavioral Changes in Older Adults

University of Rhode Island; *Endocrinology*.

University of Rhode Island researchers exposed young and old mice to varying levels of microplastics in drinking water for three weeks. The mice began to move and behave peculiarly, exhibiting behaviors akin to dementia in humans. The researchers also found alterations in immune markers in liver and brain tissues. Microplastics may decrease GFAP, a protein that supports many cell processes in the brain. "A decrease in GFAP has been associated with early stages of some neurodegenerative diseases, including mouse models of Alzheimer's disease, as well as depression," said Jaime Ross, PhD. The results were most profound in older animals.

Humans are exposed to microplastics through inhalation of particles in the air and ingestion from dust, food, and water. It is estimated that people ingest several milligrams of microplastics daily, researchers reported in *Endocrinology*.

Older Drivers with ADHD Have More Accidents

"Motor Vehicle Crash Risk in Older Adult Drivers With Attention-Deficit/Hyperactivity Disorder," led by researchers at Columbia University School of Public Health, New York City, published in *JAMA Network Open*.

Reaction time and eyesight are two factors that weaken as we age, making driving difficult for some. But there are other factors at play. According to a new study led by the Columbia University School of Public Health, older drivers (ages 65 to 79) diagnosed with attention-deficit/hyperactivity disorder (ADHD) are at significantly higher risk for dangerous driving. Although adult-ADHD is diagnosed in about 10 percent of adults, many more older adults may have undiagnosed ADHD.

The study is published in the American Medical Association's journal *JAMA Network Open*. The research team analyzed data from the Longitudinal Research on Aging Drivers (LongROAD) project collected from primary care clinics in five states: Michigan, Maryland, New York, Colorado, and California. The data included information gathered by questionnaire and by in-vehicle recording devices over 44 months of active driving.

What Adult ADHD Looks Like...

Symptoms of adult ADHD include hyperactivity, impulsivity, and inattention, all of which may contribute to unsafe driving.

ADHD is commonly considered a disorder of childhood, but about 30 percent of children (some studies have it as high as 60 percent) continue to have ADHD as adults, and for these people, ADHD is a lifetime disorder.

These symptoms must be persistent and interfere with or reduce the quality of life at school, work, and general social situations. There is no cure for adult ADHD, but symptoms can be effectively treated with education, support, psychotherapy, and in some cases with medications. Diagnosis of ADHD for older adults can be a life-changing event. It may also be a *life-saving* event.

ADHD does not start in adulthood. Diagnosis requires symptoms that start before age 12. The American Psychiatric Association did not formally recognize ADHD as a mental disorder of childhood until the 1960s. Many seniors with ADHD before the 60s grew up having their symptoms blamed on behavior or personality problems.

What the Researchers Found in Older Drivers with ADHD

Three outcomes that the team analyzed were hard braking events, traffic citations, and car crashes. There were 2,832 drivers in the study, 53 percent women, 47 percent men, with an average age of 71. Between two and three percent (75 drivers) were diagnosed with ADHD. *These were the key findings for these drivers compared to drivers without an ADHD diagnosis...*

- A 7 percent higher risk of hard braking
- A 102 percent higher risk of a traffic ticket
- A 74 percent higher risk of a car crash

The study concludes that adult ADHD is significantly associated with dangerous driving and that improved diagnosis of adult ADHD and management is important for the promotion of healthy aging, which could result in safer driving. The findings are similar to prior studies on driving dangers for adolescents and young adults. Dangers for older adults may be increased by age-related risks like impaired reaction time or mild cognitive impairment.

According to the Attention Deficit Disorder Association, the most common warning signs of ADHD in adults may include difficulty staying focused or paying attention to details, misplacing or losing things, running late or missing appointments, risky behaviors such as careless driving, inability to be patient, and being easily angered or irritated.

Seniors: Be Careful with Cannabis Products

Kenneth Finn, MD, is a physician in Colorado Springs, commenting on a study published in *Journal of the American Geriatrics Society*.

A recent 15-year period saw a 1,804 percent increase in cannabis-related ER visits by Californians age 65 and older. Dispensary cannabis is unreliable in terms of potency and contamination, and elders are vulnerable to effects on memory, cognition, and balance. Older people who tend to be on more medications risk negative interactions with cannabis. Even seemingly benign cannabinoids such as CBD have known interactions with hundreds of drugs, including over-the-counter medications.

Our Body Temperature Changes

University of Pennsylvania.

As a vital sign, temperature is an indicator of what's occurring physiologically in the body. Researchers point out that there is no universal "normal" body temperature for everyone at all times. Despite the fixation on 98.6°F, most clinicians recognize that "normal" temperatures have a range. Throughout the day, body temperature can vary by as much as 1°F, from its lowest in the early morning to its highest in the late afternoon. It also varies across the menstrual cycle and following physical activity, and tends to decrease as we age.

Digestive Health and Loneliness in the Elderly

Study titled "Loneliness and Depressive Symptoms Are High Among Older Adults with Digestive Disease and Associated with Lower Perceived Health," by researchers at the University of Michigan, published in *Clinical Gastroenterology and Hepatology*.

In May 2023, the United States Surgeon General issued an advisory calling attention to a public health crisis: loneliness and social isolation. A new study from the Division of Gastroenterology and Hepatology at the University of Michigan has found that people aged 50 and older who are living with a digestive disorder have a significantly higher risk of loneliness, depression, and social isolation. Their study is published in the journal of the American Gastroenterological Association, *Clinical Gastroenterology and Hepatology*.

Digestive diseases are very common, especially in older individuals. In fact, almost 40 percent of people report living with a digestive disorder, which can interfere with social activities and cause mental distress, called psychosocial factors.

An Endless Loop

Psychosocial factors can trigger digestive disorders or make them worse, and long-term digestive symptoms can cause mental and social stress. According to the research team, psychosocial factors are often ignored when doctors are managing digestive diseases in older adults. To learn more about the impact of these diseases on psychosocial heath, the research team designed a study to compare the frequency of loneliness and depression in older adults with and without a digestive disease.

The team used data from a study that was done from 2008 to 2016, called the University of Michigan Health and Retirement Study. This study followed about 20,000 people ages 50 and older and their spouses. The team identified a pool of about 4,000 people living with a digestive disease and about 3,000 people who had no long-term digestive health problems.

Babies and Pets Help the Aging Brain

Grandparents Who Babysit Live Longer

According to a recent finding, grandparents who babysat their grandchildren had a 37 percent lower risk for death during the 19-year study period compared with grandparents who did not babysit or adults the same age who did not have grandchildren. Babysitting keeps older people physically and mentally active while giving them a sense of purpose.

Study by researchers at University of Basel, Switzerland, The University of Western Australia and Max Planck Institute for Development, Berlin, Germany, published in *Evolution and Human Behavior*.

Seniors Who Own Pets Do Better on Cognitive Tests

Pet owners age 65 and older who had their pets for more than five years scored better on cognitive tests that measured immediate and delayed word recall compared with pet owners of the same age who owned their pets five years or less or people who did not own a pet. No such cognitive association was found among younger pet owners who owned pets more than five years...five years or less...or who did not have a pet.

Study of 1,369 seniors led by researchers at University of Michigan, Ann Arbor, published in *Journal of Aging and Health*.

These were the key findings from the study: People with a digestive disease were 25 percent more likely to report poor health than those without digestive disease. Among people with a digestive disease, there was a 43 percent risk of loneliness and triple the risk of depression, leading to greater odds of poor health. Older people with digestive disorders should be aware of the risk and seek professional help. Gastroenterologists and other health-care providers should consider screening these patients for loneliness and depression.

Physical Consequences of Social Isolation

Common long-term digestive diseases include inflammatory bowel disease (ulcerative colitis and Crohn's disease), GERD, irritable bowel syndrome, and chronic constipation. According to the Surgeon General Advisory, physical health consequences of loneliness and lack of social connection also include a 29 percent increased risk of heart disease, a 32 percent increased risk of stroke, a 50 percent increase in dementia, and a 60 percent increase in premature death.

Chapter 2

BRAIN HEALTH

Exciting Developments in Alzheimer's Research

This has been an exciting time in Alzheimer's disease (AD) research. Alzheimer's researchers have been developing theories that could completely upend conventional wisdom about the cause of the condition…welcomed a new drug that just might be the first pharmaceutical to slow AD progression…faced fraud allegations that called into question a key research paper…and much more. *Here's what you need to know now…*

The New Drug

Pharmaceutical company Eisai unveiled the results of a phase-3 trial of its new AD drug *lecanemab* in late November 2022. An 18-month study involving 1,795 patients found that participants who had been diagnosed with AD who received this drug experienced 27 percent less cognitive decline than those receiving a placebo. No previous drug has ever managed to slow AD this way. Lecanemab is an antiamyloid drug designed to remove the protein beta-amyloid that causes the formation of plaques in the brains of AD patients.

But: Questions remain about lecanemab, which was approved by the FDA in January 2023, and is sold under the name Leqembi. Two participants in the recent trial died from brain hemorrhages believed to be linked to the drug, raising the possibility that its risks might outweigh its benefits.

Medicare covers the cost of lecanemab for most patients (with the applicable co-pays and deductions)—paying for it out of pocket costs the typical U.S. patient more than $25,000 per year.

And now, some researchers are skeptical that beta-amyloid is even the correct target. In part, these doubts are because earlier attempts to target beta-amyloid have failed to slow or stop AD. One earlier beta-amyloid–targeting drug, *aducanumab,* received conditional FDA approval in 2021 and now is sold as Aduhelm—but questions remain about whether it benefits patients.

Donald Weaver, MD, research director and institute co-director at Toronto's Krembil Brain Institute. He is also a professor of chemistry, medicine, and pharmaceutical science at University of Toronto, and a clinical neurologist at Toronto Western Hospital. He has won the Prix Galien Award, considered the Nobel Prize of biopharmaceutical research. WeaverLab.ca

Researchers' opinions range from "Give it a chance" to "Why did they approve this?" The conditional approval means this drug also is not covered for most Medicare patients. Out-of-pocket costs for U.S. patients are around $28,000 per year.

Improved Detection

Currently, doctors resort to crude tests of cognitive ability—such as asking patients to spell words backwards—to diagnose AD. But a team of researchers at Germany's Cancer Research Centre and Centre for Protein Diagnostics recently developed a sensor that can identify signs of AD in patients' blood up to 17 years before clinical symptoms appear. Advances in the ability to detect AD are crucial, though generally receive less attention than new drugs. It's likely to be some time before we can be certain about the accuracy or specificity of such blood tests. When a test is claimed to identify signs of a disease 17 years before symptoms appear, it takes 17 years to confirm that those claims are correct.

Fraud Allegations

An article in *Science* in 2022 suggested that an influential 2006 AD research paper was based on suspicious data. The paper, along with others, played a key role in the theory that beta-amyloid plaques are the primary cause of AD.

Result: Some researchers suggest that the past 15 years of AD research has been built on a flawed premise.

But: The impact is not as substantial as some claimed. No one study is responsible for 15 years of research—science had largely moved on from that paper even before the allegations.

Still, these allegations have helped call attention to the growing doubts surrounding the idea that an accumulation of beta-amyloid proteins is the primary cause of AD—and that has helped focus attention on alternative ideas.

New Avenues of Research

Because AD research was focused on amyloids, proposed AD studies that lacked an amyloid focus often were rejected by grant committees. That has changed dramatically. Among the proposed alternative causes for AD...

•**Mitochondria.** A paper in *Journal of Clinical Medicine* by researchers at the European Brain Research Institute and Italy's Institute of Biomembranes, Bioenergetics and Molecular Biotechnologies is among several to identify a link between AD and dysfunction in mitochondria—the organelles that serve as cells' energy units. Intriguingly, AD patients appear to experience mitochondrial dysfunction before beta-amyloid protein builds up or other symptoms appear, hinting that the mitochondrial issue might be the trigger of the disease.

•**Synapses.** A paper in *Frontiers in Cellular Neuroscience* by researchers at the Netherlands' Utrecht Brain Center reviewed the research into the connection between synapse loss and AD. AD patients experience a loss of synapses—the ends of neurons that send messages to adjacent cells. Research suggests that this synapse loss might be related to changes that occur in patients' astrocytes—a type of cell found in the brain and spinal cord—hinting that preventing astrocyte changes could become an AD therapy.

•**Autoimmune dysfunction.** If you made a list of key AD risk factors, setting aside age and family history, it would include such seemingly unconnected dangers as repeated head trauma...infections, including dental infections...and exposure to air pollution. But there is a common thread—the immune system plays a role in helping people recover from all of them. Could AD be a result of an immune system problem? That might help explain why beta-amyloid plaques build up in AD patients' brains. Research by scientists at the Krembil Brain Institute suggests that beta-amyloid plays a role in the brain's immune system, killing off viruses and bacteria, but it struggles to differentiate between bacteria and brain cells. Perhaps AD is the result of the immune system mistakenly killing brain cells, and beta-amyloid plaques are a consequence.

What's Next?

Which of these theories will turn out to be the Holy Grail that AD researchers have been seeking for decades? Most likely none. There probably is no one solution. It probably is more likely a family of diseases that we haven't yet figured out how to differentiate. For example, there's increasing evidence that early-onset AD is different from late-onset. The ultimate solution might turn out to be a cocktail of treatments that involves more than one of these theories and others, and a treatment that targets beta-amyloids could be part of that cocktail.

Good news: After decades where no meaningful Alzheimer's treatments reached patients, a range of treatments that truly could provide improved outcomes might start to become available, perhaps in as little as three years.

Hormone-Replacement Therapy: The Earlier the Better to Protect Against Alzheimer's

Rachel Buckley, PhD, assistant professor of neurology at Massachusetts General Hospital in Boston, and coauthor of a study of 300 adults published in *JAMA Neurology.*

Timely hormone-replacement therapy does not increase the risk of Alzheimer's disease (AD). Two proteins, tau and beta-amyloid, are associated with AD. Women naturally have more tau in their brains, but researchers have found that levels are particularly elevated in women who underwent early menopause (ages 40 to 45), and in those who started hormone-replacement therapy (HT) at least five years after the onset of menopause. The good news, however, is the women who start HT soon after beginning menopause do not have elevated tau, suggesting that HT can have a protective effect, even among women who entered menopause early. Despite initial concerns after a study published 20 years ago, HT is consistently shown to be a safe and effective way to manage menopause symptoms and possibly to reduce AD risk—if it's started right away. But if not started within five years, it should not be used. One hypothesis is that after five to six years, estrogen receptors in the hippocampus, the memory center of the brain, have downregulated, so they no longer benefit from HT.

Does COVID Increase Alzheimer's Risk?

There is evidence that neurological inflammation can be a driver of AD and cognitive decline...and approximately one-third of confirmed COVID patients develop neurological symptoms. Already there is evidence that existing dementia patients diagnosed with COVID experience worsened clinical outcomes.

It will be many years before we know the true scale of this latest AD danger. At this point, we can't even say which COVID patients are at greatest risk. But there is a real chance that decades from now the pandemic that recently devastated the world could do so again, by potentially doubling global dementia rates.

—Donald Weaver, MD

Brain Health

For Cognitive Benefit, Dancing Beats the Treadmill

Study by researchers at Albert Einstein College of Medicine, Bronx, New York, published in *Journal of Aging and Physical Activity*.

A recent study showed that either walking on a treadmill or ballroom dancing for six months was associated with improvement on cognitive tests. But people who danced outperformed walkers on executive function and processing speed (the time it takes to respond to information)...and they experienced less atrophy in the hippocampus, the part of the brain that is critical to functional memory.

Possible reason: Besides providing physical exercise, dancing also has social and cognitive elements that call on a wider network of brain areas than walking.

Can You Reduce Your Risk of AD?

Yes. According to the U.S. Centers for Disease Control and Prevention (CDC), healthy aging may reduce your risk by about 40 percent. You can reduce your risk by being mentally active. Mental activities like learning a new skill, reading, doing brain teasers, and being socially active build cognitive resilience. That means that even if you have some early AD, you have built up enough brain power to combat it. Autopsy studies show that some people have significant AD in their brains but never develop symptoms of AD, due to cognitive resilience. The CDC says these other eight lifestyle changes can help reduce AD risk...

- Prevent or manage high blood pressure.
- Prevent or manage high blood sugar.
- Maintain a healthy weight.
- Be physically active.
- Don't smoke.
- Avoid alcohol or drink only in moderation.
- Prevent or correct hearing loss.
- Get enough sleep.

U.S. Centers for Disease Control and Prevention.

Take Steps to Avoid Dementia

Ronald Lazar, PhD, E.F. McKnight Endowed Chair of Learning and Memory in Aging and director of the Division of Neuropsychology at the University of Alabama at Birmingham School of Medicine.

A 2021 poll found that people over age 65 fear dementia more than any other disease. The good news is that a new study, published in the journal *Alzheimer's & Dementia*, suggests that older adults can reduce their risk and maybe their fear of dementia with a very simple strategy: taking more steps every day.

Researchers from the School of Public Health and Human Longevity at University of California San Diego compared older women who averaged less than 1,867 steps per day (just under one mile) to women who averaged about 4,000 steps (just under two miles). The women who took more steps were 64 percent less likely to develop mild cognitive impairment (MCI) and 52 percent less likely to develop dementia over a period of four years.

The study was done only on women, who tend to have a higher risk for dementia than men, mainly because they live longer. It is assumed that results would be similar for men.

MCI and dementia both cause cognitive impairment, which is the loss of mental abilities like memory, thinking clearly, understanding, communicating, and learning.

Beyond Normal Cognitive Loss

It is normal to have some age-related memory loss, which refers to cognitive loss after age 65. Most of us will have "senior moments" like taking longer to find the right word or remember a name.

About 10 to 20 percent of people over age 65 will develop MCI. MCI is a step further on the path to dementia, and most people with MCI will continue to follow the path, with about 10 to 15 percent developing dementia each year, usually diagnosed as Alzheimer's disease (AD). AD is, by far, the most common cause of dementia.

From Preclinical to Full Dementia

MCI will show up as a low score on a cognitive test. Common cognitive tests like the Mini-Mental State Exam or the Montreal Cognitive Assessment can take only 10 to 15 minutes. A low score is a significant warning of cognitive impairment. During these tests, a health-care provider may ask a person to repeat a short list of words, name objects from pictures, copy shapes from a drawing, or answer simple questions related to well-known facts.

The period before symptoms of cognitive loss are noticeable is called the preclinical phase. During this phase, the brain changes that cause MCI and AD have already started.

Protein clumps are starting to build up in the brain. The protein is called amyloid, and it can form into the tangles and plaques that destroy nerve cells called neurons, leading to eventual dementia. It can take 10 to 20 years for a preclinical brain to become a dementia brain.

MCI is diagnosed when cognitive loss is more than would be expected for a person's age, and the symptoms have become noticeable to the person or to friends and family. These symptoms will show up on a cognitive test, but they are not significant enough to affect the activities of daily living. AD is the most severe form of cognitive impairment, and the symptoms of impairment become obvious even without testing. AD is severe enough to progressively interfere with the everyday needs of living.

The Many Benefits of Exercise

Lack of exercise is one of many known risk factors for MCI and dementia. Other risk factors include older age, smoking, high cholesterol, diabetes, depression, obesity, sleep deprivation, social isolation, and a lack of stimulating mental and social activities.

Exercise, or lack thereof, is one of the most important risk factors because it is a *pleotropic* risk factor, which means it checks several of the boxes for risk reduction, including benefits for high blood pressure, high blood sugar, obesity, and sleep deprivation.

Recent research suggests that exercise has another very specific effect on amyloid plaques and tangles. Exercise increases a brain protein called brain-derived neurotrophic factor (BDNF). BDNF stimulates neurons to form more connections with other neurons. These are like new roads that allow brain signals to travel through the brain. When amyloid plaques and tangles destroy neurons in one part of the brain, connectivity offers side roads to detour around the damage, preserving cognitive health. In fact, brain imaging studies show that people who have more connectivity may have the same amount of amyloid plaques and tangles as people with AD, but none of the signs and symptoms.

There are many ways to get more steps into your day...

- **Schedule a daily walk, even if it's just for five minutes to start.**
- **Park farther from your destination.**
- **Walk to a colleague's desk instead of emailing.**
- **Walk up and down the stairs.**

Brain Health

- Pace while talking on the phone or waiting.

Every little bit counts, so look for opportunities to walk a little more.

Start Now

Researchers from the School of Public Health and Human Longevity stress that the earlier you start adding steps, the better chance you have of delaying or avoiding MCI and dementia. That is important because once you have MCI or dementia, there has been no treatment to slow, stop, or reverse the buildup of the amyloid plaques and proteins.

Promising Medications on the Horizon

That may finally be changing. On July 6, the FDA gave final approval to *lecanemab-irbm* (Leqembi), the first drug that can slow the course of AD in the earliest stages of the disease. This is a new type of drug called an anti-amyloid antibody. It attaches to and removes the amyloid proteins needed to form AD plaques and tangles. These new drugs (there are more anti-amyloid antibody drugs in the clinical trial pipeline) offer hope for people with MCI and early AD and make it more important for everyone to know the early warning signs when treatment is most effective.

Warning Signs to Discuss with Your Doctor

- Frequently repeating the same questions or stories
- Being unable to follow a conversation or the plot of a book or movie
- Losing things or missing appointments more often
- Struggling to make decisions and making more poor choices
- Getting lost in familiar places
- Having more trouble concentrating, making plans, and completing tasks.

New Risk Factors for Early Dementia

JAMA Neurology.

Orthostatic hypotension, vitamin D deficiency, high C-reactive protein (CRP) levels, and social isolation have been identified as risk factors for dementia before age 65, according to a new study of 356,052 people. Previously identified factors significantly associated with a higher risk of young-onset dementia risk were depression, alcohol use disorder, stroke, carrying two *APOE4* alleles, lower socioeconomic status, diabetes, heart disease, hearing impairment, and social isolation.

Belly Fat Link to Alzheimer's Disease

Cyrus Raji, MD, PhD, is associate professor of radiology at Washington University School of Medicine, Saint Louis, Missouri. MIR.WUSTL.edu

More belly fat suggests greater Alzheimer's risk. Increased visceral fat during midlife is linked with brain changes consistent with the development of Alzheimer's decades before symptom onset—including volume loss in memory centers and increased presence of amyloid plaque.

Inflammation leading to insulin resistance could be the driver. Visceral fat hides around abdominal organs and isn't captured by body mass index.

Rule of thumb: Your waist circumference should be less than half of your height.

Certain Vaccines Lower Alzheimer's Risk

Paul Schulz, MD, professor of neurology with McGovern Medical School at UTHealth Houston in Texas and senior author of a study of 1.6 million people published in *Journal of Alzheimer's Disease*.

Receiving certain vaccinations is associated with significantly lower risk for Alzheimer's over an eight-year period—tetanus and diphtheria, 30 percent lower...shingles, 25 percent...pneumococcus, 27 percent... influenza, 40 percent. Rather than merely preventing diseases that could contribute to Alzheimer's, these vaccines seem to bring about changes to the immune system that are protective against the disease.

Heart Health = Brain Health

Chengxuan Qiu, PhD, associate professor, senior lecturer, and assistant division head of the Aging Research Center in the Department of Neurobiology, Care Sciences and Society at Karolinska Institutet in Stockholm, Sweden. He is a senior author of the study "Association Between Behavioral, Biological and Genetic Markers of Cardiovascular Health and MRI Markers of Brain Aging," published in *Neurology*.

To keep your brain healthy as you get older, focus on your heart health now. That is the conclusion of a recent study by scientists at Karolinska Institutet in Stockholm, Sweden. We spoke with one of the study's lead researchers, Chengxuan Qiu, PhD, about the ways in which heart health directly influences how our brain ages.

In 2010, the American Heart Association (AHA) created *Life's Simple 7*—seven modifiable health metrics that can positively influence heart health and reduce risk for heart disease. Four of those metrics are behavioral—being physically active, eating a healthy diet, having a normal body mass index (BMI), and not smoking. Three are biological—normal or well-controlled total cholesterol, blood pressure, and fasting blood sugar. (*Editor's note:* The AHA added getting adequate sleep to this list after the study was underway.) You have control of all of these metrics...and taking control of them benefits your heart and supports your brain health!

The heart, the brain and the mind (or cognition) all are connected, especially during the aging process. Cognitive decline and heart disease share many risk factors, including smoking, high blood pressure, and diabetes. What's more, heart disease can contribute to cognitive decline by causing inadequate blood supply to the brain, and that sets the stage for forms of dementia. The Karolinska Institutet study looked specifically at how adhering to Life's Simple 7 could influence the structural changes of brain aging among older people.

Most of us know about the link between amyloid and tau brain lesions and dementia...and about how plaque buildup in large arteries increases stroke risk. But perhaps you are not aware that damage to micro vessels, the smaller blood vessels in the brain, can deprive the brain of vital oxygen and nutrients. Called *microvascular lesions* (MVLs) or *small vessel disease* (SVD), this damage can cause three different types of impairment—physical, such as slowed walking speed and balance problems... cognitive, including problems with memory, language, and executive function... and emotional, which can show up as symptoms of depression. The damage to these vessels shows up on brain MRI scans as a higher volume of *white matter hyperintensity*, or WMH...*lacunes,* or small deep lesions or cavities...and a new biomarker of damage, the appearance of perivascular spaces that appear outside the roots of very small vessels. Another common MRI marker of cerebral SVD are microbleeds, small areas of *hemosiderin* deposits (hemosiderin is derived from the disintegration of red blood vessels).

Study Details

To assess the protective role of Life's Simple 7 on brain health, the study followed 317 participants from the Swedish National Study on Aging and Care, a multidisciplinary study of aging and health among people 60 and older in the Kungsholmen district of Stockholm. Among the participants were people who were genetically more susceptible to metabolic risk factors, such as diabetes and high cholesterol, so researchers could determine whether having such genes increases risk for faster vascular brain aging.

The participants were followed for an average of 5.5 years. For each of the seven health metrics, they were given a score of 0, 1, or 2, depending on how well they adhered to them, with 14 being the highest total score possible.

Examples: For the metric of smoking, current smokers were given a score of 0…previous smokers who had stopped at least five years earlier got a 1…and those who never smoked, 2. People with a BMI of 30 or higher were given 0…those who were overweight, 1…and those at a healthy weight, 2. Participants' overall scores fell into three groups—unfavorable (with a mean score of 5.31)…intermediate (a mean of 7.5)…and favorable (a mean of 9.78). Participants had repeated MRI scans to measure the signs of MVLs.

Results: The findings showed the impact that cardiovascular health can have on maintaining vascular brain health in older adults. Overall, having an intermediate or favorable score was linked to slower progression of WMH volume versus having an unfavorable score. Intermediate to favorable scores on the biological metrics in particular (normal or well-controlled total cholesterol, blood pressure, and fasting blood sugar) were related to slower progression of WMH among people ages 60 to 72 years, though not among people 78 years or older. (Why the brain of a person in his/her late 70s or older doesn't respond in the same way is complicated. There may be existing damage that limits the brain's abilities. Having low blood pressure or low LDL cholesterol has been linked to increased WMH volume in old age, and low total cholesterol late in life can accelerate the brain aging process.)

Having a higher genetic predisposition to the metabolic risk factors (diabetes and high cholesterol) was linked with faster accumulation of WMH among people with an unfavorable or intermediate score but not among those with a favorable score, and in particular, with favorable scores on the behavioral metrics (not smoking, being physically active, eating a healthy diet, and having a normal BMI).

What that means: Healthy behaviors may counteract the detrimental effects of these genes and, in turn, slow the progression of vascular brain aging.

Your Action Plan

The way to keep your brain healthy is to prevent MVLs…and the way to do that is

---

Multivitamin Reduces Age-Related Memory Decline

According to a recent study, people over age 60 who took the multivitamin Centrum Silver daily outperformed those who took a placebo on memory tests by the equivalent of 3.1 years of age-related decline. Benefits were greatest for individuals who had underlying cardiovascular disease.

Adam M. Brickman, PhD, professor of neuropsychology at Columbia University in New York City and lead author of a study published in *The American Journal of Clinical Nutrition*.

to adhere to Life's Simple 7, now Life's Essential 8—being physically active, eating a healthy diet, having a normal BMI, not smoking, and getting good sleep as well as keeping total cholesterol, blood pressure, and fasting blood sugar under control.

The sooner you take action, the better. If you don't protect your heart health—say, your blood pressure isn't controlled in midlife—heart disease and stroke risk will start at a much younger age, perhaps in your 40s or 50s, and then start to affect your brain by your 70s. If you have high blood pressure, cholesterol, and/or blood sugar, controlling your numbers is essential, and that means working with your doctor on a plan and sticking to it.

Reminder: It is important for brain health to maintain or boost your cognitive reserve—that bank of cognitive abilities that you add to throughout your life with education and continued learning, mentally demanding activities at leisure time or work, and social engagement. The greater your reserve, the better your brain is able to function, even with microvascular damage.

Should You Get a Cognition Test?

Forgetting an acquaintance's name or where you left the remote is normal as we age. But certain kinds of lapses can indicate that something more serious may be going on—and you might need a test of your cognition.

Examples: Forgetting family members' names...repeatedly putting things in strange places (eyeglasses in the utensil drawer)...getting lost on familiar routes...losing the thread of conversations. If you have concerns about your cognition—or family members have expressed concern—request a cognition test at your next annual wellness check. The test takes only a few minutes. Results will help your doctor know if more extensive assessments should be done.

Sam Gandy, MD, PhD, associate director, Alzheimer's Disease Research Center, Icahn School of Medicine at Mount Sinai, New York City. MountSinai.org

---

Proceed with Caution with the Direct-to-Consumer Alzheimer's Disease Blood Test

Zaldy Tan, MD, MPH, medical director of the Jona Goldrich Center for Alzheimer's and Memory Disorders and the Carmen and Louis Warschaw Endowed Chair in Neurology at Cedars-Sinai.

In 2023 the first direct-to-consumer blood test designed to assess the risk for developing Alzheimer's disease hit the market. The test measures the level of a protein called beta amyloid, a key component of plaques that form in the brains of people with Alzheimer's disease.

Blood tests for Alzheimer's disease provide a convenient way for patients to see whether they might be developing Alzheimer's-type changes or pathology in their brain years before memory issues even begin.

The challenge here is that these brain changes do not necessarily mean that they have Alzheimer's disease, which is a clinical diagnosis.

What blood tests do is to look at traces of certain proteins that are known to develop in patients with Alzheimer's disease.

The test currently on the market has not been evaluated or approved by the FDA. Neither have any of the other, similar tests that are in development. And these blood tests should really be reserved for people who are at risk or are having early symptoms of memory issues.

These types of blood tests do not have a place for people who do not have significant risk factors for developing memory problems or are not having any functional or social issues related to cognitive change.

A blood test alone does not provide enough information to diagnose potential memory issues. Only a trained clinician can. So, for people who are interested in these kinds of blood tests, I would suggest that they first speak with their health-care professional to see if these tests are right for them.

Alternatives to these newer-on-the-market tests are things like cognitive testing, a neurologic examination, or consultation with memory specialists.

Alzheimer's Spotted During Eye Exam

Study of older adults led by researchers at Cedars-Sinai Medical Center, Los Angeles, published in Acta Neuropathologica.

Retinas of people with Alzheimer's disease (AD) have the same amyloid and tau proteins found in the brains of people with AD. Eye exams that could increase detection of AD are in development.

Scents May Boost Memory

Frontiers in Neuroscience.

A study conducted at the University of California, Irvine, suggests that fragrance can boost memory. The study involved men and women ages 60 to 85 without memory impairment. Participants were given diffusers and seven cartridges, each containing a different natural oil (rose, orange, eucalyptus, lemon, peppermint, rosemary, and lavender). The enriched group received full-strength cartridges, while the control group received the oils in small amounts. Before going to bed each evening, participants inserted a different cartridge into the diffuser, which remained activated for two hours during their sleep. The enriched group exhibited a significant improvement in cognitive performance, as measured by a standard word list memory test. Participants in the enriched group also reported improved sleep quality. Past studies have shown that exposing people with moderate dementia to multiple odors twice a day resulted in memory and language improvement, reduced depression, and enhanced olfactory capacities. The olfactory sense is directly connected to the brain's memory circuits, said Michael Yassa, PhD.

What Is Frontotemporal Dementia?

Ryan Darby, MD, assistant professor of neurology and director of the Frontotemporal Dementia Clinic at Vanderbilt University Medical Center in Nashville.

When the family of actor Bruce Willis announced that he has *frontotemporal dementia* (FTD), many Americans learned for the first time about a condition that isn't nearly as well-known as Alzheimer's disease or other brain disorders.

Up until the 1990s, even doctors were largely in the dark about FTD, which is more precisely called *frontotemporal lobar degeneration* (FTLD), because it describes a group of conditions that affect the frontal and temporal lobes of the brain.

What doctors and scientists do know today isn't enough to offer cures or slow down the damage caused by these conditions. But progress is being made. And greater public awareness may help more patients get help sooner for the life-altering symptoms that often begin in midlife and go years without appropriate diagnosis and treatment.

So, here are the answers to a few common questions...

What happens in frontotemporal lobar degeneration?

Conditions under the FTLD umbrella can cause problems with behavior, language, decision-making, and movement. The common thread is that they all involve progressive damage to brain cells in the frontal and temporal lobes of the brain. Those are the areas behind your forehead and ears. The underlying cause is likely a buildup of abnormal proteins. As the damage progresses, different symptoms may emerge, most often between ages 45 and 64. About 60,000 Americans have some form of FTLD, according to the Association for Frontotemporal Degeneration.

While some people with FTLD are initially misdiagnosed with Alzheimer's disease, the conditions differ in important ways. Memory loss is the most prominent early symptom of Alzheimer's disease, but not FTLD. Most, though not all, Alzheimer's cases are diagnosed in older people.

Doctors divide FTLD into several subtypes, based on which symptoms are most pronounced when patients are first diagnosed. These are...

• **Behavioral-variant frontotemporal dementia.** This is the most common type and often starts with socially inappropriate behaviors, such as making rude comments, shoplifting, neglecting personal hygiene, and touching strangers. A loss of judgment, which makes people vulnerable to scams and financial mistakes, is common, as are emotional changes, including a loss of warmth and concern for others. Other symptoms can include binge-eating sweets and obsessive-compulsive habits, such repeating words and phrases.

• **Primary progressive aphasia.** This type starts with problems using language to speak, read, write, or understand others. The person may struggle to produce speech, talking in a way that is increasingly hesitant and labored or, in another variation, may seem to speak almost normally while gradually losing the ability to use and understand specific words. Willis's family said he was initially diagnosed with language problems.

• **Movement and muscle disorders that may or may not involve behavior or speech changes.** These include a condition called corticobasal syndrome, which can start with problems using the hands and arms in a purposeful way, and another called progressive supranuclear palsy, which causes muscle stiffness and changes in walking, posture, and eye movements.

How are these conditions diagnosed?

These conditions often are misdiagnosed as Alzheimer's disease, other forms of dementia or, in the case of the behavioral variant, as anything from depression to bipolar disorder to a midlife crisis. Some people with movement and muscle symptoms are misdiagnosed with Parkinson's disease. It's common for symptoms to persist for more than two years before a correct diagnosis is made.

Getting a correct diagnosis will typically start with a visit to a neurologist, who will take a thorough history, relying not just on the patient, but on the people closest to them, to describe changes in behavior, speech, movement, or other possible clues. The patient also will take tests that can show language and thinking problems and undergo blood tests to rule out other conditions. The doctor will perform a physical exam, looking for altered reflexes and other possible signs of neurological damage.

Finally, the patient will undergo brain scans that look for telltale shrinkage in the frontal and temporal lobes and sometimes additional scans that show how the brain is functioning. Right now, there's no test for the underlying buildup of abnormal proteins, but that's likely coming in the future.

What's the treatment?

While there's no cure, treatment can help patients manage their symptoms and function better. For people with the behavioral variant, the mainstays are drugs that might reduce abnormal behavior and improve psychological well-being, including antidepressants, antipsychotics, and certain antiseizure drugs that have mood stabilizing effects. Medications used primarily for Alzheimer's disease haven't been found to be effective and can make symptoms worse in some people.

People with language problems can undergo speech and language therapy to work on ways to communicate more effectively. For example, someone having trouble speaking might point to pictures, words, or letters on a communication board to make themselves better understood.

People with motor problems might benefit from physical therapy and medication. Counseling for patients and families can be an important part of treatment, as well.

And there's hope for better treatments in the future. Promising research on medications that directly target genetic causes is under way.

What happens as these conditions progress?

FTLD gets worse over time and eventually leads to death. But there's a lot of variation in how quickly patients decline and how long they live. The typical life span after symptoms start is seven to 10 years, but the range is two to 20 years, studies suggest.

Who's at Risk?

About 10 percent of people with FTLD carry a known gene strongly associated with their condition. In roughly 40 percent of remaining cases, some family history suggests there might be a genetic link. Other possible risk factors, including autoimmune diseases, childhood learning disabilities, toxin exposures, and head injuries, have been studied but not proven to increase risks.

Patients who have family histories suggesting a genetic link can undergo counseling to decide if they want genetic testing. If they test positive, their families also can consider testing.

As these disorders progress, people with behavioral symptoms may also develop speech and motor problems, and people primarily affected with speech or motor problems may develop behavioral symptoms, as well. That's because larger areas of the brain may become damaged over time.

During milder stages, patients may be able to continue some normal activities and spend some time alone. Later on, people typically need close, constant supervision and help with most daily activities. Families may need to consider in-home help, adult day programs, and other services. At some point, it may make sense for the person to move to a facility that offers extra support. Memory care facilities designed for people with Alzheimer's and other more common kinds of dementia may not always be a good fit, because the needs of generally younger, more active people with FTLD can be quite different. But individual needs vary widely.

Eventually, the brain damage associated with these conditions causes physical changes such as swallowing problems, reduced appetite, and losses in strength, mobility, and control of the bowels and bladder. These changes can make people vulnerable to urinary tract and skin infections, as well as pneumonia. Many people die from one of those infections.

Coping with a Dementia Diagnosis

Elizabeth Landsverk, MD, founder of Dr. Liz Geriatrics in Lake Tahoe and author of *Living in the Moment: A Guide to Overcoming Challenges and Finding Moments of Joy in Alzheimer's Disease and Other Dementias.* DrLizGeriatrics.com

A dementia diagnosis can be received with a crushing finality. The frightening decline into late-stage dementia that lies ahead can leave patients and loved ones struggling to enjoy the present. But patients who receive a dementia diagnosis often still have many good years ahead. Seeing a therapist is, of course, one way to learn to cope with the feelings surrounding this diagnosis. Five additional strategies that can help…

•**Join a dementia support group**—with people who share your current level of dementia. Don't just join the first group you find. If the other members of that group have more advanced dementia, spending time with them will only make you more depressed. You're more likely to find the friendship and support you need in a group where everyone is more or less at your stage.

Example: The Alzheimer's Association's "early-stage social engagement programs" are for people in the beginning stages of the dementia. (On Alz.org/help-support, click "Programs and Support," then "early-stage social engagement programs.")

•**Remain active with community and religious groups unrelated to dementia.** A dementia diagnosis is neither an embarrassment nor a reason to hide from the world. An estimated one in nine Americans age 65 and older has Alzheimer's. Your fellow members of community and religious groups probably know other people who have dementia…some likely even have early-stage dementia themselves. Your continued participation not only will help you maintain beneficial social connections and a sense of normalcy, it also could encourage other people facing the same diagnosis to continue to participate as well.

•**Engage in physical activity.** Getting regular exercise appears to significantly reduce the odds of developing dementia. Less well-known is that exercise also might slow the progression of dementia among people who already have it—that was the conclusion of a recent study by researchers at University of California, San Francisco. Even something as simple as walking appears to increase the production of a protein that aids communication between brain cells.

> **Where Can Families Find Help?**
>
> Caring for a loved with FTLD is challenging, so many families find it helpful to talk to others in the same situation. The Association for Frontotemporal Degeneration has a variety of support options…
>
> •**FTD Support Forum.** FTDsupportforum.com
>
> •**Public Facebook group.** Facebook.com/TheAFTD
>
> •**Facebook group for spouses.** Facebook.com/groups/TheFTDSpouse/
>
> •**Private Facebook group.** Facebook.com/groups/52543721114/
>
> •**In-person support groups.** TheAFTD.org/sign-up/
>
> •**The Well Spouse Association.** WellSpouse.org
>
> •**Dementia Action Alliance.** DAANow.org
>
> •**Dementia Alliance International.** DementiaAllianceInternational.org

Similar: There's some evidence that shifting to a largely plant-based diet can slow cognitive decline.

•**Listen to music.** Music can help people who have dementia rediscover memories and adjust their moods.

•**Ask your doctor to review your medications.** Dementia typically is diagnosed by evaluating patients' behavior and performance on cognitive tests. The confusion, memory loss and disorientation that a doctor might assume is evidence of dementia also could be side effects of many medications, including pain meds such as Tylenol PM or Advil PM…Benadryl, an allergy med used to sedate…and bladder pills such as *oxybutynin chloride* and *trospium chloride*. Ativan, Xanax, and other sedatives work like alcohol and can make a person look confused and can lead to agitation. If you have been diagnosed with dementia, find a geriatrician to review the drugs you're taking and deprescribe any that you no longer need and/or that might be contributing to your dementia symptoms. Making medication modifications might reveal that your dementia is far less advanced than you feared...or even that you don't have dementia at all.

Don't Forgo Laxatives for Fear of Dementia

Ali Rezaie, MD, medical director of the GI Motility Program at Cedars-Sinai in Los Angeles, commenting on a study of 502,229 adults published in *Neurology*.

A recent study indicated that taking laxatives regularly was associated with significantly increased risk for dementia. But the study had severe limitations that make that conclusion unwarranted. Constipation is an early symptom of dementia, occurring years before diagnosis...and the study period was too short to conclude a causal link. Laxatives are not only safe but can be lifesaving.

Brain Health in a Bottle?

Chris Iliades, a retired surgeon and regular contributor to *Bottom Line Health*.

The most common health fear among people over age 50 is Alzheimer's disease. One solution to this angst for many people is a brain health supplement. About 25 percent of Americans over age 50 are taking at least one product that's advertised for brain health. The problem is that there is very little evidence that these products actually do anything.

You've probably seen or heard commercials for Prevagen, Neuriva, Neuro Health, or Focus Factor. It's hard to miss them. A recent review of brain health supplements in the journal *Senior Care Pharmacist* found these are some of the most common brands. It also found that many of these brands have similar ingredients, such as ginkgo biloba, B vitamins, huperzine-A, Bacopa monnieri, and phosphatidylserine. Fish oil (omega-3 fatty acid), curcumin, and vitamin E are also popular ingredients.

Brain health supplements are not inexpensive. Fifty Neuriva gummies may cost you well over $50.

What the Science Says

Supplement studies are hard to do, and there is very little research for most ingredients. Pharmaceutical companies and major health organizations are not investing in studies on supplements like huperzine-A and Bacopa monnieri, but there is some research on ginkgo biloba, omega-3 fatty acids, B vitamins, and vitamin E.

•**Ginkgo biloba** has been studied in some big and well-funded clinical trials. In a trial of 3,000 older adults, it failed to reduce the risk of dementia or Alzheimer's disease. Some smaller trials found that it improved cognitive function in patients with Alzheimer's, but not enough to improve quality of life. There is also some small-trial evidence for improvement in people with early cognitive impairment. These studies conclude that more research is needed.

•**Omega-3 fatty acids.** According to the National Center for Complementary and Integrative Health, omega-3 fatty acids show consistently good results in studies—but those benefits show up only when looking at high omega-3 diets. Diets high in fish, like mackerel or salmon, are consistently linked to better brain health. Supplements don't show the same benefits.

According to the Harvard School of Public Health, the reason vitamins and other nutrients—even antioxidants—have benefits in whole foods but not supplements is due to nutrient synergy. Nutrients from foods are absorbed in a balanced mix of vitamins, minerals, phytochemicals, and antioxidants. Pulling out one nutrient and giving it as a high-dose supplement is like pulling one instrument out of a symphony orchestra.

- **Vitamin B.** A 2022 review of 95 studies, including about 50,000 people, concluded that vitamin B supplements may slow cognitive decline. However, an earlier review of five studies with about 900 people did not find any benefits for people over age 50 with or without Alzheimer's disease.
- **Vitamin E** studies have been less hopeful. A 2021 review of five studies including over 14,000 people found no benefits for people with or without AD.

Other Supplements

This is what we know about the other supplements...

- **Curcumin** is the active ingredient in the spice turmeric, and it has a long history of use as medicine for its anti-inflammatory effects. A 2019 review found some benefits for mind health, but not consistently.
- **Huperzine** is a Chinese herb used to treat Alzheimer's disease in China. A review of 20 clinical trials with close to 2,000 patients found that huperzine may have beneficial effects for AD, but the trials were small and inconsistent, with more research needed.
- **Phosphatidylserine** is an important fatty substance needed in animal nerve cells. Supplements made from cow brains were stopped due to fear of mad cow disease. Today this supplement is made from soybeans or cabbage, and support for cognitive health is limited.
- **Bacopa** monnieri is an Asian herb used in India for memory. Research is scarce. A review of six small studies found that people without dementia had some improved memory performance when taking it.
- **Apoaequorin** is found only in Prevagen, and it is the only active ingredient in Prevagen. The only research supporting the product was done by the manufacturer, and there is no evidence that this supplement reaches the brain.

Some brain health supplements may help, but no supplement has the kind of support that would be required for FDA approval. Fortunately for supplement makers, the FDA does not approve supplements for safety, content, or effectiveness. That is why, no matter what a supplement claims to do, the label must say that the product has not been evaluated by the FDA and that the product is not intended to diagnose, treat, cure, or prevent any disease.

What Really Works

There is a lot of research on preventing dementia through lifestyle changes. The Finnish Geriatric Intervention (FINGERS) Study to Prevent Cognitive Impairment and Disability was a three-year trial that included more than 1,200 older adults. It found that exercise, diet, social activity, and challenging brain activities (cognitive stimulation) improved memory by 40 percent and cognition by 25 percent. The study continues today as the Worldwide FINGERS study.

Two recent studies presented at the Alzheimer's Association International Conference followed close to 2,000 older adults for about 14 years. Those who had healthier diets, more exercise, and more cognitive stimulation had a 60 percent lower risk of developing dementia than others in the study.

Proven Ways to Protect Cognition

- **Eat a brain-healthy diet,** such as the Mediterranean, MIND, or the DASH diet.
- **Exercise regularly.**
- **Keep your brain active.**
- **Be socially active.**
- **Get at least seven hours of sleep every night.**
- **Don't smoke, and limit or avoid alcohol.**
- **Maintain a healthy weight.**
- **If you experience depression,** talk to your doctor about treatment options.

Brain Health

The bottom line: Try a supplement if you want, but don't ignore the proven ways to improve mind health and reduce your risk of dementia.

Most supplements are harmless, and some people do swear by them. The main danger of taking a supplement is that you may think you are doing all you can for brain health. That would be a mistake because there are other things you can do that science more strongly supports.

Saunas May Help Head Off Alzheimer's

Study by researchers at University of Eastern Finland, Kuopio, published in *Age and Ageing*.

According to a recent finding, men who spent time in saunas four to seven times a week had a 65 percent lower risk for Alzheimer's disease over 20 years compared with men who used saunas once a week. Saunas reduce inflammation and prompt the body to make proteins that are good for the brain. Saunas also give the heart a workout, much as exercise does. And since going to the sauna is usually a social experience—at least in Finland, where the study was done—saunas counteract depression and social isolation, known risk factors for dementia.

Another Promising Alzheimer's Drug

Eli Lilly.

Eli Lilly and Co. reported that a clinical study showed promising results for its experimental Alzheimer's disease drug, *donanemab*. In the 18-month trial, early-stage Alzheimer's patients who received infusions of donanemab experienced a 35 percent slower decline in cognitive abilities than people given a placebo, according to a press release. Donanemab is designed to target and eliminate beta-amyloid, a sticky protein that accumulates in the brain and forms plaques that are a hallmark of Alzheimer's disease. Donanemab poses a risk of brain swelling or small brain bleeds, which caused the death of three study participants. The study results have not yet been reviewed by independent experts.

Positive Thinking May Reverse Mild Cognitive Impairment

Yale School of Public Health.

People who have positive cultural beliefs about aging are 30 percent more likely to regain normal cognition after experiencing mild cognitive impairment than people with negative beliefs, according to Yale researchers.

"Most people assume there is no recovery from MCI, but in fact half of those who have it do recover," says Becca Levy, PhD.

Dr. Levy's previous research found that positive age beliefs reduced stress and improved cognitive performance.

Traumatic Brain Injury May Become a Chronic Condition

American Academy of Neurology.

People with traumatic brain injury (TBI) may continue to show changes across a range of areas for years. In a study of more than 1,000 people, 29 percent of people with mild TBI and 23 percent of people with moderate to severe TBI declined in their abilities over two to seven years. But other people showed improve-

How Diet Affects Your Brain

Dietary Magnesium Boosts Brain Health

People who eat plenty of magnesium-rich foods, such as leafy green vegetables, legumes, nuts, seeds, and whole grains, have less brain shrinkage as they age. That translates to better cognitive function and a lower risk of dementia, researchers reported in the *European Journal of Nutrition*. The neuroprotective effects appear to be stronger in women, particularly those who are postmenopausal. The study looked only at magnesium-rich foods and did not examine the role of magnesium supplements.

European Journal of Nutrition.

Eat a Mediterranean Diet to Lower Dementia Risk

A study that analyzed data from more than 60,000 people found that those who ate a diet that was rich in fruits, vegetables, whole grains, and healthy fats had a 23 percent lower risk of developing dementia. Even people with a genetic predisposition for dementia benefited from the healthy eating plan.

BMC Medicine.

A Low-Flavanol Diet Is Linked to Age-Related Memory Loss

According to researchers from Columbia University and Brigham and Women's Hospital, older adults with low flavanol intake showed memory decline, and replenishing these nutrients improved performance on memory tests. Flavanols, particularly epicatechin, enhance memory by promoting the growth of neurons and blood vessels in the hippocampus.

Columbia University.

Junk Food Changes the Brain

If you consistently eat high-fat and high-sugar foods, your brain "rewires itself" to want more of the same. Researchers found that people who ate a daily high-sugar, high-fat pudding for eight weeks had elevated activity in the dopaminergic system, which is responsible for motivation and reward. "Through these changes in the brain, we will unconsciously always prefer the foods that contain a lot of fat and sugar," explained Marc Tittgemeyer, PhD, who led the study.

Max Planck Institute for Metabolism Research in Cologne and Yale University.

ments over that time period, including 22 percent of those with mild TBI and 36 percent of those with moderate to severe TBI.

Freezing Up: What Does It Mean?

Louis J. Marino, MD, chief of medical staff and medical director of geriatric services at Sheppard Pratt Health System.

When Senator Mitch McConnell had a sudden dead-space moment while delivering remarks on Capitol Hill, he seemed frozen in time and unresponsive for about 30 seconds. He was experiencing a neurological event called an altered or sudden change in mental status. Although the senator's aides blamed the episode on just being overtired, some medical experts questioned why the senator wasn't taken to the hospital for observation and a mental status exam.

The phrase mental status refers to a global assessment of a person's cognitive and behavioral state. When mental-health providers do a global assessment of functioning (GAF), they look at three major areas of function: social, occupational, and psychological. The GAF attempts to quantify a person's overall functioning with a score ranging from 1 to 100. The lower the score, the worse the function. A mental status exam is a formal examination that considers several factors, including mood, mental and physical functioning, clarity of thought, orientation, speech, ability to use language, judgment, and memory.

A sudden change in mental status often refers to a sudden loss of usual functioning due to a change in one or more of these areas. A change in mental status may also be accompanied by a loss in physical functioning.

The press described the senator's change in mental status as blanking out or freezing. When physicians refer to freezing, they are describing an episode in which the patient is unable to act. It could be an episode of silence or staying motionlessness or very still while staring into space.

Episodes of freezing may also be accompanied by symptoms of sudden change in mental status, such as confusion, severe anxiety, and disorientation.

Freezing can cause loss of speech, as happened with the senator. The inability or unwillingness to speak is referred to as mutism. Mutism can have many causes, such as severe anxiety, called selective mutism, or involuntary loss of speech due to an inability to emotionally process a traumatic event. Aphasia is another medical term for loss of ability to speak or understand speech. Aphasia is usually used to describe a physical rather than an emotional cause.

Many Possible Causes

While the cause of Senator McConnell's sudden change in mental status is unknown, there are many possibilities.

•**Brain injury or diseases.** About four months before his sudden change in mental status, the senator had suffered a severe fall causing broken ribs and a concussion. A concussion is a traumatic brain injury that affects your mental status. Brain injury can result in temporary or permanent disability. A brain injury from a stroke, for instance, can permanently affect the speech centers of the brain.

Chronic degenerating brain diseases such as Parkinson's disease and related illnesses like amyotrophic lateral sclerosis, multiple sclerosis, or Alzheimer's disease can also be associated with freezing. In people with Parkinson's disease, freezing is commonly seen in patients with advanced disease. Patients may find themselves suddenly but temporarily unable to move or speak for a few seconds to a few minutes. The patient is typically aware of the deficits. Although the freezing goes away, other Parkinson's symptoms persist.

•**TIA.** Mental health experts speculated that a transient ischemic attack (TIA) or seizure could be possible causes. A TIA causes temporary stroke symptoms due to a brief disruption of blood flow to the brain. The symptoms are limited to the parts of the body controlled by the affected brain area. Typical symptoms include weakness or numbness on one side of the body affecting the face, arm, or leg, loss of vision, loss of the ability to speak or to speak clearly, or sudden dizziness. A TIA lasts a few minutes, and the patient may or may not be aware of the deficit. A considerable percentage of patients who experience a TIA eventually go on to develop a stroke.

•**Seizures.** A type of seizure called an absence seizure is caused by abnormal electrical activity in the brain, resulting in a temporary loss of consciousness. An observer may note that the person has suddenly stopped their usual movement for 10 to 30 seconds, can't speak, but can stand without falling, and is manifesting some simple repetitive motor movements such as lip smacking, chewing, small hand

Don't Delay, Call 911

If a person freezes up and blanks out, the best thing to do is to visit an emergency room for evaluation. It's best not to wait it out and assume it was nothing to worry about if it goes away. That could be a serious mistake. A new episode of freezing always requires an emergency medical evaluation.

movements, or fluttering eyelids. The person typically reverts to normal functioning without awareness of the event.

Emergency Evaluation

Although there are many causes of freezing and blanking out, any sudden and new change in mental status is a red flag for a serious problem. Freezing is seen in a broad range of psychiatric, medical, and neurologic diseases and requires a comprehensive evaluation to determine the underlying cause. There are serious and less serious causes of freezing, some of which are recurrent, while others are restricted to a single episode.

Even for a skilled observer, like a neurologist, psychiatrist, or emergency physician, it is usually not possible to know the cause of freezing without additional information from testing and a physical examination.

The examination includes a thorough review of the events leading to the episode, as well as details about the areas of disability and time course of the symptoms. In many cases, the most valuable information comes from someone who had observed the event. For example, Senator McConnell could not tell what happened to him or how long it lasted but many observers could.

A neurological examination of sensory (sensations and feeling) and motor (movement and strength) systems can identify any remaining symptoms or deficits. The findings in a routine physical examination may help the doctor's understanding of possible causes, and a careful psychiatric evaluation can clarify if there are underlying emotional or behavioral issues complicating or causing the episodes of freezing.

With the data from these evaluations, a physician can identify which, if any, of the many available tests and studies would be appropriate to further confirm a cause of the episodes.

Important tests to evaluate altered mental status include brain imaging studies, electrocardiograms (EKG), and electroencephalograms (EEG), which is the best test for seizure. The best treatment depends on finding the right cause.

Mediterranean Diet May Improve Memory in People with MS

American Academy of Neurology.

People with multiple sclerosis (MS) who follow a Mediterranean diet may have a lower risk for problems with memory and thinking skills than those who do not follow the diet, according to a preliminary study presented at the American Academy of Neurology's 75th Annual Meeting. The Mediterranean diet includes a high intake of vegetables, legumes, fruits, fish, and healthy fats such as olive oil, and a low intake of dairy products, meats, and saturated fatty acids. The study involved 563 people with MS. People completed a questionnaire to show how closely they followed the Mediterranean diet. They were assigned a score of zero to 14 based on their responses, with higher scores given to those who more closely followed the diet. Researchers then divided participants into four groups based on their diet scores, with the lowest group having scores of zero to four and the highest group having scores of nine or higher. Participants also took three tests assessing their thinking and memory skills. The researchers found that people who more closely followed the Mediterranean diet had a 20 percent lower risk for cognitive impairment than people who did not follow the diet. Among those in the lowest diet score group, 43 of 133 people, or 34 percent, had cognitive impairment compared with 13 of 103, or 13 percent, of people in the highest diet score group. The relationship was stronger among people with progressive MS, in which

Brain Health

the disease steadily worsens, than among those with relapsing-remitting MS, in which the disease flares up and then goes into periods of remission.

Traffic Noise Increases Risk of Tinnitus

University of Southern Denmark Faculty of Health Sciences.

In a new study with data from 3.5 million people, researchers found that the more traffic noise residents are exposed to in their homes, the more they are at risk of developing tinnitus. For every 10-decibel increase in noise, the risk of developing tinnitus increased by 6 percent. In 2021, the same team found a correlation between traffic noise and dementia.

Turn Down the Volume on Tinnitus

Bradley Kesser, MD, professor of otology and neurotology at The University of Virginia, Charlottesville. He is vice chair of UVA's Otolaryngology–Head and Neck Surgery department. UVAHealth.com

Few things are as frustrating as an annoying sound that won't stop…or as disturbing as the realization that the sound is coming from inside your own head.

Tinnitus—a condition that causes a persistent ringing, buzzing, hissing, whooshing or comparable sound that only the individual can hear—affects around 15 percent of the U.S. population. For some, the sound is just an annoyance…but for others, it's so loud that it can't be ignored and interferes with the ability to sleep and concentrate.

The bad news: There is no cure for tinnitus—in fact, there isn't even scientific consensus about why it occurs.

But there is good news—tinnitus is rarely a sign of a serious underlying health issue…it tends to fade substantially over time—often within roughly three to four months, though this varies…and there are ways to reduce the impact it takes on your life.

Who Gets Tinnitus—and Why?

Tinnitus is very poorly understood, but we do know that certain things can be triggers. The most common culprit is hearing loss—either age-related or stemming from long-term exposure to loud noise such as machinery, power tools, firearms, or blaring music. The pitch of the sound that a tinnitus sufferer hears in his/her head tends to match the pitch that his ears have lost the ability to hear.

Example: If hearing loss has deprived someone of his ability to hear high-frequency sound, the ringing or buzzing of his tinnitus is likely to be similarly high-pitched. One potential explanation for this is that tinnitus might be caused by the brain trying to fill in the frequency of sound that has been lost.

Even onetime exposure to very loud noise, such as being in the vicinity of a large explosion or sitting near the speakers at a loud rock concert, can trigger tinnitus. Tinnitus caused by a onetime exposure is likely to be relatively short term, generally lasting only a few days to a few weeks.

But loud-noise exposure and hearing loss aren't responsible for all tinnitus. A wide range of other tinnitus triggers and contributing factors have been identified, including earwax buildup…infections, including sinus infections and the flu… stress…and the use of certain drugs, including over-the-counter painkillers. In some cases, the type of sound the tinnitus sufferer hears hints at a potential cause—particularly when this sound is not the ringing or buzzing that most tinnitus sufferers experience. *Examples…*

•**The sound of a heartbeat.** Called pulsatile tinnitus, this tends to be caused by issues related to the blood vessels near the ear. The sound itself usually is not a beat but rather a whooshing that keeps pace with the person's pulse. It is similar to the sound parents hear when an ultrasound allows them to hear their unborn child's heart. Seek medical attention for this form of tinnitus—CT and/or MRI scans typically can pinpoint the problem, and most of the conditions that lead to pulsatile tinnitus can be treated, likely reducing or ending this tinnitus. Examples of treatable pulsatile tinnitus include a malformation of blood vessels in a part of the brain near the ear, a loss of bone over one of the large blood vessels that delivers blood from the brain back down to the heart, and elevated intracranial pressure.

•**Clicking or thumping.** Potential causes here include spasms of the tiny muscles in the middle ear...contractions in the soft palate (the flexible part of the roof of the mouth)...or issues related to the eustachian tubes—the passages that connect the middle ear to the back of the nose. The eustachian tubes make a clicking sound every time we swallow, but we generally don't notice it. A blockage or infection might make this sound more noticeable. Treatments are available for many of the underlying conditions that lead to clicking/thumping tinnitus.

•**Any tinnitus sound only or largely in one ear.** This could be caused by a vestibular schwannoma, a noncancerous tumor that may affect both hearing and balance. Options for managing vestibular schwannomas include observation with serial MRI imaging, radiation, or surgical removal. Any of these treatment options can put hearing and balance functions at risk. Many times, doctors who treat patients with these tumors recommend observation—they are benign and very slow-growing.

What Can You Do?

An ear, nose and throat doctor might be able to identify a treatable underlying issue, such as excessive wax buildup in the

> ### Can CBD Help Tinnitus?
>
> Cannabidiol (CBD), a compound found in marijuana that does not cause impairment, is occasionally mentioned as a potential treatment for tinnitus. That makes some sense—it has been hypothesized that tinnitus might be a form of sensory epilepsy, and CBD has anti-epileptic properties.
>
> ***But:*** The research that has been done has not produced encouraging results. A 2015 study on rats by researchers at New Zealand's University of Otago suggested that CBD might make tinnitus worse... and a 2019 study by Stanford University researchers found that habitual marijuana use appears to increase risk for tinnitus. Several small studies have concluded that CBD does nothing to make tinnitus better or worse.
>
> Given these findings, it is not reasonable to recommend CBD as a tinnitus treatment.
>
> —Bradley Kesser, MD

ears. But there are some DIY strategies that can reduce tinnitus—or at least reduce the impact it takes on your life...

•**Cover the tinnitus with outside sound.** Options worth trying include white noise from a fan, a sound machine, or a white noise phone app, such as Rain Rain (available for iOS, Android, or Amazon devices)...YouTube background noise videos, such as "Are Cricket Sounds the New Cure for Tinnitus?"...or simply letting a TV or radio play in the background. There also are in-ear hearing-aid–like devices called "tinnitus maskers" designed specifically for this purpose—these typically are programmed by an audiologist to mask the precise frequency of the patient's tinnitus. Some hearing aids offer a tinnitus-masking function as well.

Helpful: Tinnitus sufferers who own hearing aids should consider wearing those hearing aids more often. Being able to hear more outside sound tends to make tinnitus less troublesome.

• **Seek stress reduction.** Stress can trigger or worsen tinnitus. Some sufferers even end up trapped in a tinnitus/stress spiral—the endless noise and sleep problems caused by the tinnitus increases their stress…which increases their tinnitus…and so on.

Potential stress treatments: Yoga, cognitive behavioral therapy, and/or antianxiety medications—the same treatments that might be used to treat stress unrelated to tinnitus.

Also: The treatment tinnitus retraining therapy combines cognitive behavioral therapy with a noise-canceling device such as those mentioned above. Studies have found that this provides some relief for most people who try it.

Warning: Do not take any supplements that claim to cure tinnitus. No supplement has ever been proven to provide any tinnitus benefit beyond the placebo effect.

• **Reduce use of caffeine, nicotine, alcohol, and/or certain painkillers.** Heavy use of any of these can contribute to tinnitus, and cutting back could provide significant relief—or potentially make tinnitus disappear entirely.

Helpful: When you need pain relief, lean toward Tylenol. Nonsteroidal anti-inflammatory drugs (NSAIDs) such as *ibuprofen* (Motrin or Advil), *naproxen,* and aspirin, may cause or worsen tinnitus. Tylenol is not an NSAID and does not seem to contribute to tinnitus.

• **Ask your dentist if you might have a TMJ disorder.** Problems with the temporomandibular joint (TMJ)—including chronic clenching of the jaw, a misaligned bite, or other conditions that involve the muscles and ligaments of the jaw joints—sometimes lead to tinnitus. Other TMJ symptoms include jaw pain, headaches, difficulty opening the mouth, or clicking sounds when the mouth is opened or shut. If TMJ is the cause of your tinnitus, a dentist should be able to propose treatments. A bite guard can be helpful for those who grind their teeth at night.

Ultrasound May Treat Parkinson's Symptoms

Study of 94 adults led by researchers at University of North Carolina, Chapel Hill, published in *The New England Journal of Medicine.*

Focused ultrasound ablation (sound waves) directed at a cluster of brain neurons was linked to improved motor function and reduced involuntary movements in 69 percent of Parkinson's patients for three months after treatment… and for 77 percent of patients who had improvements, the effects lasted nine months.

Parkinson's Disease Linked to Mitochondria

University of Copenhagen.

Researchers have discovered that Parkinson's disease may be caused by damaged mitochondria. When mitochondria are damaged, small fragments of DNA can be released into the cell. When the fragments are misplaced, they become toxic to the cell, and those toxic fragments spread throughout the brain. The researchers hope that a blood test could be developed to detect early disease development.

Head Pain When Bending Down

Alan Rapoport, MD, clinical professor of neurology, The David Geffen School of Medicine, UCLA, Los Angeles, California.

If you experience an uncomfortable pressure in your head when bending down, be sure to discuss this condition with your doctor. Although it is unlikely that there is any serious problem going on, especially if you have no other symptoms, such as nausea, visual problems, or severe pain, a doctor can assess whether there is some change in pressure in the brain upon changing head position. Irregularities in cerebral spinal fluid pressure, lack of cerebral spinal fluid flow, or structural abnormalities in the back of the brain all can be possible problems. The good news is that, most of the time, nothing serious is found after a thorough evaluation. It is possible that the pain, pressure, or light-headedness you feel is due to a sinus problem. Or your symptoms might be a sign of high or low blood pressure, which can be easily treated with medication and lifestyle changes.

Brain-Computer Interface Translates Brain Signals to Speech

University of California San Francisco.

A woman who was paralyzed after a brainstem stroke can now speak through a digital avatar, thanks to the development of a brain-computer interface. Researchers implanted electrodes onto the surface of her brain that intercept the brain signals. A cable connected the electrodes to a bank of computers that learned to associate brain activity patterns with parts of

Bad Air Affects Brain Health

Short-Term Smoke Exposure Can Cause Lingering Brain Health Issues

Exposure to wood smoke from a nearby forest fire every other day for two weeks caused significant inflammation-related changes to cerebrovascular endothelial cells in the brains of mice during laboratory tests. The mice also experienced changes in the hippocampal region of the brain, suggesting that smoke exposure negatively affects cognitive function and mood. These neural consequences persisted for weeks following the exposure to smoke. In human brains, similar exposure theoretically could increase dementia risk. More research is needed.

Study by researchers at University of New Mexico, Albuquerque, published in *Journal of Neuroinflammation*.

Pollution Exposure May Be Linked to Parkinson's Risk

People living in areas with the highest concentrations of fine particulate matter had 25 percent greater risk for Parkinson's than those living where concentrations were lowest. "Hotspots" were found in the Rocky Mountain region, Lake County, Colorado…and Mississippi-Ohio River valleys of Tennessee and Kentucky.

To reduce exposure: Use an air purifier and avoid outdoor exertion during periods of low air quality.

Brittany Krzyzanowski, PhD, postdoctoral research fellow at Barrow Neurological Institute, Phoenix, and leader of a study presented at the American Academy of Neurology annual meeting.

words. Altogether, the system translated the woman's brain signals into a talking animated character.

Internet Use Is Linked to Lower Dementia Risk

Study of 18,154 adults by researchers at New York University, New York City, published in *Journal of the American Geriatrics Society*.

A recent study showed that adults 50 and older who use the Internet regularly have 62 percent of the risk for dementia as people of similar age who are not regular Internet users. This finding holds true even after controlling for factors such as education level, gender, and signs of cognitive decline at the start of the study. It may be that the social and cognitive engagement offered by the Internet reduces dementia risk.

But: Dementia risk is slightly higher when Internet use for this age demographic is more than two hours per day—compared with those who use it less than two hours.

Controlling Light Exposure May Help Sundowning

Heather Ferris, MD, PhD, assistant professor of medicine, University of Virginia, Charlottesville, Virginia.

Enhanced light sensitivity may contribute to the worsening of Alzheimer's disease symptoms late in the day. Light therapy, recent research suggests, might be an effective tool to help manage what's called sundowning. Controlling the kind of light and the timing of light exposure could reduce circadian disruptions in Alzheimer's disease.

Chapter 3

CANCER BREAKTHROUGHS

How to Catch Cancer Early

The COVID-19 pandemic itself was bad enough, but it had a negative effect that few anticipated: more cases of advanced cancer.

That's because during the pandemic many people couldn't visit their primary care physicians for so-called elective procedures. As a result, they weren't routinely screened for breast, prostate, colon, lung, or other deadly cancers; weren't referred to oncologists because of suspicious findings; and weren't scheduled for further diagnostic tests.

A 2023 study from researchers at the American Cancer Society, published in *Lancet Oncology,* tells the sad story: After the initial shutdowns in March 2020, monthly cancer diagnoses plummeted by 50 percent, from 70,000 to 35,000. But overall in 2020, the risk of being diagnosed with advanced stage 4 cancer—when undiagnosed cancer has spread (metastasized) beyond its original location to distant sites in the body—rose by 26 percent. Stage 4 cancer is far more deadly than stage 1 cancer. For example, the five-year survival rate for stage 1 lung cancer is 56 percent, but for stage 4 lung cancer, it's 5 percent. That trend of more advanced cancer continues, according to Hannah Hazard-Jenkins, MD, director of the West Virginia University Cancer Institute.

"In the breast cancer world, last year [2022], we had a profound amount of advanced disease—numbers of advanced disease I haven't seen in 15 years," she told *STAT* magazine.

Four cancers account for 50 percent of all new diagnoses in the United States: breast (15 percent), prostate (15 percent), lung (12 percent), and colorectal (8 percent). Here are important ways to catch those cancers early.

Breast Cancer

The USPSTF recommends every-other-year mammograms for women ages 50 to 74. However, they give the relatively low grade of "C" to starting mammography in women younger than 50, saying it

---

Yuri Fesko, MD, a board-certified oncologist, assistant consulting professor in the Department of Medicine at the Duke University School of Medicine, and Vice President of Medical Affairs and Medical Oncology for Quest Diagnostics.

leads to many false positives and unnecessary biopsies, while preventing a relatively small number of deaths. On the other hand, the American Cancer Society says women ages 40 to 44 should have the option to start yearly mammograms, women ages 45 to 54 should get yearly mammograms, and women ages 55 and older can switch to a mammogram every other year.

But there's one thing that most of the top experts on breast cancer agree on: If a mammogram shows dense breasts—more fibrous tissue and glands than fat, which occurs in nearly half of women over age 40—a women should consider further testing to detect a possible cancer. That's because dense breasts make it much harder to see cancer on a mammogram. Plus, dense breasts are themselves a risk factor for breast cancer.

The test recommended by most breast imaging experts, a 3D mammogram (digital breast tomosynthesis), produces more visual clarity, reduces the likelihood of a false positive result (leading to an unnecessary biopsy), and better identifies the size and growth of a possible tumor. If you have dense breasts, your future mammograms should be 3D, if available.

You should also talk with your doctor about whether or not you need more tests, including genetic testing, which depends on your level of risk, taking into account risk factors like dense breasts, the BRCA gene, a family history of breast cancer, and obesity after menopause. You can calculate your risk level at BCRiskTool.Cancer.gov.

If you're at high risk, you should have a yearly breast MRI in addition to your mammogram.

If you have dense breasts and you're not at high risk, talk to your health care professional about screening tests in addition to a 3D mammogram, like a breast MRI or ultrasound. If you've had breast cancer, you should have a yearly mammogram and breast MRI—especially if you have dense breasts or were diagnosed before age 50.

Prostate Cancer

It's difficult for a man to know what to do about the early detection of prostate cancer. In most cases, it is a slow-growing disease that is not life-threatening, but it also kills 50,000 men yearly.

The main screening tool is the prostate-specific antigen (PSA) test. But there's a reason why the U.S. Preventive Task Force (USPSTF)—a widely respected consortium of scientists that evaluates preventive services used to recommend against prostate cancer screening. Now it recommends that men ages 55 to 69 engage in a shared decision-making process with their doctors about the pros and cons of screening.

Research shows that it requires 1,000 men to have a PSA test in order to prevent one death from prostate cancer. But of those 1,000 men, between 150 to 200 will have a worrisome PSA test (a level higher than 4) that will lead to a biopsy of the prostate—an invasive procedure that can cause blood in the urine, infections, and a high rate of hospitalization in the month after the procedure.

Of those biopsied, 30 to 100 will be treated for prostate cancer, and between one-third to one-half of those men will become impotent. Another 20 to 30 percent will become incontinent.

The overdiagnosis, overtreatment, and treatment complications should lead you and your doctor to carefully consider the risks and benefits of PSA testing, says the USPSTF.

The USPSTF also recommends no PSA testing for men 70 and older because the chance of dying from prostate cancer is lower than the chance of dying from another cause.

The problem is, with fewer men receiving PSA tests, there is now an increasing incidence of metastatic prostate cancers, with the rate doubling from 2011 to 2023, according to a new report from the American Cancer Society.

Fortunately, there are several newer types of blood tests (such as the 4kScore,

Prostate Health Index and IsoPSA) that are used to augment PSA. A study published in *Urology Practice* showed that these tests can reduce recommendations for biopsies by 55 percent.

These testes are included in the guidelines from the National Comprehensive Cancer Network (NCCN), an alliance of 33 leading cancer centers. If you have a high PSA, ask your doctor about this test.

Lung Cancer

About 80 to 90 percent of people who develop lung cancer are smokers or former smokers. The best way to detect their cancer early is with yearly low-dose computed tomography (LDCT) screening. The USPSTF added this screening to their recommendations in 2021. The problem is that only 5 to 6 percent of the people who should be getting LDCT screening are actually getting it. *You should definitely get the screening if you meet these criteria...*

- **Current smokers or those who have quit within the past 15 years**
- **Adults ages 50 to 80**
- **A 20-pack-year smoking history** (one pack a day for 20 years or one-half pack a day for 40 years).

The earlier lung cancer is detected, the greater the chance of successfully fighting the disease and adding years to your life.

Colorectal Cancer

Colorectal cancer—the second-biggest cancer killer in the United States—is being detected more commonly in people under age 50. In fact, people born in 1990 have *double* the risk of colorectal cancer as people born in 1950. No one knows the reason why, but it's probably environmental factors like obesity, sedentary lifestyle, or a diet low in fruits and vegetables and high in processed meats.

A study in the *Journal of the National Cancer Institute* found that people under age 55 are nearly 60 percent more likely to be diagnosed with stage 4 colorectal cancer than older adults. In response, both the American Cancer Society and the USPSTF now recommend that colorectal cancer screenings begin at age 45, which is five years earlier than their previous recommendations.

You can screen for colorectal cancer with a stool-based test, such as a fecal immunochemical test (FIT), or a colonoscopy. If a stool-based test is positive, you need a colonoscopy.

After your first test, you should get a screen once every five to 10 years, depending on your level of risk. Talk to your doctor about your risk level. If you

---

The Next Generation in Screening: Multi-Cancer Early Detection Tests

The latest development in cancer detection is the multi-cancer early detection test, or MCED (also called a liquid biopsy), a blood test that can help detect cancer cells from a tumor by identifying certain biomarkers circulating in the blood. This type of blood test undercuts many of the problems with conventional screening: lack of knowledge about what screens are recommended when, anxiety about false positives from the procedure, and generally low adherence. The tests measure genetic mutations linked to cancer, cancer-associated proteins, and cancer signals, allowing the detection of multiple cancers from a single blood draw. Currently, there's a bill in congress called the The Multi-Cancer Early Detection Screening Coverage Act that would ensure Medicare patients have coverage for the MCED. At this time, the only test available from your doctor is the GRAIL Galleri test. There are no current guidelines as to when and how the test should be used. But stay tuned for more news on this cutting-edge development in early detection.

have a higher-than-average level of risk, talk to your doctor about whether you should get a screen every five years. If precancerous polyps are detected and removed during a colonoscopy, you need a screen every five years. You may not need any more testing after you turn 75 or 80.

Air Pollution Increases Breast Cancer Risk

"Ambient Fine Particulate Matter and Breast Cancer Incidence in a Large Prospective US Cohort," by researchers at the National Institute of Environmental Health Sciences, published in the *Journal of the National Cancer Institute*.

It's no surprise that air pollution is bad for our bodies, especially respiratory systems. But what about cancer? A recent study from researchers at the National Institutes of Health (NIH) is one of the largest to look at the link between outdoor air pollution levels and breast cancer. The results raise concern and demand attention to air quality.

Fine particulate-matter air pollution is a mixture of toxins in the air that are microscopic (equal or less than 2.5 microns in size). Also called *ambient fine particulate matter*, these toxins can be deeply inhaled into the lungs where they enter the blood stream and disperse through the body. A growing amount of research evidence suggests that fine particulate matter exposure is associated with an increased risk of breast cancer. One review of six European studies found an increased breast cancer risk of about six percent.

What the NIH Air Pollution Study Looked At

The NIH team used data on air pollution exposure for close to 200,000 women who were enrolled in the NIH-AARP Diet and Health Study, which began in 1995. They matched breast cancer diagnosis rates with levels of particulate-matter air pollution in six states (California, Florida, Pennsylvania, New Jersey, North Carolina, and Louisiana) and two cities, Atlanta and Detroit. This study is the first to include exposure risk starting 10 to 15 years before the study began. Other studies have only looked at exposure during the years of the study. This study also breaks down the risk by the type of breast cancer.

The average age of the women in the study was 62. During about 20 years of follow-up, there were 15,870 breast cancers diagnosed. A 10-microgram increase in particulate-matter air pollution was associated with an 8 percent increase in breast cancer incidence. Eight percent is a significant increase, and a risk factor shared by all women exposed to this type of air pollution. All the areas surveyed had an increase in breast cancer linked to particulate matter air pollution. The highest increase was for Atlanta at 22 percent. For the states, California had the lowest risk at 6 percent and North Carolina, the highest at 26 percent.

Pollution Is an Estrogen Disrupter

This study also broke down the cancers by estrogen receptor status. Most breast cancers are sensitive to the female hormone estrogen, called ER-positive cancers. These tumors use estrogen to help them grow. The increase in breast cancer diagnosis was in ER-positive cancers. This may explain how particulate matter air pollution increases breast cancer risk. Many of the toxins included in particulate matter are estrogen disruptors, meaning they may increase estrogen production in the body.

Particulate matter is a mixture of solid and liquid particles or droplets in the air from motor vehicle exhaust fumes, burning of oil or coal, industrial waste, or smoke from burning wood or vegetation. Airborne toxins that are estrogen disruptors include polybrominated diphenyl ethers, phthalates, and metals. Other possible carcinogenic particles can include organic compounds, ammonium, nitrate, ozone, sulfate, and others.

Breast cancer is the most common cancer in women, other than skin cancer. Known risk factors for breast cancer are family history (genes), reproductive history, alcohol intake, estrogen medications, and obesity. Reducing and avoiding air pollution may be a way women can reduce their risk of breast cancer. The U.S. Environmental Protection Agency provides a website called Air Now (AirNow.gov) where you can enter your zip code and find out about air quality and the level of particulate-matter air pollution in your area.

Artificial Intelligence Can Predict Breast Cancer Chemotherapy Outcomes

University of Waterloo.

Neoadjuvant chemotherapy is a presurgical treatment that, in some women, can shrink breast cancer tumors to reduce the need for major surgery. In a project at the Vision and Image Processing (VIP) Lab, artificial intelligence software was trained with images of breast cancer made with a new modality called synthetic correlated diffusion imaging (CDI). With knowledge gleaned from CDI images of old breast cancer cases and information on their outcomes, the AI can predict if preoperative chemotherapy treatment would benefit new patients based on their CDI images.

A False-Positive Is a Cancer Warning

Study titled "Breast Cancer Incidence After a False-Positive Mammography Result," by researchers at the Karolinska Institutet, Stockholm, Sweden, published in *JAMA Oncology*.

Breast cancer screening with mammography reduces the risk of dying from breast cancer by 20 percent by finding cancer early when it can be treated more effectively. In the U.S., about 10 percent of mammography exams result in callbacks. When the follow-up visit reveals no cancer (either through another mammogram or a biopsy), it's known as a false-positive result.

No Cancer Now, But Maybe Later

False-positive mammograms create mental stress and may discourage a woman from future screenings. But they may be an important risk factor for a future breast cancer diagnosis. Previous studies have hinted at this risk, but in 2015, a very large review that included over one million women confirmed that a false-positive mammogram increases the risk of a future breast cancer significantly over the following 10 years. Now, a new study has found that the risk extends out to 20 years.

The new study, from Sweden, compared more than 45,000 women with a false-positive mammogram to more than 450,000 women who had a negative mammogram at the same age and on the same year. These women were followed for up to 20 years to compare breast cancer rates and other risk factors that might add to or explain the association between a false-positive mammogram and breast cancer. The study is published in the *Journal of the American Medical Association (JAMA) Oncology*. These were two key findings...

- **Over 20 years,** about seven percent of women with a negative mammogram developed breast cancer, compared to about 11 percent of women with a false-positive result, an overall increased risk of about 60 percent.
- **Women who had a false-positive mammogram had an overall 84 percent higher risk** of dying from breast cancer than women who had a negative result.

Among those women who developed breast cancer...

- **Being age 60 to 75 at the time of the false-positive exam doubled the risk.**
- **Women with lower-density (less fat and breast tissue) breasts had a four to five times higher risk.**
- **Women who had a biopsy to rule out cancer had a nearly 80 percent higher risk.**
- **The future breast cancer was two to three times more likely to occur** in the first four years after the false positive.

Changes in Breast Tissue Can Affect Readings

The reasons why false-positive mammograms increase breast cancer risk are not completely understood. It is possible that cancers occurring in the same breast within four years were missed on the follow-up exam. However, many future cancers occurred many years later and in the opposite breast, which suggests changes in breast tissue that make mammograms slightly abnormal or harder to read may be warning signs of a future cancer. Increased risk after biopsy may be due to tissue changes caused by the biopsy.

In the U.S., about half of women will have at least one false-positive result after 10 screening mammograms. The American Cancer Society guidelines suggest a yearly mammogram for women ages 40 to 54, and every two years for women age 55 and older.

The researchers conclude that women with a history of a false-positive result should be considered at higher risk than other women, especially if they have added risk factors like older age (60 to 75), low-density breasts, and a history of a negative biopsy. They and their health-care providers may consider more frequent breast exams in the first four years, and these exams may continue to be yearly after age 55. Women with a false-positive mammogram should talk to their health-care providers about risk prevention strategies.

Which Women Benefit Most from Medication for Breast Cancer Prevention

Study titled "Effect of Baseline Oestradiol Serum Concentration on the Efficacy of Anastrozole for Preventing Breast Cancer in Postmenopausal Women at High Risk: a Case-Control Study of the IBIS-II Prevention Trial" led by researchers at Queen Mary University of London Wolfson Institute of Population Health, published in *The Lancet Oncology*.

Certain drugs can help prevent breast cancer in women who are high risk. From previous studies, breast cancer researchers know that a class of drugs called aromatase inhibitors (AIs) are the most effective medications to prevent estrogen receptor-positive breast cancer in women after menopause. These breast cancers make up 80 percent of all breast cancers. The female hormone estrogen fuels cancer cell growth and development.

A new study from Queen Mary University of London's Wolfson Institute of Population Health finds that measuring estrogen with a blood test is a simple and inexpensive way of predicting which women will benefit the most from AIs. This is important because these medications can have side effects. By knowing who may benefit, women and their doctors can have a more reliable way of measuring the risks versus advantages of treatment.

What Makes a Woman High Risk

Currently, the UK's National Institute of Clinical Care and Excellence (NICE) recommends AIs for postmenopausal women at high risk for breast cancer. According to the American Cancer Society, two AIs have been shown in studies to lower breast cancer risk: *anastrozole* (Arimidex) and *exemestane* (Aromasin). AIs work by blocking an enzyme that converts other hormones into estrogen. They do not block the ovaries from producing estrogen, so they work best in postmenopausal women.

High risk may include a previous breast biopsy that was suspicious or precancerous but not cancer, or a strong family history of breast cancer. The new study is published in the journal *The Lancet Oncology*. The research team analyzed data from a large breast cancer prevention study that included women from 18 countries.

Significant Benefit from AIs

There were more than 3,800 women in the study. All the women had risk factors for breast cancer but had never been diagnosed. All the women were postmenopausal with ages ranging from 40 to 70. They were equally divided into two groups. One group received one dose of oral anastrozole every day for five years. The other group received a placebo pill. Neither the women nor the researchers knew who was given which pill until the end of the study. The women were followed for an average of about 11 years.

Based on their estrogen blood levels drawn at the start of the study and during the follow-up period, the women were divided into four groups from the lowest 25 percent to the highest 25 percent of estrogen levels. *These were the key results…*

- **There were 85 cases of breast cancer diagnosed in the AI group** compared to 165 in the placebo group.
- **For women in the highest 75 percent of estrogen blood levels** the risk reduction from AI was 55 percent compared to women not taking the AI.
- **For women in the bottom 25 percent of estrogen blood level,** the risk reduction was not significant.

The most common side effects of AIs include symptoms that are similar to menopausal symptoms and may include hot flashes, vaginal dryness, headache, and fatigue. More serious but less common risks are osteoporosis, high cholesterol, and joint or muscle pain.

The researchers conclude that testing estrogen blood levels should be included in the weighing of the risks versus benefits of AI intake for breast cancer prevention. Women with low levels of estrogen are less likely to benefit, in which case the risks would most likely outweigh the benefits.

Why Breast Cancer Survival Has Improved

Study titled "Analysis of Breast Cancer Mortality in the US—1975 to 2019," led by researchers at Stanford University School of Medicine and the Cancer Intervention and Surveillance Modeling Network, published in *JAMA*.

More breast cancer cases are being diagnosed, but fewer women are dying. The yearly number of new breast cancers has been rising steadily from about 200,000 in 2000 to about 270,000 in 2019, according to the Centers for Disease Control and Prevention. However, a new study in the *Journal of the American Medical Society, (JAMA)*, reveals that deaths from breast cancer have decreased by 58 percent between 1975 and 2019.

The study was led by Stanford Medicine researchers in collaboration with the Cancer Intervention and Surveillance Modeling Network (CISNET). CISNET was established by the National Cancer Institute in 2000 to study and report on the impact of screening, treatment, and mortality of common cancers in the United States.

The team used breast cancer screening and treatment data collected from observational studies and clinical trials to learn how much screening and treatment contributed to improved survival. They also analyzed how estrogen receptor (ER) and HER2 (also known as ErbB2) status effect treatment and survival.

Early Intervention and Targeted Therapy Help Survival

Breast cancer screening with mammography has been recommended by the American Cancer Society since 1976 and remains the most reliable way to screen for breast cancer. Mammography finds breast cancer at an early stage before signs or symptoms develop.

ER status is positive if breast cancer cells are found to have proteins that bind to the female hormone estrogen. These cancers are more aggressive due to this estrogen binding. Along with standard cancer treatments, ER-positive cancers can be treated with hormone therapy to reduce estrogen or block the receptors. HER2 is a protein found in some breast cancer cells that make cancers more likely to grow quickly and spread. HER2-positive cancers can be treated with cancer drugs that target HER2, called targeted therapy.

These were some of the study's key findings on breast cancer from 1975 to 2019...

- Deaths from breast cancer decreased by 58 percent.
- Improved treatment of early-stage cancer (stages 1-3) accounted for 47 percent of the decrease in deaths.
- Improved screening for early-stage cancer accounted for 25 percent of the decrease in deaths.
- Improved treatment of advanced (stage 4) cancer accounted for 29 percent of the decrease in deaths.

Women with Stage 4 Cancer Living Longer

Advanced cancers that have spread to other parts of the body (called metastatic disease) are generally not curable, but the 29 precent improvement was an indication that women with stage 4 breast cancer are living longer. ER and HER2 status have had a recent impact on treatment and survival of metastatic breast cancer from 2000 thru 2019...

- Patients with HER2-positive and ER-positive cancers had an increased survival of two to three years.
- Patients with HER2-negative and ER-positive cancers had an increased survival of one to two years.
- Patients with ER-negative and HER2-negative had an increased survival of one to two-and-a-half years. These figures are based on simulations.

The researchers say that this type of study reinforces the value for routine screening, the success of early cancer treatment, and the benefits of new treatments that can help patients with metastatic cancer live longer. They

---

Artificial Sweetener May Increase Cancer Risk

The World Health Organization (WHO) has classified aspartame as possibly carcinogenic to humans. More research is needed, but ethical considerations associated with putting human subjects at risk make that challenging. There already are good reasons to avoid artificial sweeteners, including that they fuel sugar cravings.

Maya Adam, MD, director of health media innovation at Stanford School of Medicine, Stanford, California, commenting on assessment of risk by the International Agency for Research on Cancer (IARC), the World Health Organization (WHO), and the Food and Agriculture Organization (FAO) Joint Expert Committee on Food Additives (JECFA). Med.Stanford.edu

expect that deaths from breast cancer will continue to go down as new developments in diagnosis and treatment become available.

Get a Second Opinion for Cancer Diagnosis

Study of 2,000 patients from 140 cancer centers around the U.S. by researchers at the National Heart, Lung and Blood Institute, Bethesda, Maryland, published in *Blood Advances*.

A second opinion is especially important for diagnoses of rare cancers—few clinicians are able to detect these accurately.

Recent finding: Expert pathologists who examined bone-marrow samples taken by local doctors found that 20 percent might have been misdiagnosed…did not have the type of cancer identified…or the patients were incorrectly given a clean bill of health.

Does Eating Organic Foods Protect You from Cancer?

Bottom Line Health.

According to the Centers for Disease Control and Prevention, more than 85 percent of Americans have pesticides and other chemicals in their bodies. Studies have shown that when people eat organic food, bodily pesticide levels decrease.

A study published in the *Journal of the American Medical Association* suggests that this may reduce the risk of cancer. The study looked at close to 70,000 people (mostly women) and found the biggest drop was in lymphomas and postmenopausal breast cancers. But these results aren't so clear cut. The study is being criticized for having a poor design that makes the conclusions untrustworthy. One of the concerns is that the researchers did not control for all factors that may affect cancer risk. That is not to say that eating organic foods doesn't lower the risk of cancer, only that this study does not prove the link.

Red Meat and Dairy Appear Protective Against Cancer

Jing Chen, PhD, a cancer researcher at The University of Chicago and a senior author of a study published in *Nature*.

Hundreds of food-derived metabolites—blood nutrients—were screened for antitumor activity, the most robust tested on both human T cells and on mice with cancer. The metabolite with the strongest immune response was *transvaccenic acid* (TVA), a long-chain fatty acid found in red meat and dairy. Overconsuming red meat and dairy still is not healthy…but these results underscore the value of including both in a well-balanced diet.

Weight-Loss Surgery in Women Reduces Blood Cancer Risk

Study titled "Long-Term Incidence of Haematological Cancer After Bariatric Surgery or Usual Care in the Swedish Obese Subjects Study: A Prospective Cohort Study," by researchers at the University of Gothenburg, Sweden, published in *The Lancet Healthy Longevity*.

It's well known that obesity increases your risk for heart disease and diabetes. In recent years, many studies have also found that it increases risk for cancer. In fact, past research has shown that 13 different cancers have a direct link to obesity.

But there's good news: several previous studies have found that significant weight loss may reduce obesity-related cancer risk.

The only hematologic cancer (blood cancer) to be recognized as obesity related is multiple myeloma. Obesity researchers at Gothenburg University in Sweden wanted to find out if bariatric surgery would reduce the risk of other common hematologic cancers. These are cancers that start in cells of the immune system or in blood-forming cells. The most common hematologic cancers are leukemias and lymphomas. The researchers used bariatric surgery (weight-loss surgery) as the most reliable way to achieve substantial long-term weight loss.

The research team enrolled patients from the Swedish Obese Subjects study—a long-term study that follows obese patients after bariatric surgery. To be considered for this research, which began in 1987, men needed to have a body mass index (BMI) of at least 34 and women a BMI of 38. Age had to be between 37 and 60. Any BMI over 30 is considered obese.

Women Fared Better with Weight Loss

The results of the study are reported in the medical journal *The Lancet Healthy Longevity.* Just over 4,000 people with obesity were enrolled in the study between 1987 and 2001. About 2,000 people had bariatric surgery and about 2,000 had usual care for obesity, but no surgery. These people served as the control group. Most of the participants were women, about 70 percent. The follow-up time was up to 33 years and averaged about 25 years. During that time, these were the key results of the study...

- **In the control group, weight loss never exceeded 3 kilograms (kg).** One kg is a little over two pounds. In the surgery group, average weight loss was 28.5 kg after two years, 20.8 kg after 10 years, and 21.2 kg after 15 years.

- **During the study, there were 85 hematologic cancers diagnosed—**34 in the surgery group and 51 in the control group—a risk reduction of 40 percent for the surgery group.

- **There were 13 cancer deaths in the control group and three in the surgery group,** a risk reduction of about 70 percent.

- **The most common cancers were lymphomas.** Risk for lymphoma was reduced by about 55 percent.

- **Although women had reduced risk for all hematologic cancers after bariatric surgery,** the same was not found for men. Men had no risk reduction compared to the control group.

Theory on Obesity and Cancer Risk

Why obesity increases cancer risk is not known for sure, but the main reasons most likely include the effects of obesity on the body, including inflammation and high blood sugar. Why weight reduction did not reduce cancer risk in men is also unknown, but probably has to do with the increased production of the female hormone estrogen. Previous studies have found a higher rate of blood cancers in women and a lower risk linked to bariatric surgery.

Specifically, the researchers concluded that bariatric surgery is associated with a reduced risk of hematologic cancers in women. Their findings support obesity as a significant risk factor for these cancers. Along with exercise and diet to lose weight, bariatric surgery may be considered as a primary treatment for people with obesity. They also note that the recently approved weight loss drugs should be evaluated in future studies to see if they also reduce cancer risk.

How to Survive the No. 2 Cause of Death in America

Timothy Burns, MD, PhD, associate professor of medicine in the division of hematology-oncology at the University of Pittsburgh and UPMC Hillman Cancer Center, and a specialist in the treatment of lung cancer.

Approximately 127,000 Americans die from lung cancer each year, making it the most deadly cancer by far and the second leading cause of death in the United States. (Cardiovascular disease is the first.) But if you or a loved one is diagnosed with lung cancer this year, don't despair. Medical breakthroughs are dramatically extending the lives of patients with lung cancer—particularly people with non-small cell lung cancer (NSCLC), which accounts for 85 percent of all lung cancers.

Two classes of new drugs have proven themselves very effective at extending life.

•**Checkpoint inhibitors.** These immunotherapy drugs (also called monoclonal antibodies) energize the immune system to kill cancer cells by blocking one of two cancer-encouraging proteins, PD-1 or PDL-1. These drugs include *pembrolizumab* (Keytruda), *nivolumab* (Opdivo), and *ipilimumab* (Yervoy). They are now often used as first-line therapy before or with chemotherapy.

•**Targeted therapy.** These drugs turn off one of several genetic mutations (oncogenes) that can drive NSCLC, like EGFR, EML4-ALK, ROS1, and KRAS. About 50 percent of NSCLC patients have a "targetable" mutation. These drugs include *crizotinib* (Xalkori), *osimertinib* (Tagrisso), and *alectinib* (Alecensa). They're very effective.

The average survival time in lung cancer that has metastasized (spread beyond the lungs, typically to the brain, bones, or liver) is 12 to 14 months after treatment. But 70 to 80 percent of metastatic NSCLC patients who have the ALK-positive mutation respond to *crizotinib* (Xalkori) or similar drugs. Among them, 62 percent are alive five years later.

Another breakthrough: If a patient becomes resistant to a gene-modulating drug—which commonly happens within a year—there are now second- and third-generation drugs.

In one of the latest scientific papers on targeted therapy—published in the *Journal of Clinical Oncology*, researchers from across the world studied 682 patients with NCSLC and the EGFR mutation who'd had their tumors surgically removed.

Investigators divided the patients into two groups: One group received osimertinib and the other received a placebo. Over four years, 73 percent of the patients taking osimertinib had disease-free survival, compared with 38 percent in the placebo group. Among the placebo group, 60 percent had a

---

Liquid Biopsy for Lung Cancer

Anyone with suspected lung cancer should receive a biopsy before starting therapy. In many cases, however, a tissue biopsy isn't possible. That's where a liquid biopsy comes in.

This blood test, which was approved by the FDA in 2016, is as accurate as a tissue biopsy, and it can be routinely used where a tissue biopsy is not an option.

A five-year study published in the March 2023 issue of *Clinical Lung Cancer* showed that a liquid biopsy is, in many ways, superior to tissue biopsy. Results came back 26 days sooner. The liquid biopsy was more accurate than the tissue biopsy in identifying biomarkers for treatment—76 percent of the time for liquid, 55 percent for tissue. And there was no difference in treatment outcome, progression-free survival (the length of time after receiving treatment when the disease does not progress), or overall survival (the time between receiving treatment and death).

If it's time for a biopsy, talk to your oncologist about this option.

recurrence of lung cancer, compared with 27 percent in the osimertinib group. The osimertinib group also had fewer metastases.

Drugs for KRAS mutation

A new development in gene-modulating medications is a class of drugs that target the KRAS G12C genetic mutation. This is the most common, smoking-linked genetic mutation in NSCLC, occurring in 12 to 15 percent of people with the disease. (Never-smokers can also have this mutation.) Until recently, there have been no gene-modulating medications for this form of the disease.

On May 28, 2021, the FDA approved *sotorasib* (Lumakras) for KRAS G12C-mutated NSCLC that is either locally advanced (spread into nearby tissues or lymph nodes) or metastatic (spread beyond the lungs). The drug was approved for people who already had one type of systemic therapy, like chemotherapy or hormonal therapy.

In December 2022, the FDA approved *adagrasib* (Krazati) for KRAS G12C-mutated NSCLC for any case of locally advanced or metastatic cancer.

Genetic Testing

Unfortunately, only 50 to 60 percent of patients who are newly diagnosed with NSCLC receive genetic testing to see if they are a candidate for a gene-modulating drug. But among those tested, about half are candidates.

The testing is FDA-approved, and Medicare and most other insurance cover both the testing and the gene-modulating drugs. So, why is there such a low rate of testing for a gold standard therapy?

There is a disconnect between the scientific findings on these newer classes of cancer drugs and routine care in community, nonacademic cancer centers.

Bottom line: If you're diagnosed with NSCLC, testing for your mutation status is a must to ensure the most effective treatment. Talk to your oncologist about your options.

If you don't have a genetic mutation, then you should be offered immunotherapy, along with surgery and/or chemotherapy. About 40 percent of patients who do not have a genetic mutation respond to immunotherapy. Talk to your oncologist about this approach.

Early Diagnosis

The majority of people who develop lung cancer are smokers or former smokers. About 10 to 20 percent of cases occur in never-smokers. The best way to detect their cancer early is with low-dose computed tomography (LDCT) screening, conducted yearly.

In March 2021, the U.S. Preventive Service Task Force revised the screening guidelines to recommend annual LDCT screening for people who meet the following criteria...

• **Adults ages 50 to 80**

• **A 20-pack-year smoking history** (one pack a day for 20 years, or one-half pack a day for 40 years)

• **Current smokers or those who have quit within the past 15 years.**

If you meet these criteria, talk to your primary care physician about getting a yearly LDCT for your lungs. This screening is crucial to your longevity because the earlier lung cancer is detected, the greater the likelihood you can successfully fight the disease.

Mortality Risk from Lung Cancer May Be Cut in Half

Study of 682 patients ages 30 to 86 in 26 countries by researchers at Yale University, New Haven, Connecticut, presented at the recent annual meeting of the American Society of Clinical Oncology.

The drug *osimertinib* (Tagrisso) is standard therapy when lung cancer returns after surgery to remove tumors.

Recent finding: Taking the drug after surgery, without waiting to see if the cancer returns, led to a 51 percent reduced death risk among patients with non-small cell lung cancer (NSCL)—the most common form of the disease. All patients studied had a mutation of the EGFR gene, which is found in about one-quarter of global lung cancer cases. After five years, 88 percent of patients who took *osimertinib* daily after surgery were still alive—compared with 78 percent of patients who took a placebo. The survival benefit was seen regardless of whether patients had prior chemotherapy. The drug is available in the U.S. and elsewhere.

Nail-Gel Dryers Boost Cancer Risk

Nail-gel manicures are dried under a UV lamp. Up to 70 percent of human and mouse skin cells exposed to similar radiation for three 20-minute sessions died... and the remaining cells underwent damage consistent with skin cancer.

Self-defense: Limit gel manicures...before having one, apply high-SPF sunscreen to your hands and around the nails...consider wearing fingerless gloves.

Maria Zhivagui, PhD, post-doctoral scholar in cellular and molecular medicine at University of California, San Diego, and leader of a study published in *Nature Communications*.

Skin Cancer— Not a Deadly Diagnosis Anymore

Julie K. Karen, MD, assistant professor at NYU in the Ronald O. Perelman Department of Dermatology, New York City. She and her sister, Elizabeth Hale, MD, practice at CompleteSkinMD and are board-certified dermatologists who specialize in the diagnosis and treatment of skin cancer. CompleteSkinMD.com

It is a frightening statistic—one in five of us will develop skin cancer by the time we turn 70, according to the Skin Cancer Foundation. That's despite the fact that we all know the basics about protecting our skin by always wearing sunscreen and a hat...avoiding the sun when it is at its strongest...checking our skin regularly for anything that looks suspicious...and, of course, never using tanning beds.

Yet, skin cancer is the most common type of cancer in the U.S. and around the globe.

Even worse: The rates of the three major types of skin cancer—basal cell carcinoma (BCC), squamous cell carcinoma (SCC) and melanoma—have been rapidly rising in recent decades. These alarming increases are attributed to several factors, including depletion of the ozone layer, which translates into greater and more potent UV exposure...increased longevity (skin cancer is more common in older adults)...more frequent travel to tropical destinations...and use of indoor tanning devices.

But there is good news: The likelihood of dying from skin cancer is declining, due to increased awareness about how to prevent the disease (sunscreen, sunscreen, sunscreen!) and early detection.

Even better: There have been advances in treatments that are helping to squash this deadly disease.

What Is Skin Cancer?

Skin cancer occurs when abnormal cells grow rapidly in the outer layer (epidermis) of the skin as a result of damage to DNA and subsequent genetic mutations. This damage typically is caused by UV radiation from the sun.

BCCs and SCCs generally pose little risk for death, but melanoma can be deadly, especially if it's not caught early.

Reason: Melanomas tend to grow more rapidly and are much more likely to invade the bloodstream and lymphatics and spread to regional lymph nodes and ultimately distant organs.

But: If caught and treated early, 99 percent of people with melanoma will still be alive in five years.

Lighter vs. Darker Skin

Lighter-skinned people with naturally blonde or red hair, light-colored eyes, and freckles are most at risk for skin cancer because their skin contains relatively less pigment (melanin), which is protective against UV-induced damage. Lighter-skinned people tend to get skin cancer on body parts that are often exposed to the sun—both those more chronically exposed (face, chest, and tops of the hands), as well as those areas subject to acute, intermittent "sunburst" exposure (the back and shoulders in men and the lower legs in women).

But that doesn't mean that people with olive, brown, or black skin can't get melanoma and other skin cancers. In fact, the death rate from skin cancer is higher among darker-skinned people because awareness of the risk is low and because diagnosis and, ultimately, treatment may be delayed.

Recent finding: Skin cancers among darker-skinned people are less linked to sun exposure and demonstrate different genetic mutations than skin cancers in their fair-skinned counterparts. Melanomas in darker ethnicities are more commonly seen in sun-protected areas of the skin, such as the palms and soles (a specific subtype known as acral lentiginous melanoma), the mucosa (for example, inside the mouth and the genital region) and beneath the nail bed. These lesions often evade detection and are diagnosed at a later stage.

Immunotherapy Is the Word

The immune system has a natural ability to attack tumors, but when our immune system's ability to look for and correct DNA damage is impaired (due to UV-induced immunosuppresion, local or systemic infections, or unrelated malignancies), genetic mutations accumulate and skin cancers emerge.

For decades, surgery, chemotherapy, and sometimes radiation therapy have been the staples of skin cancer treatment. These still are effective in many cases, but chemotherapy, in particular, can cause many debilitating side effects, including fatigue, rash, bruising, diarrhea, and hair loss.

Reason: Chemotherapy drugs target rapidly dividing cells—the hallmark of cancer—but they do so nonspecifically and so also damage healthy cells that divide rapidly such as those of the skin, gastrointestinal tract, and hair follicles.

Enter immunotherapy with revolutionary drugs known as checkpoint inhibitors that specifically target cancerous cells. Im-

> ### The ABCs of Melanomas
>
> Keep an eye out for these signs...
>
> • **Asymmetry.** A mole looks different on one side versus the other.
>
> • **Border irregularity.** A mole has an irregular (not round) shape with jagged or indistinct borders.
>
> • **Color variation.** A mole has different colors within a single lesion.
>
> • **Diameter or Dark.** Lesions that are bigger than one-quarter of an inch (the size of a pencil eraser) and/or darker than other lesions on an individual warrant closer attention.
>
> • **Evolving.** A lesion that changes in color, size, shape, texture and/or symptoms (scabbing or bleeding) warrants prompt evaluation.
>
> Darker-skinned people should look for the ABCDEs of melanoma as well as signs of acral lentiginous melanoma, signaled by...
>
> • **Black or brown spots** on the palms of the hands, soles of the feet or nail beds.
>
> • **A spot that bleeds,** doesn't heal and/or grows bigger over time.

munotherapy revs up the body's own immune system to attack tumors and acts on certain proteins and specific pathways (or checkpoints) that block the body's ability to fight cancers. Research has shown this treatment can lead to long remissions and extend survival for people with advanced melanomas. Recent studies demonstrate that both alone and in combination, checkpoint inhibitors such as *ipilimumab* (Yervoy) and *nivolumab* (Opdivo) can suppress melanoma tumors that have spread to other organs, such as the brain, for years.

Downside: These drugs don't work for all melanomas and the drugs themselves may lead to skin, kidney, and lung damage in addition to other side effects that may limit their efficacy.

Until the advent of immunotherapy, survival had typically been measured in only months for people with advanced melanomas. Eventually, these types of drugs and combinations may be able to cure melanomas completely even when they have spread to other organs.

Thousands of studies are being conducted worldwide using immunotherapy for advanced skin cancer as well as other cancers—and there are other types of immunotherapies beyond checkpoint inhibitors that are being studied. In the past, immunotherapy would be offered only after chemotherapy had failed, but today many oncologists believe it should be used as an initial treatment for advanced melanomas.

Therapeutic Vaccines

We typically think of a vaccine as a way to prevent disease, but there are some vaccines being developed to treat tumors and prevent them from coming back after they've been surgically removed. The vaccines work by helping the immune system remember what to do if it detects melanoma cells in the future.

> By enabling doctors to predict which tumors are more susceptible to specific therapies, biomarkers lead to more successful outcomes while minimizing side effects.

Example: Pharmaceutical company Moderna recently announced that its experimental mRNA melanoma vaccine successfully reduced the risk for relapse or death from melanoma when it was combined with the checkpoint inhibitor *pembrolizumab* (Keytruda). The vaccine is customized for the patient to target a specific tumor and genetic mutation.

Will It Spread?

Unfortunately, even if a melanoma is completely removed or eradicated, it still can come back in the same or a different body part.

Good news: Tests have been developed that can help doctors assess how likely a recurrence is.

Example: Researchers at Newcastle University in the UK have developed the AMBLor test, which uses biopsied tissue of an early-stage melanoma to reliably predict if the melanoma is likely to recur, indicating that more frequent screenings and potentially adjuvant therapy are appropriate.

Ultra-Processed Foods Linked to Higher Cancer Risks

University of Bristol and the International Agency for Research on Cancer.

Ultra-processed foods (UPFs) are associated with a higher risk of developing cancers of the mouth, throat, and esophagus. The association may be partially explained by the inclusion of additives, such as emulsifiers and artificial sweeteners, as well as contaminants from food packaging and the manufacturing process. However, the researchers also found evidence of an association between higher UPF consumption and increased risk of accidental deaths—which shows that association does not prove causation.

"Whether underlying factors such as general health-related behaviors and socioeconomic position are responsible for the link, is still unclear," said George Davey Smith, FRS, MD, DSc, MSc, coauthor of the paper.

Food Wrappers Contain Dangerous Chemicals

Test by researchers at *Consumer Reports.* ConsumerReports.org

Many restaurant chains and supermarkets have pledged to reduce use of products containing polyfluoroalkyl substances (PFAS).

Recent finding: Half of samples of packaging used by 24 restaurant chains (including Arby's, Burger King, and Nathan's Famous restaurants) and supermarket chains (including Kroger, Stop & Shop, and Trader Joe's) for 118 products contained unacceptably high levels. PFAS have strong chemical bonds that make them virtually indestructible. They also have grease-resistant properties, which is why they are used in food packaging.

Growing concern: PFAS leach into foods...and are linked to a growing list of health issues, including immune problems, lower birth weights, and some cancers.

Cancer Treatment Gets Personal

Harold J. Burstein, MD, PhD, a professor of medicine at Harvard Medical School and a medical oncologist at Dana-Farber Cancer Institute and Brigham & Women's Hospital. Dr. Burstein is a consultant editor for cancer education at the *Journal of Clinical Oncology.*

Cancer treatment has come a long way since Hippocrates proposed that it was caused by a buildup of black bile. Remedies ranged from powdered worms and ground elm poultices to, as recently as 150 years ago, bloodletting. With the advent of surgery, chemotherapy, and radiation, many cancers have evolved from almost certainly fatal to quite treatable and even curable.

Personalized Patient Care

But only in the last several decades have oncologists moved from a "one-size-fits-all" approach to being able to truly personalize patient care, using information about an individual's tumor to tailor treatment. Just as we all have different fingerprints, personalities, and DNA, cancers possess distinctive features that reveal so much about how they operate. Called biomarkers—shorthand for biological markers—these are proteins, genes, or genetic mutations found in a person's tumor, blood, or other body fluid that, thanks to pioneering research, clinical trials, and real-world practice, have revolutionized cancer treatment.

If one or more biomarkers are detected, it offers vital information as to what is driving the cancer, such as a specific mutation or cancer-fueling protein. That, in turn, reveals vulnerabilities in the cancer that medical oncologists can use to plan an attack using biomarker-based therapies like immunotherapy or targeted therapy. Five patients with, say, breast cancer, might each undergo different treatment protocols based on their cancer's distinctive characteristics—and all of them could be successful.

Targeted Therapy

For example, up to 20 percent of breast cancer patients have a mutation that results in excess amounts of a cancer-accelerating protein called HER2. If a person's tumor is found to have this mutation, their cancer is considered HER2-positive. These tumors are highly susceptible to HER2 inhibitors (also called anti-HER2 therapies) such as *trastuzumab* (Herceptin) and *pertuzumab* (Perjeta), which, when infused or taken orally, hunt down and attack HER2-positive cancer cells with missile-like precision. (These are often used in combination with other treatments, like surgery, chemotherapy, or radiation.) HER2-negative patients, on the other hand, would not benefit from these medications. Depending on the presence or absence of other biomarkers, like ER (estrogen receptor) or PR (progesterone receptor), they would want to follow a different protocol. The use of medications that take specific aim at genetic abnormalities in a patient's tumor is called targeted therapy.

Immunotherapy

Another class of biomarker-based treatment, immunotherapy, doesn't directly pursue cancer cells, but rather harnesses the power of the immune system to wage an attack. Ordinarily, the immune system recognizes and disables foreign invaders, including viruses, bacteria, and precancerous cells, but certain biomarkers act like camouflage for cancer cells, allowing them to avoid destruction by hiding in plain sight. If a patient's cancer shows elevated levels of one of these biomarkers, they would benefit from immunotherapeutic drugs that unmask the cancer cells, allowing the immune system to take action. Examples of immunotherapy include immune checkpoint inhibitors, monoclonal antibodies, T-cell transfer therapy, immune system modulators, and treatment vaccines.

Better Outcomes

By enabling doctors to predict which tumors are more susceptible to specific therapies, biomarkers lead to more successful outcomes while minimizing side effects. According to the American Cancer Society, the risk of dying from cancer dropped 32 percent between 1991 and 2019, meaning that about 3.5 million cancer deaths were prevented. Biomarker-based treatments are an important contributing factor. (Others include reduced rates of smoking, enhanced screening protocols, and the use of post-surgical chemotherapy for colon and breast cancer.)

In addition to fine-tuning treatment, biomarkers are used to determine where a tumor is located, how advanced it is, and whether or not it has spread to any lymph nodes; to help predict how aggressively a cancer will act; and to provide insight into how a cancer is responding once treatment is underway, as well as whether it might recur after treatment.

Biomarkers are also a critical component of certain cancer screenings, meaning they're tested before any cancer symptoms have developed. Even if you've never had cancer yourself, you're likely familiar with some of these. BRCA 1 and BRCA2 and prostate-specific antigen (PSA), for instance, are biomarkers that, when detected, offer clues about a person's future risk of developing breast or prostate cancer, respectively. (PSA and BRCA are also used when weighing treatment options after cancer has been diagnosed.)

Biomarker testing is typically one of the first steps to occur following a cancer diagnosis. It may even be performed on tissue sampled during a biopsy. It's almost always covered by insurance. Some patients may be retested in the future, as biomarker levels can change with time.

> ### Common Biomarkers
>
> - **Breast cancer:** Estrogen receptor (ER) protein, progesterone receptor (PR) protein, HER2, BRCA1 and BRCA2
> - **Colorectal cancer:** EGFR, KRAS, BRAF, NRAS
> - **Melanoma:** BRAF
> - **Non-small cell lung cancer:** KRAS, ALK, EGFR, ROS1, BRAF, RET, MET, PD-L1
> - **Ovarian:** KRAS, BRAF, EGFR, BRCA 1 and BRCA2
> - **Hodgkin lymphoma:** TNFAIP3, CIITA, KLF4, CD30

Cancer Breakthroughs

The Thymus Is Important After All

New England Journal of Medicine.

The thymus gland is often regarded as nonfunctional and sometimes removed during cardiac surgery. But new research has uncovered evidence that it is important to overall health as well as preventing cancer. Researchers looked at 1,146 adults who had their thymus removed during surgery and 1,146 who underwent similar cardiothoracic surgery without thymectomy. Five years after surgery, those who had a thymectomy had a 2.9-times higher risk of death. They also had double the risk of developing cancer.

Alternatives to Colonoscopy

Robert Bresalier, MD, gastroenterologist in the department of gastroenterology, hepatology and nutrition, Division of Internal Medicine, and Bridie J. and Lydia J. Resoft Distinguished Professor in Gastrointestinal Oncology at University of Texas MD Anderson Cancer Center, Houston. MDAnderson.org

Colon cancer screening guidelines from the U.S. Preventive Services Taskforce, the American Cancer Society and gastroenterology organizations call for most adults to get screened starting at age 45 and continuing through age 75.

The most accurate screening test is colonoscopy, which is 94 percent accurate. It is recommended for people who are at high risk for colon cancer because of family history, personal history of polyps in the colon (which can turn into cancer) or a genetic predisposition to colon cancer.

Problem: Despite the guidelines—and the fact that screening saves lives—40 percent of eligible people don't get screened. Why? Many of them don't want to go through the onerous bowel-cleansing regimen the night before the procedure.

There are other easier—although less accurate—options available. But if the results of one of these tests are positive, you'll still need to have a colonoscopy.

•**Fecal immunochemical test (FIT).** This test looks for hidden blood in your stool, which suggests polyps or even cancer. Your doctor will give you a FIT test kit to use at home. You take a small sample of stool, and mail it to a lab to be analyzed. You don't need to do any prep. The cost of the annual test is covered by insurance and Medicare. FIT has an almost 80 percent accuracy rate for detecting colon cancer, but it detects only about 28 percent of advanced polyps that might turn into cancer.

•**Cologuard.** This screening kit looks for hidden blood as well as altered DNA in stool. Your doctor will order the test, and you will receive the collection kit in the mail. You do the test at home every three years and send stool samples to Cologuard via UPS. No special prep or change to your diet or medication schedule is required. Cologuard, which is covered by Medicare and most insurers, detects 92 percent of colon cancers but only 42 percent of large precancerous polyps. It also may provide a false-positive—indicating that you might have cancer when you don't.

•**Blood test.** In 2016, the Food and Drug Administration approved the Epi proColon test that looks for circulating DNA and markers of colon cancer in blood. This "liquid biopsy" is offered to people who refuse other forms of screening. While relatively sensitive for detecting late-stage cancer, the test's sensitivity for detecting early-stage cancer or polyps in the colon is low. For this reason and because of its high false-positive rate, this test is not recommended in the screening guidelines, and the cost is not covered by Medicare or private insurers.

Colorectal Cancer Is Skewing Younger

Rebecca Siegel, MPH, cancer epidemiologist at the American Cancer Society in Atlanta, commenting on a report published in *CA: A Cancer Journal for Clinicians.*

One in five patients diagnosed with colorectal cancer is under age 55—versus one in 10 in 1995, according to recent research. Obesity, poor diet, and lack of exercise may be factors but do not fully explain the trend. Young people can use low-cost, at-home screening tools... those with a family history of colorectal cancer should alert their doctors and inquire about colonoscopy. Rectal bleeding, abdominal pain, and/or changes to bowel habits should prompt a doctor visit.

New Diabetes Drugs Can Reduce Risk of Colon Cancer

Study titled "GLP-1 Receptor Agonists and Colorectal Cancer Risk in Drug-Naive Patients with Type 2 Diabetes, With and Without Overweight/Obesity," led by researchers at Case Western Reserve University School of Medicine, Cleveland, published in *JAMA Oncology.*

Trulicity, Ozempic, Victoza, and Rybelsus...you've probably heard of at least a few of these brand-name drugs on TV. They're a relatively new class of drugs first approved by the FDA in 2005 to treat type 2 diabetes. Since then, these drugs have been found to reduce blood sugar, increase sensitivity to insulin, reduce hunger, promote weight loss, and reduce heart disease risk. Now, a new study is the first to link these drugs to a significant reduction of colorectal cancer risk.

How These Multitasking Drugs Work

The drugs are glucagon-like peptide 1 (GLP-1) agonists. GLP-1 drugs increase the production of insulin by the pancreas in response to eating. Insulin is the hormone that helps your cells use glucose for energy. Since the first GLP-1 was approved in 2005, these drugs have also been found to promote weight loss by curbing hunger and slowing digestion. The combination of weight loss and lower blood sugar has resulted in a decreased risk for cardiovascular disease.

Because both diabetes and obesity are risk factors for colorectal cancer, researchers from Case Western Reserve University wanted to know if GLP-1 drugs reduce the risk of colon cancer, the third most commonly diagnosed type of cancer and the second-leading cause of cancer deaths, according to the American Cancer Society.

The researchers reviewed the medical records of 1.2 million Americans between 2005 and 2019. They looked at anyone with type 2 diabetes newly started on a diabetes medication. The other two most-used medications are insulin and metformin. The study is published in the American Medical Society journal *JAMA Oncology.*

Patients who started insulin, metformin, or a GLP-1 agonist were matched for age, sex, weight, smoking, alcohol use, family history and other colorectal-cancer risk factors, and then compared to see who would develop colorectal cancer over 15 years. These were the key results for 1.2 million patients matched...

•**Patients on a GLP-1 drug were 44 percent less likely** to be diagnosed with colorectal cancer than those taking insulin.

•**Patients on a GLP-1 drug were 25 percent less likely** to be diagnosed with colorectal cancer than those taking metformin.

•**Patients who were obese or overweight and on a GLP-1 drug** had a 50 percent lower risk of colorectal cancer than those on insulin and a 42 percent lower risk than those on metformin.

Obesity is a known risk for colorectal cancer, but the study found that the reduced risk was seen in both obese and normal weight patients. This shows that GLP-1 agonists may have a yet unknown protective activity against cancer. More research is needed to explore the effects of these drugs on colorectal cancer as well as other obesity-related cancers.

Now Approved for Weight Loss Only

Early GLP-1 agonists were approved to only treat type 2 diabetes, with weight loss as an added benefit. But if you don't have diabetes and are struggling to lose weight, talk to your doctor about GLP-1 drugs. Because these new drugs continue to show significant success in the weight-loss department, the FDA has approved Wegovy for obesity without type 2 diabetes. The newest GLP-1 drug is Zepbound and has also been approved for obesity management with or without type 2 diabetes. Zepbound has demonstrated weight loss in clinical trials of 34 to 58 pounds, depending on the dose.

For Treating Some Cancers, Less May Be More

Julie Gralow, MD, chief medical officer, executive vice president, American Society of Clinical Oncology (ASCO), Alexandria, Virginia. ASCO.org

Cancer doctors are increasingly pursuing a strategy called *de-escalation,* in which they cut back on certain therapies to improve their patients' quality of life without jeopardizing survival.

Examples: Less invasive surgery appears just as effective for some cervical and pancreatic cancer cases, and giving less radiation to some patients with rectal cancer or Hodgkin's lymphoma also seems to provide equal benefit without as many side effects. HPV-related head and neck cancers also have had recent successful de-escalation trials.

Don't Trust ChatGPT for Cancer Information

Brigham and Women's Hospital.

Researchers from Brigham and Women's Hospital warn that ChatGPT, the artificial intelligence chatbot, provides inappropriate recommendations for cancer treatment about one-third of the time. Danielle Bitterman, MD, and colleagues asked ChatGPT to provide treatment recommendations for breast, prostate, and lung cancer. Nearly all responses (98 percent) included at least one treatment approach that agreed with guidelines from the National Comprehensive Cancer Network (NCCN), but 34 percent of these responses also included one or more recommendations that were only partially correct. In 12.5 percent of cases, ChatGPT produced treatment recommendations that were entirely absent from NCCN guidelines. These included curative therapies for incurable cancers.

"Patients should feel empowered to educate themselves about their medical conditions, but they should always discuss with a clinician," said Dr. Bitterman. "ChatGPT responses can sound a lot like a human and can be quite convincing. But, when it comes to clinical decision-making, there are so many subtleties for every patient's unique situation. A right answer can be very nuanced, and not necessarily something ChatGPT or another large language model can provide."

Chapter 4

DIABETES BREAKTHROUGHS AND BLOOD SUGAR CONTROL

How to Reverse Prediabetes

More than 96 million American adults—more than one in three of us—have prediabetes: blood sugar levels that are lower than type 2 diabetes but higher than normal. Prediabetes is not a pre-problem: It puts you at increased risk for the same chronic conditions that are linked to diabetes, and for diabetes itself.

The good news: Decades of scientific research shows that reversing prediabetes by restoring your blood sugar to normal levels is possible if you make a few lifestyle changes. The Diabetes Prevention Program (DPP), a three-year-long study with more than 3,000 participants, showed that lifestyle changes like improving diet and increasing activity levels (exercising moderately for 30 minutes, five days a week) can cut the risk of developing type 2 diabetes by 58 percent—and 71 percent for people ages 60 and older. People who participated in the DPP also had lower cholesterol and triglyceride levels, healthier blood pressure, and less chronic inflammation.

Start Today

Prediabetes has no symptoms, but there are clues. It's more likely you have prediabetes if you have excess weight, smoke, are inactive, sleep poorly, or have high blood pressure, high triglycerides, low HDL (good) cholesterol, or heart disease. However, the only foolproof way to diagnose prediabetes is through testing. If you have one or more of the risk factors for diabetes, you should be tested sooner rather than later. Prediabetes is progressive, and every day, the window of opportunity to stabilize or reverse blood sugar levels closes ever so slightly.

If you discover that you have prediabetes, research shows you should improve your diet, increase your activity, and lose a little weight (if you have excess weight to lose). Here are some proven ways to do just that.

Improve Your Diet

There is no "best" diet to stabilize and lower high blood sugar. Not keto. Not vegan. Not

---

Jill Weisenberger, MS, RDN, CDCES, a registered dietitian nutritionist, certified diabetes care and education specialist, and author of four books on health and nutrition, including *Prediabetes: A Complete Guide (Second Edition).* JillWeisenberger.com

low carb. Not low fat. All those diets require willpower and deprivation, which work until you inevitably run out of willpower or rebel against deprivation. Rather, you should emphasize nutrient-dense foods that you enjoy—foods that keep you energized and satisfied, and that you can stick with. Nutrient-dense foods deliver high levels of nutrients and a relatively small amount of calories—like fruits, vegetables, whole grains, beans, nuts, seeds, lean meats, fish, and low-fat and nonfat dairy products. By eating more nutrient-dense foods, you'll inevitably eat fewer foods that are less nutritious.

> ### Testing for Prediabetes
>
> If you have one or more risk factors for prediabetes—like obesity or high blood pressure—you should ask your doctor to test your blood sugar levels. There are three tests for prediabetes and diabetes. If a test confirms higher-than-normal levels, your doctor will either repeat that same test or use a second type of test.
>
> •**Fasting plasma glucose.** Your blood glucose is measured first thing in the morning after having consumed nothing but water for eight to 12 hours. A result of 100 to 125 milligrams per deciliter (mg/dL) is prediabetes; 126 or higher is diabetes.
>
> •**2-hour oral glucose tolerance test.** You consume nothing but water for eight to 12 hours, then drink a glucose-containing beverage, and your blood glucose is measured two hours later. A result of 140 to 199 mg/dL is prediabetes; 200 or higher is diabetes.
>
> •**AIC.** This test measures the percentage of blood glucose that is adhering to your hemoglobin molecules (a component of red blood cells). It is indicative of long-term blood glucose levels. A result of 5.7 to 6.4 percent is prediabetes; 6.5 percent or higher is diabetes.

There is one category of food you should avoid: sugar-sweetened beverages, including soft drinks, fruit drinks, energy drinks, sports drinks, sweetened ice teas, and coffee beverages with added sugar or flavored syrups. Research links these beverages to insulin resistance, prediabetes, diabetes, and obesity (a leading risk factor for prediabetes and diabetes).

Plate Method

To help you emphasize whole, nutrient-dense foods, use the plate method—one of the easiest, most flexible tools to help you build a wholesome meal…

•**Start with a 9-inch plate and draw an imaginary line down the middle.** Fill one-half of the plate with non-starchy vegetables like broccoli, cabbage, tomatoes, carrots, or string beans.

•**Draw another imaginary line across the other half of your plate,** so you have two sections equal to one-quarter plate. Put a protein-rich food like lean beef, salmon, black beans, or low-fat cottage cheese in one section.

•**Put a starchy food like corn, peas, quinoa, potato, or brown rice in the last section.**

This method delivers variety and balance—the keystones of healthy eating. Eat three meals a day, and eat wholesome snacks—like an apple with peanut butter or hummus and whole-grain crackers—whenever you're hungry.

Increase Activity

Developing the habit of being active is more important than the immediate physical benefits of exercise because a habit will help you realize those benefits next month, next year, and all the years to come. If you enjoy walking, set aside at least five minutes every day rather than longer periods just two or three times weekly. A daily behavior is more likely to become a habit. Gradually increase the daily time you spend walking, until you're walking about 20 to 30 minutes every day.

Ideally, you want three components of an exercise plan: aerobic (daily), muscle-strengthening (twice weekly), and flexibility (twice weekly). You could also add balance exercises twice weekly.

Use FITT principles to guide your routines: frequency (how often you will do a particular kind of exercise), intensity (how vigorously you will exercise), time (how many minutes you will perform the exercise), and type (what type of exercise you will do). *For aerobic fitness, your FITT goals might look like this...*

F: at least five times per week
I: at a moderate intensity (at this pace, you can hold a conversation)
T: for at least 10 minutes
T: walking.

As your fitness level improves, you can increase the frequency, intensity, and/or time.

Sleep Deeply

Getting at least seven hours sleep a night is a must for good health—including healthy blood sugar levels. Sleep deprivation is a risk factor for obesity, which increases the risk of prediabetes and diabetes. Too little sleep and poor sleep also affect glucose metabolism, increasing insulin resistance. *Some good ideas for getting sufficient and restful sleep...*

•**Create a routine.** Go to bed and wake up at approximately the same time each day, even on weekends.

•**Mind the light at night.** Avoid light from TV, tablets, and computers shortly before bed. Keep your room dark for sleeping, too.

•**Cool off.** Dial down the temperature to a cool 60 to 67° F.

•**Don't fret.** Instead of watching the clock, relax with deep breathing exercises or meditation.

•**Cut off the caffeine.** Consuming caffeine six hours or less before bedtime can hinder good sleep.

•**Lose a little weight.**

> **The Cause of Prediabetes**
>
> Prediabetes is a problem with insulin, the hormone that normally ushers blood sugar out of the bloodstream and into cells. In prediabetes, you might have insulin resistance—your cells don't react normally to insulin, and blood sugar levels rise. Or you might have fewer insulin-producing beta cells of the pancreas, leading to impaired production of insulin and poor blood sugar control. (Research shows that people with prediabetes have lost about 30 percent of their beta cells.) Or you might have both. The result is slowly rising blood sugar levels—until prediabetes becomes diabetes.

Usually (but not always), prediabetes is accompanied by extra body fat. If you carry excess weight, losing even a few pounds can help. In one study, people at high risk for developing type 2 diabetes who lost just 5 percent of their body weight improved the function of their pancreas beta-cells and decreased insulin resistance.

Controlling portions (which automatically controls calories) is an excellent strategy for weight loss...

•**Use small dishes.** Serve lunch and dinner on nine-inch plates. Ladle soups into cups that hold about one cup. Look for half-cup dishes for desserts.

•**Eat from a dish.** No reaching into a bag or box.

•**Treat yourself to foods in single-serving portions.** Skip the half-gallon containers of ice cream in favor of a small cone or cup.

•**Try a low-calorie, portion-controlled meal.** Meal replacements and portion-controlled meals can help you relearn appropriate portions.

Red, Purple, Blue Foods Reduce Risk of Diabetes

Journal of Agricultural and Food Chemistry.

The red, purple, and blue pigments in fruits, vegetables, and tubers (called anthocyanins) can reduce the risk of diabetes by affecting energy metabolism, gut microbiota, and inflammation. Purple potatoes, purple sweet potatoes, radishes, purple carrots, and red cabbages are particularly beneficial, as they contain supercharged pigments, called acylated anthocyanins.

Easy, Delicious Low-Carb, Low-Sugar Recipes

Linda Gassenheimer, an award-winning author of several cookbooks, including *The 12-Week Diabetes Cookbook* and *Delicious One-Pot Dishes*. Listen to her *Food News and Views* podcast. She writes a syndicated newspaper column, "Dinner in Minutes/Quick Fix." DinnerInMinutes.com

A diabetes-friendly diet doesn't mean eating just steamed vegetables and broiled fish all the time. Following the guidelines from the American Diabetes Association to manage your blood sugar means eating lots of the right kinds of foods in moderate amounts—healthy carbs such as fruits, vegetables, whole grains, legumes, and low-fat dairy products...good fats like avocados, nuts, and canola, olive, and peanut oils...and fish as well as moderate amounts of chicken and beef. In fact, eating this way is healthy for almost everyone—it helps to reduce risk for cardiovascular diseases and certain types of cancer.

We asked cookbook author Linda Gassenheimer for her favorite diabetes-friendly meals that can be made in just minutes. Each meal below makes two servings.

Bronzed Chicken Breasts Over Red, Green, and Brown Rice

Brozed Chicken Breasts
2 tablespoons Cajun or blackened spice seasoning mix
1 tablespoon flour
¾ pound boneless, skinless chicken breast cutlets
2 teaspoons canola oil

Mix the Cajun or blackened seasoning and flour together. Spoon one tablespoon of the spice mixture onto one side of each chicken breast cutlet, pressing it into the flesh.

Heat a medium-sized nonstick skillet over high heat and add the canola oil. When the skillet is very hot—you can tell the skillet is ready when a few drops of water sizzle—add the chicken breasts, seasoned side down. Spread the remaining one tablespoon of the spice mixture on the top side of each cutlet.

Cook until the underside is bronze in color, two to three minutes. Cook the second side three to four minutes or until cooked through. A meat thermometer should read 165°F. Keeping your skillet hot will make the coating of this bronzed chicken golden and caramelized.

Per serving: 260 calories, 9 g fat, 1.5 g saturated fat, 100 mg cholesterol, 37 g protein, 5 g carbohydrates, 0 g dietary fiber, 0 g sugars, 615 mg sodium.

Red, Green, and Brown Rice
½ cup water
½ cup no-added-salt tomato juice
1½ cups brown rice (microwavable)
2 cups washed, ready-to-eat spinach
1 teaspoon canola oil
Salt and freshly ground black pepper

Bring the water and tomato juice to a boil in a medium-size saucepan over high heat.

Microwave the rice according to the package instructions. Add the rice and spinach to the tomato juice.

Mix well until the spinach begins to wilt. Add oil and salt and pepper to taste.

Per serving: 209 calories, 4 g fat, <1 g saturated fat, 0 mg cholesterol, 5 g protein, 39 g carbohydrates, 3 g dietary fiber, 5 g sugars, 33 mg sodium.

Mediterranean Steak with Minted Couscous

You can make this sautéed steak flavored with the bounty of the Mediterranean—olives, walnuts, and capers—in just 15 minutes.

Mediterranean Steak

½ pound beef tenderloin steak (¾-inch thick)
Pinch cayenne pepper (about ⅛ teaspoon)
Olive oil spray
1 tablespoon chopped walnut pieces
8 sliced pimento stuffed green olives
Salt and freshly ground black pepper

Remove any visible fat from the steak, and sprinkle it with cayenne pepper.

Heat a small nonstick skillet over medium-high heat. Spray the skillet with olive oil spray, and add the steak. Brown the steak for one minute. Flip it over, and brown the other side for one minute.

Sprinkle walnuts and olives over the steak and into the skillet.

Lower heat to medium, and cook two minutes for medium rare. A meat thermometer should read 135°F. Cook a thicker steak two minutes longer. Add salt and pepper to taste.

Per serving: 227 calories, 116 calories from fat, 12.9 g total fat (3.4 g saturated fat, 5.5 g monounsaturated fat), 72 mg cholesterol, 246 mg sodium, 1.4 g carbohydrate, 0.7 g dietary fiber, 0.1 g sugars, 25.8 g protein.

Minted Couscous

1 cup water
½ cup whole-wheat couscous
1 cup fresh diced tomatoes
¼ cup chopped fresh mint
Salt and freshly ground black pepper

Bring water to a boil over high heat, then remove from heat. Add couscous and tomatoes. Cover with a lid and let stand five minutes. When ready, fluff up with a fork. Add mint and salt and pepper to taste.

To serve, place couscous on two dinner plates, slice the steak and place on top. Spoon pan juice over the steak.

Per serving: 179 calories, 4 calories from fat, 0.5 g total fat, (0.1 g saturated fat, 0.1 g monounsaturated fat), 0 mg cholesterol, 9 mg sodium, 37.0 g carbohydrate, 3.3 g dietary fiber, 2.4 g sugars, 63 g protein.

Mushroom Pesto Pasta with Pimento Pepper Salad

Add some meaty sautéed portobello mushrooms to a healthy store-bought pesto sauce to make this flavorful pasta dish in the time it takes to boil pasta.

Mushroom Pesto Pasta

½ tablespoon olive oil
¼ pound portobello mushrooms, thinly sliced (2 cups)
¼ cup reduced-fat prepared pesto sauce (such as Buitoni Reduced Fat Pesto with Basil)
1 tablespoon pine nuts
¼ pound fresh linguine (or dried linguine if fresh is unavailable)
Salt and freshly ground black pepper

Bring three to four quarts of water to a boil in a large pot.

Heat one-half tablespoon of olive oil in a small nonstick skillet over medium-high heat. Sauté the mushrooms for five minutes. Remove them from skillet and chop. Place the mushrooms in a bowl, and add pesto sauce and pine nuts. Mix well.

Cook the linguine in the boiling water for three minutes or until it's cooked but still firm. (If dried linguine is used, follow package directions for how long to cook until firm—usually about eight minutes.)

Drain and toss with the pesto sauce and mushrooms. Add salt and pepper to taste.

Per serving: 441 calories, 145 calories from fat, 16.2 g total fat (3.0 g saturated fat, 9.4 g monounsaturated fat), 8 mg cholesterol, 227 mg sodium, 50.0 g carbohydrate, 3.7 g dietary fiber, 4.0 g sugars, 14.1 g protein.

Pimento Pepper Salad

4 cups washed, ready-to-eat Italian-style salad
1 cup canned drained sliced sweet pimento
2 teaspoons olive oil
2 teaspoons balsamic vinegar
Salt and freshly ground black pepper

Arrange salad leaves on two dinner plates. In a small bowl, mix the pimento, olive oil and vinegar together. Add salt and pepper to taste. Spoon over lettuce.

Per serving: 83 calories, 46 calories from fat, 5.1 g total fat (0.7 g saturated fat, 3.3 g monounsaturated fat), 0 mg cholesterol, 23 mg sodium, 8.9 g carbohydrate, 38 g dietary fiber, 4.5 g sugars, 2.2 g protein.

High Doses of Vitamin D Slash Diabetes Risk

Michael F. Holick, PhD, MD, professor of medicine at Boston University School of Medicine, commenting on a meta study published in *Annals of Internal Medicine*.

Prediabetes patients who maintained high blood levels of 25-hydroxyvitamin D (at least 50 ng/mL) were 76% less likely to develop diabetes, according to a recent meta study.

Best: Food and sunlight are insufficient sources—most people should supplement with 4,000 to 6,000 international units (IU) of vitamin D daily...double that if you're obese (prior research shows this is safe).

Caution: Check with your doctor before taking vitamin D supplements, especially if you are being treated for a medical condition.

Phthalate Exposure Is Associated with Diabetes, Endocrine Disorders

University of Michigan School of Public Health.

Phthalates are chemicals widely used in plastics such as personal care products, children's toys, and food and beverage packaging. A new study reports that white women who were exposed to high levels of some phthalates had a 30 to 63 percent higher chance of developing diabetes. The chemicals were not linked to diabetes in Black or Asian women.

To reduce your exposure to phthalates, avoid products that list phthalates or fragrance in their ingredients, avoid plastic wrap and plastic food containers made from PVC, which carries the recycling label #3. Choose glass or stainless-steel food containers instead. And don't reheat food or beverages in plastic containers.

Women Who Are "Night Owls" Are at Higher Risk for Diabetes

Study titled "Chronotype, Unhealthy Lifestyle, and Diabetes Risk in Middle-Aged U.S. Women: A Prospective Cohort Study," by researchers at Brigham and Women's Hospital, published in *Annals of Internal Medicine*.

The medical term for someone who burns the midnight oil is evening chronotype or evening circadian preference, or in everyday language, "night owls." Morning circadian preference or a morning chronotype is usually called a morning person or "early bird." It seems to be simply a matter of choice, and if people are getting enough sleep, what difference does it make?

Apparently it makes a significant difference when it comes to averting disease, according to a new study from researchers at Brigham and Women's Hospital in Boston. Researchers there found that chronotype impacts healthy lifestyles and type 2 diabetes. The study is published in the prestigious journal *Annals of Internal Medicine*. It draws on data collected from 63,676 female nurses, ages 45 to 62. These women are part of an ongoing study called the Nurses' Health Study II.

Biggest Study on Women's Health Spans Close to 50 Years

The Nurses' Health Study II is a joint effort of Brigham and Women's Hospital and the Harvard T.H. Chan School of Public Health. The first part of the study began in 1976 and has been called the most significant study ever done in women's health. As part of the study, women have been asked to report on many aspects of their health and lifestyle with health questionnaires every two years.

One of the questionnaires is the Morningness-Eveningness Questionnaire. It asks questions about preferred time for sleeping, highest energy time during the day, and when you start to feel sleepy in the evening. Other lifestyle factors that were measured include diet, physical activity, alcohol and smoking, and body weight by body mass index (BMI). None of the nurses had type 2 diabetes at the start of the study and they were followed for about seven years. These were the key results…

• **Women who scored high as evening chronotype** were 54 percent more likely to report unhealthy lifestyle factors.

• **Compared with women who scored high on morning chronotype,** the evening chronotype women were 72 percent more likely to be diagnosed with type 2 diabetes during the study period.

• **Compared with women who were neither evening nor morning chronotypes (intermediate type),** the evening chronotypes were 21 percent more likely to be diagnosed with type 2 diabetes.

Because the unhealthy lifestyle habits in themselves are risk factors for type 2 diabetes, the researchers wanted to know if the chronotype alone affected type 2 diabetes risk (an independent risk factor). To find out, they adjusted for the lifestyle risk factors. Without the other risk factors, women who were just evening chronotypes still had a 19 percent greater risk for type 2 diabetes than the morning chronotypes.

More of Us Are Night Owls

According to previous surveys for all people, about 20 percent are night owls, and 10 percent are early birds. The rest of us fall somewhere in between. The chronotype may change with age. Teens are more likely to be night owls and elderly people are more likely to be early birds. However, studies have also found that chronotype is partly genetic and may be hard to shift.

The study concludes that middle-aged nurses with evening chronotype may be at increased risk of both unhealthy lifestyle and type 2 diabetes.

It makes sense: Late nights encourage unhealthy snacking and lots of sitting in front of blue light from laptops and smartphone screens (which, according to the Sleep Foundation, can hinder sleep). The team plans to expand their study to find out if chronotype is associated with heart disease.

Just a Little Sleep Loss Affects Diabetes Risk in Women

Study titled, "Chronic Insufficient Sleep in Women Impairs Insulin Sensitivity Independent of Adiposity Changes: Results of a Randomized Trial," by researchers at Columbia University, New York, published in *Diabetes Care*.

One third of American adults say they are not getting the recommended seven to nine hours of sleep. And in recent years, researchers have been focusing in on just how much sleep deprivation impacts health. Studies show that poor sleep can increase your risk of dementia, stroke, and obesity, and weaken your immune system.

Past studies have found that severe sleep loss in men increases the risk of type 2 diabetes, the most common type of diabetes. A new study is the first to find that only 90 minutes of sleep loss over just six weeks may increase the risk of diabetes in women. The study is published in the American Diabetes Association's journal *Diabetes Care*.

Researchers from Columbia University's Center for Excellence for Sleep & Circadian Research wanted to know if prolonged mild sleep restriction, resembling what occurs in most people who complain of not getting enough sleep, is associated with insulin resistance, which is a risk factor for type 2 diabetes.

Women Experience More Sleep Disruption

The researchers chose to study women since they tend to experience sleep disruptions more often than men due to lifestyle factors that include bearing and caring for children and menopause. Studies suggest that sleep loss may affect women's health more than men.

The 12-week study out of Columbia University involved two phases of research. In one phase, women were asked to maintain their normal sleep time for six weeks and then, in the other six-week phase, they went to bed 90 minutes later than normal. A wearable device confirmed sleep times. All the women in the study were healthy and accustomed to getting seven to nine hours of sleep.

Thirty-eight women, ages 20 to 75, completed the study, including 11 women who were postmenopausal. At the end of each phase, blood tests were done to measure blood sugar (glucose), fasting insulin levels, and insulin resistance.

Why Insulin Resistance Matters

Insulin is the chemical messenger (hormone) released by the pancreas to help fat, muscle, and liver cells absorb and store glucose to use as energy. Insulin resistance is a condition that causes those cells to become less responsive to insulin. This results in the pancreas needing to work harder and produce more insulin to keep blood sugar normal. Over time the pancreas wears out, leading to higher levels of blood sugar and diabetes.

These were they key results of the study...

- Compared to normal sleep time, reducing sleep by 90 minutes over six weeks increased fasting insulin levels by more than 12 percent in premenopausal women and 15 percent in postmenopausal women.

- Compared to normal sleep time, reducing sleep by 90 minutes over six weeks increased insulin resistance by 15 percent in premenopausal women and 20 percent in postmenopausal women.

- Blood sugar levels did not change, but the researchers note that over a longer period this amount of insulin resistance would put enough stress on the pancreas to cause insulin-producing cells to fail and lead to diabetes.

The researchers conclude that promoting healthy sleep and sleep time can be another way to reduce the risk of diabetes, along with diet and exercise, especially in postmenopausal women. Sleep may be added to other known causes of insulin resistance such as obesity, heart disease, poor diet, lack of physical activity, and liver disease.

The Skinny on Sugar

Dr. Mahmud Kara, MD, founder and CEO of KaraMD, a company that offers natural remedies that target digestive health, heart health, reducing inflammation, increasing natural energy, weight management, and more.

It has become popular to say that "sugar is bad for you," but what exactly is sugar?

What are the different types? And can any of it be good for you? Let's take a closer look.

- **Natural sugars** exist in certain foods like fruits, vegetables, or dairy products. Under the umbrella of natural sugars, there is glucose, which is found in starchy vegetables, fructose, found in fruits and vegetables, and lactose, which naturally occurs in dairy products. Sucrose is a combination of glucose and fructose that forms table sugar.
- **Added sugars** are most often found as sweeteners or flavors in drinks and packaged foods. When most people think of added sugar, they think of cookies or soda, but there can also be added sugar in foods that don't taste sweet, like salad dressing, bread, and pasta sauce. On food labels, added sugar can go by many different names: agave nectar, barley malt syrup, brown sugar, brown rice syrup, cane juice, cane sugar, coconut sugar, corn syrup, corn syrup solids, evaporated cane juice, evaporated corn sweetener, high fructose corn syrup, honey, invert sugar, malt syrup, maltodextrin, maple syrup, molasses, palm sugar, raw sugar, or rice syrup.
- **Artificial sugars.** These sugars are man-made in a lab and are most often found in sugar substitutes or sweeteners that claim to be "low calorie" or "zero calorie" while also adding flavor to a specific food item. These include aspartame (NutraSweet, Equal, SugarTwin), acesulfame potassium (Equal), saccharin (Sweet'N Low, Sugar Twin, Necta Sweet, Equal Saccharin), xylitol (XyloSweet, Lite&Sweet, Xyla, and Global Sweet), and sucralose (Splenda, Equal Sucralose).

I would classify stevia as a natural sweetener or sugar substitute, as it is harvested from the stevia shrub. Monk fruit would also be considered a natural sugar because the taste comes primarily from the fructose, glucose, and mogrosides in it. Erythritol is a sugar alcohol or polyol and should be considered an artificial sweetener.

Body's Response to Sugar

At the very basic level, when natural or added sugars are consumed, it triggers the body to create insulin. Over time, if there is a consistent demand for insulin, for example due to repeatedly eating too much sugar, it can place increased pressure on the body and its systems to perform properly and can lead to issues like insulin resistance, weight gain, low energy, increased risk for disease, and other problems. When it comes to artificial sugars specifically, more studies need to be conducted to determine the immediate effects of whether these sugars specifically raise insulin levels; however, there is some evidence to support that consumption of these artificial sweeteners can lead to insulin resistance in the same way that sugar does.

Furthermore, studies have suggested that sugar affects the reward system in the brain. When you consume sugar, the pleasure system is activated, causing you to crave more sugar in the future. This is where the idea that sugar is addicting comes from.

When it comes to artificial sugars specifically, studies have shown that daily consumption can lead to numerous health issues, including increased risk for disease, obesity, imbalance of the gut microbiome, and more.

Fruit Sugar Is Fine

When it comes to sugar, the largest concern is eating processed food items rather than eating natural fruits and vegetables. In general, it is fine to consume fruit, despite its sugar content, because of the natural sugars. Fruit also contains fiber and other nutrients that we need to be healthy. Hav-

The healthiest way to indulge in a sweet tooth is by choosing organic fruits and sweeter vegetables instead of indulging in processed and packaged items.

ing said that, don't allow fruits to displace vegetable consumption. You should be eating more vegetables than fruit. It is always best to shop organically whenever possible to avoid any harmful additives or pesticides and to also ensure that you are getting the actual nutrient value of the produce.

Role of Artificial Sweeteners

In an ideal world, there would not be a place for artificial sweeteners in a healthy diet. However, artificial sweeteners can be helpful for people who are transitioning into a healthier lifestyle. For example, if you are used to eating highly processed, sugary foods and drinks, then replacing them with artificial sweeteners in the beginning can be helpful when it comes to building the foundation for your healthy habits. In the long-term, it would be best to stick with natural sugars and limit the amount of artificial sweeteners in your diet.

Healthy Sweet Tooth Options

The healthiest way to indulge in a sweet tooth is by choosing organic fruits and sweeter vegetables instead of indulging in processed and packaged items. Try Greek yogurt with mixed fruits, homemade granola bites with fruit, or dried fruit chips, preferably made at home using a dehydrator.

If you don't have a dehydrator, you can use an oven or an air fryer to make baked snacks using organic fruits and vegetables. Furthermore, if you do not have access to any appliances but still have a sweet tooth, the best alternatives are simply eating fruits and vegetables whole.

Furthermore, honey and maple syrup can be good toppings to add a little bit of sweetness to things like fruit, oats, or yogurt. Try to stick with organic options when it comes to honey or maple syrup to ensure you are getting the nutrients and not adding any harmful preservatives to your diet.

Non-Sugar Sweeteners Won't Help You Lose Weight

Abigail Raffner Basson, PhD, RD, an NIH-funded instructor in the department of nutrition at Case Western Reserve University in Cleveland commenting on new guidelines from the World Health Organization.

Replacing sugar with non-sugar sweeteners doesn't reduce body fat among non-diabetics, according to a recent finding—and might increase risk for type 2 diabetes or cardiovascular disease. Neither synthetic nor naturally occurring non-sugar sweeteners are beneficial.

Best: Consume less sweet food...opt for fruit over other sweets. Coconut sugar and date syrup are the least-unhealthful options to add sweetness.

Are Sugar Alcohols Safe for Diabetics?

Franca B. Alphin, MPH, RD, assistant clinical professor, department of community and family medicine, Duke University, Chapel Hill, North Carolina.

Most sugar-free products contain sugar alcohols. Are these safe for diabetics?

More Evidence of Sugar's Harm

A meta-study of 73 reviews documented significant links between eating too much sugar and 45 health problems, including diabetes, heart attack, cancer, and early death.

Self-defense: Stay below 25 grams of sugar a day. Avoid processed food and soda...wean yourself off desserts and sugar in your coffee.

Maya Adam, MD, director of health media innovation at Stanford School of Medicine in California, commenting on a study published in *The BMJ*.

Sugar alcohols are a type of nutritive sweetener. The most common types are mannitol, sorbitol, and xylitol. They each contain about one-half to one-third fewer calories than regular sugar. Because sugar alcohols don't cause sudden increases in blood sugar, candy,cookies, soft drinks, and other products that contain sugar alcohols are safe for people with diabetes. However, eating sugar alcohols can cause bloating and gas. In some people, they can also cause diarrhea.

What You Drink Has a Major Health Impact

Qi Sun, MD, ScD, associate professor in the departments of nutrition and epidemiology at Harvard TH Chan School of Public Health in Boston and lead author of a study of 15,500 adults published in *BMJ*.

According to a recent study, adults diagnosed with diabetes who drank four cups of coffee per day had 26 percent lower risk for death over an 18-year study. Other beverages also lowered risk—water (23 percent), tea (21 percent), and low-fat milk (12 percent).

But: Sugar-sweetened beverages raised risk of dying over the same period—by 20 percent for those who drank more than one drink per day.

Type 2 Diabetes Can Directly Cause Lung Complications

University of Surrey.

In the largest-ever genetic study exploring how genes affect blood sugar levels and health outcomes, researchers concluded that lung disorders should now be considered a complication of type 2 diabetes. Previous studies have shown that lung conditions are more common in people with type 2 diabetes, but until now, it was not known whether type 2 diabetes directly causes damage to the lungs or if other factors common to both conditions are responsible. In this study, analysis revealed that high blood sugar levels in people with type 2 diabetes directly impaired lung function. Modeling of the study data showed that an increase in average blood sugar levels from 72 mg/dL to 216 mg/dL could result in a 20 percent drop in lung capacity and function.

Bariatric Surgery Improves Neuropathy

University of Michigan Health.

Researchers followed more than 120 patients who underwent bariatric surgery for obesity. Over two years, all metabolic risk factors for developing diabetes, such as high glucose and lipid levels, improved. Patients also showed improvements in peripheral neuropathy, a condition marked by damage to the nerves that go from the spinal cord to the hands and feet. Skin biopsies showed that nerve fiber density improved in the thigh and remained stable in the leg.

Afternoon Exercise Is Better for Blood Sugar

Jingyi Qian, PhD, instructor in medicine, division of sleep and circadian disorders, Brigham and Women's Hospital, Massachusetts.

Investigators analyzed physical-activity data from the Look AHEAD study, which included more than 2,400 participants. They found that people who engaged in moderate or vigorous physical activity in the afternoon had a greater reduction in blood glucose levels compared with people who exercised at other times of day. Afternoon exercisers also had the highest chance of stopping their glucose-lowering/diabetes medications.

COVID Still Increases Diabetes Risk

Alan Kwan, MD, cardiologist at Cedars-Sinai Medical Center, Los Angeles, and leader of a study of 23,709 patients published in *JAMA Network Open*.

COVID still increases diabetes risk, although now it's milder.

Recent finding: People recovering from COVID had a 58 percent higher risk for a new diabetes diagnosis compared to before their infection...and risk was higher among recovering COVID patients who were unvaccinated at the time they caught the infection. The mechanisms driving the results are unclear, but it may be that inflammation disrupts glucose regulation.

Older Diabetes Patients Face Growing Cancer Risk

Suping Ling, PhD, assistant professor in epidemiology at London School of Hygiene & Tropical Medicine, UK, and leader of a study of 137,000 adults published in *Diabetalogia*.

Deaths fell for patients with type 2 diabetes who were followed for eight years...but deaths due to cancer at ages 75 and 85 increased by 1.2 percent and 1.6 percent per year, respectively. Patients with type 2 diabetes faced twice the risk for death from colorectal, pancreatic, liver, and endometrial cancers versus the general population.

Plastic Chemicals Are Linked to Diabetes Risk

Sung Kyun Park, ScD, associate professor of epidemiology at University of Michigan in Ann Arbor and leader of a study published in *The Journal of Clinical Endocrinology & Metabolism*.

Phthalates, compounds used to soften plastics and bind fragrances in cosmetics and lotions, are known to disrupt the body's endocrine system.

Recent finding: A study of midlife women found that high exposure to phthalates is associated with up to 63 percent increased risk for a type 2 diabetes diagnosis.

Self-defense: Avoid food and drinks sold in plastic packaging...and opt for phthalate-free toiletries.

Diabetes and Frozen Shoulder

Meta analysis of eight studies of a total of 5,388 adults led by researchers at Keele University, Newcastle-under-Lyme, UK, published in *BMJ Open*.

Also called adhesive capsulitis, frozen shoulder is a condition characterized by stiffening and thickening of the connective tissue surrounding the shoulder, which leads to restricted movement.

Recent finding: Having either type 1 or type 2 diabetes makes the odds of developing frozen shoulder 3.69 times higher compared with people who don't have either condition. While the link to diabetes is not understood, this is another reason to stay on top of treatment and discuss with your doctor strategies, such as certain exercises, to reduce your risk.

Stress Link to Metabolic Syndrome

Studied titled "Inflammatory Biomarkers Link Perceived Stress with Metabolic Dysregulation," by researchers at The Ohio State University, Columbus, published in *Brain, Behavior, & Immunity—Health*.

Many of us are living in a danger zone. About 33 percent of U.S. adults have metabolic syndrome, which is a group of five conditions that are risk factors for heart disease, type 2 diabetes, and stroke. According to researchers at The Ohio State University, prolonged stress and inflammation may both be risk factors for metabolic syndrome, but studies looking at the relationship between stress, inflammation and metabolic syndrome are few, and the results have been mixed.

The Risk Factors for Metabolic Syndrome

According to the American Heart Association, to diagnose metabolic syndrome a person must have three or more of these risk factors...

- High blood sugar
- Low levels of good (HDL) cholesterol
- High levels of triglycerides
- High blood pressure
- A large waist circumference due to belly fat

The research team at The Ohio State University started with a hypothesis that the pathway from stress to metabolic syndrome includes inflammation; stress causes inflammation which leads to an increased risk of metabolic syndrome. To test their theory, they used data obtained from the Midlife in the United States Study (MIDUS). MIDUS is a long-term study started in 1995 to study the biological, psychological, and social factors that influence health and aging.

A subset of participants in the MIDUS study had blood samples taken that included testing for inflammation and metabolic syndrome. These participants also provided a self-reported questionnaire that measured stress, called the Perceived Stress Scale (PSS), and they all had a physical examination that included any signs of metabolic syndrome. Anyone who was already diagnosed with cardiovascular disease or diabetes was excluded.

To measure body (systemic) inflammation, the team conducted blood tests that measure levels of inflammation, including the proteins associated with inflammation C-reactive protein (CRP), IL-6, and fibrinogen. Blood tests to diagnose metabolic syndrome included glucose, cholesterol, and triglycerides. The PSS test uses 10 questions to measure perceived stress over the past month. The physical exam included blood pressure, height and weight for BMI, and waist circumference.

Stess Equals Inflammation

The results of the study are published in the journal *Brain, Behavior, & Immunity—Health*. The study included 648 participants equally divided between male and female with an average age of 52. To measure the relationship between the three conditions,

---

Can Foot-Warming Socks Relieve Foot Neuropathy?

Neuropathy—the tingling, burning pain, or numbness that's often a side effect of diabetes, medications, or autoimmune disease, is caused by nerve damage. Foot-warming socks can help soothe this type of nerve pain. Some foot-warming socks are heated in the microwave, while others are battery-powered. Prices range from $20 to $40. To prevent burns, test microwaved socks before putting them on, and do not sleep in battery-powered socks.

Janice F. Wiesman, MD, FAAN, associate clincal professor of neurology at New York University School of Medicine, New York City.

> **Your Voice May Indicate Diabetes**
>
> Electronically comparing smartphone recordings revealed that differences in pitch, breathiness, hoarseness, and voice roughness are 75 percent accurate in men and 70 percent accurate in women at predicting type 2 diabetes.
>
> Study of 267 adults by researchers at Klick Applied Sciences, Klick, Inc., Toronto, Ontario, Canada, published in *Mayo Clinic Proceedings: Digital Health*.

the team used a statistical model called structural equation modeling. The most important finding, according to the researchers, was that high levels of stress were significantly associated with high levels of metabolic syndrome, and in 61.5 percent of cases, the association was explained by inflammation.

The conclusion of the study, according to the team, is that inflammation is a probable explanation for the relationship between stress and metabolic syndrome and that stress reduction interventions could be a cost-effective treatment option for reducing the risk of inflammation and metabolic syndrome.

Known ways to reduce the risk or manage metabolic syndrome are weight loss, maintaining a healthy weight, eating a heart-healthy diet, getting at least 150 minutes of moderate intensity exercise per week, and working with a health-care provider to control blood pressure and blood sugar. If other studies support the findings of this study, stress may be added as an important risk factor, and stress reduction as a way to prevent or manage metabolic syndrome.

Chapter 5

EMOTIONAL RESCUE

A Better Marriage Means Better Health

A happy marriage is like a tonic for your health. People who feel loved, respected, supported, and connected to their spouse enjoy everything from enhanced heart health and a stronger immune system to a longer life span. Research even shows that healthy, joyful relationships have a stronger influence on health than exercise does.

On the flip side, chronic marital stress can negatively impact physical and mental health. Relationship ups and downs are inevitable, of course, but when partners begin to ignore each other's needs or when criticism or contempt begin creeping in, the health benefits of marriage start to wane.

What Recent Research Shows

Researchers from Ohio State University and the University of Southern Mississippi recently reexamined data from a 2005 study that found that the stress caused by a fleeting marital argument was powerful enough to impact immunity to the point where wound healing slowed. In revisiting the data, the researchers found that in couples where one partner tended to criticize or nag their spouse, causing the other partner to grow defensive or withdraw from the argument, both spouses experienced delayed wound healing. Essentially, they found that chronic and acute negativity "is particularly bad for couples' emotions, relationships, and immune functioning," according to the new study, published in the journal *Psychoneuroendocrinology*.

This research, which looked exclusively at heterosexual couples, found that while men and women both suffer from hostile communication, women tend to bear the brunt of it.

Communication Is Key

Criticizing, blame, and withdrawal are common relationship tactics, but they're incredibly destructive. Psychologist John Gottman, PhD, the nation's most preeminent marriage researcher, actually refers to contempt as "sulfuric acid for love." There are far more constructive, kind ways to

---

Kerry Lusignan, LMHC, Certified Gottman Method Couples Therapist, Certified Daring Way Facilitator, and founder of the Northampton Couples Therapy Center (NCCT) in Northampton, Massachusetts, which has treated more 2,000 couples. Learn more about Lusignan at NorthamptonCouplesTherapy.com.

communicate with your spouse. Here are three evidence-based strategies that foster interconnectedness and growth…

Strategy #1: Sliding door moments

Your day is filled with opportunities to show your partner that you care about him or her. These can seem insignificant—passing each other in the hallway, being asked to turn up the TV volume—but each one has the potential to nurture or erode your relationship. Consider these two examples of sliding door moments…

Scenario A: You're relaxing on the couch, reading a great book, when your partner asks if you can help them with a quick home repair. You really want to see what happens next in this chapter. You could say, "Not right now, I'm reading," or you could put the book down and prioritize your partner. Both choices seem fairly inconsequential in the moment, but when they accumulate over months and years, they shape how loved and valued the other person feels.

Scenario B: You're doing a crossword puzzle in the kitchen when your partner walks in and starts venting about an upsetting event at work. You could put the pencil down and listen attentively, or you could snap, "Not again. I don't have the energy to hear you complain about this anymore."

As you can see, sliding door moments, and the way we react to them can be subtle or overt. But each involves one partner expressing a need and trusting the other one to acknowledge and respond to it.

When a partner consistently turns away, it pushes the couple toward a state where they feel they're living parallel lives instead of sharing their life with one another. It's these small interactions, micro-moments really, that can make or break a marriage much more than the occasional blow-up. Think of them as deposits in your marriage's emotional bank account.

Strategy #2: Take a break from an argument

In the heat of the moment, your nervous system enters fight-or-flight mode. Heart rate quickens, blood pressure rises. Your body is primed for battle, and healthy communication goes out the window as you tend to argue in circles, prematurely shut down the other person's point of view, or push your partner past their threshold, which often causes them to shut down and withdraw.

Here's where a time-out can be a beautiful thing. Time-outs are a chance to calm down on a physiological level as well as consider your partner's position. But you must use them wisely. There's no point in taking a break if you spend the next hour ruminating or complaining to friends. Both will keep your nervous system ramped up and prevent you from seeing the argument from both sides. And there are almost always two sides to every disagreement.

It's not easy, but if you sense your dispute escalating with no end in sight, calmly explain that you feel overwhelmed, and reassure your spouse that while you care about what they are saying and want to keep discussing it, you need to take a break. You could even say, "I think we need a time-out." Next, change your environment and give your mind a break by taking a walk, working on a project, or organizing a junk drawer.

If your mind wanders into the land of anger, blame, or contempt, try to let it go and genuinely attempt to see the argument from your spouse's viewpoint.

Once you feel more centered, it's time to re-initiate the discussion. Preferably, this should be on the same day. Any longer and you run the risk of increasing anger and resentment. Think of it as a "do-over" and not your chance to prove you were right.

Changing gears like this in the heat of the moment is difficult but incredibly beneficial. It takes practice. You can also rehearse it during couples therapy. Which brings us to the next strategy.

***Strategy #3:* Couples therapy**

Couples therapy has a reputation for being a last-resort option for couples that are somehow broken. But couple's therapy is an indicator of health, not of dysfunction, offering a chance to examine your relationship as its own entity. (There's you, there's your partner, and then there's your relationship.) You can use it to work on anything from improving communication to balancing the emotional labor of the household to cultivating compassion and empathy. It requires vulnerability and a willingness to look at how you—yes, you—have contributed to your marriage's struggles.

When interviewing therapists, ensure they have substantial experience working with couples. About 85 percent of therapists say they can do couples therapy, but only 5 percent have undergone the advanced training necessary to excel at it. One option is a Gottman-trained therapist who specializes exclusively in couples therapy. Find providers by visiting the Gottman Referral Network at GottmanReferralNetwork.com

The ideal therapist practices "state-dependent" work, which safely guides you and your partner into the same stressful state you experience at home when arguing. This offers a window into how you communicate, both verbally and nonverbally, and allows the therapist to help you learn to use new skills when you need them the most. I use heart rate monitors to track my clients' emotional dysregulation (doing so helps me learn about their communication patterns and also allows me to call attention to their physiology, so they can learn along with me) as well as to determine when it's time to take a time-out.

Be prepared to commit to weekly sessions that last 75 to 90 minutes. Any less and you risk leaving the session overaroused and more likely to fight on your way home.

Only 19 percent of couples seek marriage counseling, but of those who do, it has an 85 percent success rate.

More to Try...

- **Online relationship workshops.** Seek out classes that are tailored to your marriage's pain points. My digital "Crisis to Connected" class, for instance, focuses on how to handle gridlock, that painful space where you get stuck on the same issues, arguing again and again about seemingly insignificant details that unravel your connection. Other classes are aimed at surviving infidelity or another major painful event, reigniting passion, and the like.

- **Relevant books and podcasts.** I frequently recommend *Developing Habits for Relationship Success* by Brent Atkinson, *Daring Greatly* by Brené Brown, *Codependent No More* by Melody Beattie, and the audiobook *Your Brain on Love* by Stan Tatkin.

–Kerry Lusignan, LMHC

Oh, Brother (or Sister)

Fern Schumer Chapman, author of *Brothers, Sisters, Strangers: Sibling Estrangement and the Road to Reconciliation* and *The Sibling Estrangement Journal: A Guided Exploration of Your Experience through Writing*. She offers coaching to people struggling with estrangement issues and is a blogger for *Psychology Today*. FernSchumerChapman.com

Siblings are often our first playmates, companions, and closest confidants. In recent years, there has been a growing recognition of the importance of sibling relationships and how they shape our lives.

Warm sibling relationships in later life are associated with less loneliness and greater well-being, according to a study published in the *Journal of Family Psychology*. They may even help you live longer, notes the American Sociological Association. We spoke with Fern Schumer Chapman, the author of two books on sibling relationships, to learn more.

> **Gardening Lifts the Spirits**
>
> When healthy women participated in gardening classes or art classes, both groups saw improvements in their mood...but the gardening group got an extra benefit in the form of reduced anxiety.
>
> Study of 32 women led by researchers at University of Florida, Gainesville, published in *PLOS One*.

When Things Are Chilly

Not all sibling relationships are warm. In fact, sibling estrangement is more common than one might think, with approximately one in three people experiencing apathetic, strained, or estranged relationships with their siblings. Several factors can contribute to sibling estrangement...

•**Family trauma.** Shared experiences of family trauma, such as the death of a parent, can strain a relationship.

•**Parental favoritism.** When parents show favoritism towards one child, it can lead to resentment and jealousy among siblings.

•**Poor communication skills.** Inadequate communication within the family can hinder the ability to navigate conflicts and misunderstandings.

•**Differing values and choices.** Siblings may have divergent values, beliefs, and life choices.

•**Lifestyle, cultural, and financial differences.** Differences in lifestyle, income, social class, and cultural backgrounds can create barriers within sibling relationships.

•**Political differences.** Ideological disparities can strain sibling bonds, especially in polarized times.

•**Addiction and mental health.** Siblings grappling with addiction or mental health issues may face challenges in maintaining relationships.

In some cases, you may want to try to save a relationship, while in others, there may be factors that make it unwise to do so.

Healing a Broken Relationship

If you'd like to reconnect with an estranged sibling, it can be a difficult—but worthwhile—journey.

•**Examine your reasons for wanting to reconcile.** Has something changed that leads you to think that relations will be better now and in the future? Is it your choice or are others pressuring you? How do you really feel about reconciling? Why is the relationship important to you—not to your family or to anyone else, but to you?

•**Establish your expectations.** What kind of relationship are you seeking? Do you want a limited connection that will allow you to spend special occasions together comfortably? Are you hoping to communicate easily whenever you want to? Are you looking for support from your estranged relative? Can you offer support to them? Do you and your sibling have enough in common, including a desire to make this effort worthwhile? Can you set aside the anger, pain, and/or resentment that led to the break in order to change the pattern of relating? Do you want to resume the relationship if you discover that neither of you has changed? Do you have the resources (time, energy, emotional resilience, support of other loved ones) to reconcile and rebuild the relationship? Will you compromise too much of yourself if you try to sustain a relationship?

•**Make a plan.** Plan to meet in a local, quiet, neutral place, and set a time frame, around one to three hours, for the discussion. Set aside specific times for talking, and then have some fun together. Do not have friends or other relatives present. Decide in advance what topics to discuss, starting with those that aren't too highly charged, as well as any topics you will avoid. You may need to agree that you have different values, and neither of you will raise those issues.

•**How to approach the discussion.** Start softly, and don't try to cover too many topics in one sitting. Try to focus on the present and future, including accepting your sibling as they are now. Seek common ground, and don't try to prove that you are right. Give your sibling the benefit of the doubt and consider that past injustices may be the result of the way you were both parented, rather than something your sibling intended to be hurtful. Avoid your sibling's triggers. Research shows that siblings are most competitive about appearance, achievement, and intellect.

After each of you speak, repeat what the other person said to make sure you are listening to each other. Use non-confrontational "I" messages, such as, "I feel so much less accomplished than you," rather than provocative "you" statements, "You always looked down on me," which can make a sibling feel defensive.

Remember that a single meeting won't solve everything. Celebrate small successes and be patient. We can't control our sibling's behavior, but we can control how we see ourselves in relation to them and how we approach them. Achieving reconciliation and changing the relationship into one that's functional will, first and foremost, require you to change.

When to Limit or Let Go

In some cases, a relationship may be too toxic to reconcile. If you find yourself in such a situation, it's essential to prioritize your well-being.

Limited relationships, where interactions with a difficult sibling are kept superficial—such as seeing each other only at holiday gatherings—can be a workable solution for maintaining peace within the larger family. This approach involves disengaging from conflict and avoiding confrontation.

But in some cases, you may choose to end contact completely, such as in the case of lifelong abuse or neglect, mental illness, drug or alcohol abuse, criminal behavior, reckless or dangerous behavior, or narcissistic behavior.

On the positive side, going no-contact may provide a sense of peace, stability, and freedom. You may respect yourself more and feel you are living authentically. Your self-esteem and self-confidence may improve. You may feel a sense of self-control, self-reliance, and agency.

But there are negatives as well. You may find that you grieve for the sibling you wish you had or have feelings of guilt and remorse, loneliness, anxiety, and depression. You will likely experience backlash and pressure from your family.

Sibling relationships are complex and evolve over time, influenced by various factors. They can be a source of love, support, and companionship, but they can also be fraught with challenges. Recognizing the importance of sibling bonds and making efforts to strengthen or reconcile them can lead to more fulfilling family dynamics and personal growth. Whether close or distant, these relationships play a significant role in shaping our identities and experiences throughout life.

Drug Add-on Boosts Antidepressant Effects

Washington University School of Medicine in St. Louis.

For older adults with clinical depression that has not responded to standard treatments, adding the drug *aripiprazole* (brand name Abilify) to an antidepressant they're already taking is more effective than switching from one antidepressant to another, according to a new multicenter study led by Washington University School of Medicine in St. Louis. Aripiprazole originally was approved by the FDA in 2002 as a treatment for schizophrenia but also has been used in lower doses as an add-on treatment for clinical depression in patients who do not respond to antidepressants alone. Augmenting an antidepressant with aripiprazole helped 30 percent of patients with treatment-resistant depression, compared with only 20 percent who were switched to another solo antidepressant, results of the study show.

Emotional Rescue

Seven Habits to Fight Depression

University of Cambridge.

By examining data from almost 290,000 people, researchers found seven healthy lifestyle factors that are linked with a lower risk of depression. *Getting seven to nine hours of sleep* reduced the risk of depression, including single depressive episodes and treatment-resistant depression, by 22 percent. *Frequent social connection* reduced the risk of depression by 18 percent. *Moderate alcohol consumption* decreased the risk of depression by 11 percent, *healthy diet* by 6 percent, *regular physical activity* by 14 percent, *never smoking* by 20 percent, and *low-to-moderate sedentary behavior* by 13 percent.

Nondrug DIY Treatments for Depression All Backed by Research

Richard O'Connor, PhD, a practicing psychotherapist with offices in New York City and Sharon, Connecticut. He is former executive director of the Northwest Center for Family Service and Mental Health and author of *Undoing Depression: What Therapy Doesn't Teach You and Medication Can't Give You.*

There's a problem with traditional treatments for depression. They don't work for many patients—and studies back that up. A 2022 review of more than 200 trials of drugs prescribed for depression concluded that only around 15 percent of patients experience substantial antidepressant effects above that of a placebo. And a 2021 review of more than 200 trials of psychotherapy as a depression treatment found that it was effective for only around 41 percent of patients.

But there is good news for patients whose depression doesn't respond to these treatments. Recent research suggests that certain activities and lifestyle modifications—things that people can do on their own—often can ease or eliminate depression. Richard O'Connor, PhD, author of *Undoing Depression,* offers these do-it-yourself depression treatment strategies…

•**Sit up straight.** A 2017 study by researchers at New Zealand's University of Auckland found that people suffering from mild-to-moderate depression felt greater positivity and less fatigue and focused less on themselves when they were in an upright posture.

Reason: The mind takes mood cues from the body. Earlier research found that forcing a smile when feeling sad can make you feel happier. Hunching over is a common symptom of depression, so it makes sense that sitting and standing up straight might help convince your mind that you are not depressed.

•**Gardening.** Horticulture therapy significantly reduces depressive symptoms among older adults, according to a 2023 review of 13 studies by researchers in China and Australia. Engaging in any hobby can lift a depressed mind out of its rumination and allow it to focus on a pleasant activity for a while. But gardening could be especially beneficial because it is done outdoors and encourages close contact with nature—two things that have been shown by numerous studies to reduce anxiety and depression. A 2023 study at Tianjin Medical University in China found that spending around 1.5 hours per day in outdoor light is associated with significantly reduced depression rates.

Several studies also point to the depression-reducing benefits of immersing oneself deep in nature, such as by taking hikes in the woods, but that isn't always an option. Caring for a backyard or window-box garden might provide some of that back-to-nature benefit. A Korean study found that the simple act of repotting a plant made people feel more comfortable and soothed than performing a non-nature–based task.

Warning: The first five minutes spent engaged in a hobby—or in any other activity that requires effort—can be extremely challenging for someone who is depressed. But when depressed people manage to will themselves through this first five minutes, they often become caught up in the flow and the hobby begins to generate its own momentum.

- **Make yourself presentable.** People suffering from depression sometimes neglect their grooming, wardrobe, and even basic hygiene. Such things can seem inconsequential when you are struggling with larger issues. When you are depressed, it can be difficult to find the energy to do something as seemingly simple as brushing your hair or teeth. But neglecting grooming and hygiene can further damage a depressed person's already low self-esteem and sense of self-worth…and make it even more difficult to socialize, note researchers at Australia's Griffith University in a recent paper. Putting a little effort into grooming and wardrobe isn't just vanity when you are suffering from depression—it truly can improve the odds of recovery.

- **Cook.** Surprisingly, cooking and baking are among the leisure activities most associated with reduced depression among older Americans, according to a large study by researchers at the UK's University College London. Like any hobby, cooking can be a useful diversion, disrupting the ruminations of a depressed mind. But cooking has additional upsides—home-cooked food often is more healthful than packaged foods, and eating right is beneficial for people who are depressed. Cooking also requires you to regularly head to the store for ingredients, so it provides a modest amount of social interaction. And unlike many hobbies, cooking offers an almost immediate payoff and sense of achievement—within a few minutes or hours, the cook gets to enjoy the prepared food. Eating that food is like giving yourself a present, and it serves as a much needed reminder that you have the power to make your life better.

- **Eat right.** Eating junk food increases rates of depression, according to many recent studies…and eating a healthful diet reduces rates of depression.

One way to do it: Adhering to the Mediterranean diet, which is rich in vegetables, fruits, whole grains, fish, and legumes, is associated with a reduction in depressive symptoms. That's according to multiple studies, including a 2013 study by researchers at Rush University Medical Center in Chicago…a 2020 review of earlier studies by Italian researchers…and a 2021 study by researchers in Sweden and China. Why eating right reduces depression is not entirely clear—perhaps the nutrients in a healthful diet combat depression…or the added sugar in junk food contributes to depression…or taking steps to improve your diet provides a sense of accomplishment… or a healthful diet makes you look and feel better. Science doesn't have a conclusive answer yet. What matters is that eating right truly could help if you are depressed.

- **Attend a religious service.** Religious faith and spirituality seem to be linked to reduced rates of depression symptoms. Among the more than 150 studies reviewed by researchers at Duke University and in the Netherlands, 49 percent identified a significant benefit from attending services, while an additional 41 percent found some benefit, though not enough to be considered statistically significant. Feeling a connection with a higher being appears be helpful for those who are depressed, as does the socialization offered by attending religious services.

Caution: People who do not feel comfortable attending religious services should not do so simply as a potential depression treatment.

- **Get some sleep—but not too much.** Being depressed can make it difficult to get a good night's sleep, but recent research suggests that it works the other way, too—getting insufficient sleep increases the odds of depression. The lack of sleep and depression can become a vicious cycle, with each problem feeding upon the other.

Another twist in the sleep/depression connection: Getting more sleep doesn't always reduce depression. The association between hours slept and depression is U-shaped—if you're getting less than six hours or so of sleep per night, getting more is indeed likely to reduce your odds of depression…but if you're already sleeping at least eight hours per night, more sleep is associated with increased depression, according to a study by Japanese researchers. Irregular sleep times and durations also are associated with increased depression, according to a 2021 study by University of Michigan researchers.

•***Get some exercise—even if it's not very much.*** We know that physical exercise reduces the odds of depression—but it might come as a surprise just how effective a depression-fighter exercise can be. In 2023, researchers at University of South Australia concluded that exercise is 50 percent more effective than either medication or cognitive behavior therapy, based on an analysis of more than 1,000 trials and nearly 100 papers. It's also noteworthy that lengthy and strenuous exercise is not necessary to enjoy at least a portion of this benefit. Just 20 minutes five days per week of moderate activity, such as brisk walking, is associated with a 16 percent lower rate of depressive symptoms and 43 percent lower risk for major depression, according to a 2023 study by researchers at Ireland's University of Limerick and Trinity College Dublin.

Can Probiotics Help Depression?

Allan Young, MB, PhD, director of the Centre for Affective Disorders at Institute of Psychiatry, Psychology & Neuroscience, King's College London, and coauthor of the probiotics study published in *JAMA Psychiatry*. KCL.ac.uk

Adding probiotic supplements to a depression treatment plan has the potential to boost the effectiveness of the treatment, according to a recent study.

Study details: 49 participants received either four capsules daily of probiotics with two billion live bacterial microorganisms per capsule…or a placebo. The probiotic supplement, Bio-Kult Advanced, contained 14 bacterial strains that had shown antidepressant effects in previous studies.

Results: After eight weeks, participants who received the probiotic supplement experienced greater improvements in their depressive and anxiety symptoms compared with those who took the placebo. These findings represent an important step in our understanding of the role of probiotics in mood and mental health.

How the gut affects the brain: The brain and the gut communicate through various pathways including neuronal connections, the immune system and hormonal signaling, all of which are involved in major depressive disorder (MDD). Now a growing body of evidence, including this new study, has shown that the gut microbiome—the vast bacterial community residing in our digestive tract—is a key player in this complex network.

Result: A surge in microbiome-targeted solutions for mental well-being, including probiotics for depression. Bio-Kult Advanced is available over the counter—discuss taking it with your doctor or therapist who can help you assess its benefits.

The Rising Risk of Suicide

Dan Reidenberg, PsyD, FAPA, managing director at National Council for Suicide Prevention.

Suicide rates have reached an all-time high, and rates among seniors are rising faster than any other group.

Seniors from the baby boomer and silent generations tend to be hesitant about seeking mental health support, as mental health was a taboo topic over much of their lifetimes. But a growing number of options and innovations are making it more comfortable for everyone to benefit from the expertise of professionals who want to help.

If you're feeling hopeless, sad, or losing interest in things you previously enjoyed, talk to your primary care doctor about being screened for depression. Treatments such as talk therapy, medications, and even lifestyle changes can make a big difference in helping you feel like yourself. Grief counselors are trained to help people of all ages manage loss. There is also an anonymous and free support line that you can call any time to talk to a counselor. Just dial or text 988 to be routed to a network of more than 200 state and local call centers. In 2022, the lifeline answered nearly 5 million calls, texts, and chats.

Manage Illness

Physical health can affect mental health in many ways. A large study published in 2017 found that back pain, traumatic brain injury, cancer, congestive heart failure, chronic obstructive pulmonary disease (COPD), HIV/AIDS, migraine, renal disease, and sleep disorders are associated with an increased risk of suicide.

- **Chronic illness.** A person with chronic pain or a terminal illness may feel hopeless or too uncomfortable to enjoy life. Support groups can help you connect with other people who have similar feelings and experiences. They're also a good way to learn what is helping other people cope with their health concerns.

Tools such as cognitive behavioral therapy, acupuncture, exercise, CBD, and other alternative methods may provide relief or a feeling of control over illness. When medical science can't eliminate pain or discomfort, psychological professionals can often teach people how to manage or better live with it.

- **Medication use.** A variety of medications have been linked to depression, including those used to treat high blood pressure

---

Watch for Your Loved Ones

If you are concerned about a spouse or loved one, there are a few warning signs to look out for...

- **Withdrawing**
- **Not participating in the same activities**
- **Lack of interaction**
- **Tearfulness, sad mood, depression, sense of unhappiness, negative attitude and outlook on life, irritability, anger**
- **Talking about having no reason to live or no purpose in life**
- **Talking excessively about death or dying, talking about writing or rewriting their will**
- **Watching shows and movies or reading books with only death or suicide-related themes**
- **Giving away personal items**
- **Neglecting health or grooming**
- **Expressing little concern for safety**
- **Increased use of drugs or alcohol**
- **Decreased use of prescription medications because they seem futile.**

If you suspect a loved one may be suicidal, you can take steps to help them...

- **Ask if they are considering suicide.** Simply talking about it can reduce suicidal thinking.
- **Reduce access to firearms or large quantities of potentially lethal pills.**
- **Be present for them to increase social connection.**
- **Help them seek assistance from a health-care provider or the 988 Lifeline.**
- **Understand that men likely need more of a push to seek mental health support.**

and high cholesterol. Multiple classes of prescription insomnia medications are associated with suicidal thinking and behaviors.

Increase Your Sense of Purpose

One of the biggest issues that seniors, particularly those over age 75, struggle with is the loss of a sense of purpose as they retire from careers, see their children grow up and grow busy with their own lives, and face barriers to participating in activities they previously enjoyed.

Having a sense of purpose is associated with more than happiness: People who have a greater sense of purpose tend to have slower rates of mental decline and decreased mortality.

One of the most significant ways to increase a sense of purpose is to volunteer. Volunteers provide essential and meaningful services for the community, which can strengthen a sense of purpose, particularly when volunteer activities are aligned with something meaningful to the participant. Volunteering also increases social interaction, helps build a support system based on common interests, improves physical health, and lowers rates of depression and anxiety, especially for people 65 and older.

A study in the *American Journal of Preventive Medicine* reported that people who volunteered for more than 100 hours per year had a reduced risk of mortality and physical functioning limitations, higher physical activity, and better mood, optimism, and purpose in life. A study published in *BMC Psychiatry* reported that prosocial activity is associated with a lower risk of suicide among people with good mental health.

There are countless volunteer opportunities in the community, including in schools, animal shelters, hospitals, literacy programs, social service programs, and much more. You can visit VolunteerMatch.com to start looking for ideas.

Seniors also play a powerful role as historians. Through talking or writing, you can share valuable information, wisdom, and experience with your own families, the community, and local historical societies.

Find Ways to Engage and Learn

There are countless ways to talk yourself into staying in and watching television, but that's a recipe for loneliness and disengagement. Instead, look for activities that you enjoy—or ones that you've never tried to see if you enjoy them.

People sometimes feel that learning and growing stops at a certain age, but nothing is farther from the truth. Try attending a lecture at a local college (many colleges offer free or low-cost courses to seniors), taking an art or craft class, or learning a musical instrument.

New activities stimulate the mind, improve cognitive ability, provide socialization, boost community engagement, and give people a chance to learn from others' perspectives.

Learn to Love Technology

Technology is a double-edged sword for seniors. It can be a powerful way to engage in conversations and activities with people anywhere in the world—including tech-savvy children and grandchildren—but it falls short of many seniors' desire for face-to-face interaction. People ages 65 and older generally connect by being in person, while those under that age often prefer technological tools.

Learning how to use technology can make it less fearsome and more of a tool for seniors to connect with family, friends, and people with similar interests. If it feels intimidating, look for classes at the local library or through your school district's adult-education program to learn how to use the new tools of communication.

Bonus: Learning new skills boosts engagement.

Set Goals

You don't have to be 25 to have goals in life. What would you like to accomplish?

What have you always wanted to do? It could be anything from attaining a college degree to lifting a specific weight at the gym to learning a new language. Setting goals reminds us that we can improve over time, and it gives us motivation to move forward.

Finding the Mental Health Help You Need... When You Need It

Ken Duckworth, MD, chief medical officer of the nonprofit National Alliance on Mental Illness, Arlington, Virginia, and author of *You Are Not Alone: The NAMI Guide to Navigating Mental Health.* NAMI.org

It is a sad fact—people struggling with mental health concerns often end up struggling to find a therapist to help them. In fact, it's not uncommon these days to call every in-network therapist in a geographical area and not be able to find a single one who is accepting new patients. Many therapists were stretched thin even before depression and anxiety rates shot up during the COVID pandemic.

But don't give up. Ken Duckworth, MD, chief medical officer of the National Alliance on Mental Illness, says there are ways to find the help that you need...

•**Be persistent with your insurance provider.** The first step is obvious—call therapists in your area who are in your insurance or Medicare Advantage plan network. Don't just call one or two—work your way down the list of local mental health providers on the insurer's website, calling everyone who seems appropriate for your needs. If you have Original Medicare, use Medicare.gov to search for therapists who accept Medicare-approved payments.

If you can't get in the door with any of these therapists: Contact your insurance provider or Medicare Advantage plan and ask for help finding an appropriate mental health professional who can take you as a new patient. Insurers have a responsibility to provide their policyholders with access to necessary health care.

If this fails: Reach out to local providers who are not in-network and ask if they are willing to take you as a new patient. Then file a formal appeal with your insurer requesting that it cover your treatment from this out-of-network provider as if he/she were in network. This written appeal should explain why you require care and detail your unsuccessful attempts to obtain it from the insurer's in-network providers, including your failed attempt to have the insurer locate a provider for you.

If this request is rejected: Ask how you can appeal the rejection, then try again. Appeals are not always successful but considering the high cost of paying for therapy out of pocket, it is always worth trying.

•**Ask your primary care physician for help.** Your doctor's practice might have a social worker on staff to deal with patients' mental health needs and/or have contacts among local mental health providers. He/she also might be able to provide some basic mental health services, such as prescribing antidepressant medications, if appropriate.

Options Worth Trying

The following can provide useful support, though they might not fully replace a therapist...

•**Call volunteer support "warmlines."** These free services let callers chat with trained volunteers, not therapists.

The National Alliance on Mental Illness (NAMI) HelpLine is available across the US (800-950-NAMI)...or ask your local NAMI chapter if there are additional warmlines or other resources available in your area. To find your local chapter's contact information, visit NAMI.org/findsupport. Your local NAMI chapter also might recommend therapists in your area who are taking new patients.

Emotional Rescue

Warning: Warmlines are not crisis hotlines. If you are having a mental health crisis, dial 988, the suicide and crisis lifeline... or go to an emergency room.

- **Speak to a pastoral counselor.** Many religious organizations offer counseling, but the quality varies—not all pastoral counselors have extensive training. Ask your faith leader what his/her experience is with counseling people who have had similar experiences and symptoms. They often can work in concert with traditional mental health providers.

- **Join a peer support group.** Mental health organizations including NAMI (NAMI.org), Mental Health America (MHA.org), and the Depression and Bipolar Support Alliance (DBSAlliance.org) offer in-person or Zoom-based peer support groups that are similar to the well-known Alcoholics Anonymous meetings.

- **Contact psychology clinics at local universities.** Academic centers that train psychologists and psychiatrists often offer therapy from therapists in training. These trainees lack extensive experience, but they typically are overseen by experienced instructors. Before signing up, ask how closely the trainees are supervised and who provides that supervision.

- **Consider online therapy services—but be aware of their issues.** Services such as Talkspace (Talkspace.com) and BetterHelp (BetterHelp.com) connect patients with licensed therapists over the Internet. But the effectiveness of these services has not yet been well-established...and they've had some troubling privacy lapses.

Example: BetterHelp recently paid a $7.8 million fine for sharing its customers' data for advertising purposes.

New Therapy for Depression—ADepT

Barney D. Dunn, PhD, professor of clinical psychology and chief investigator for the ADepT project at the Mood Disorders Centre of University of Exeter, UK. Exeter.ac.uk

A new form of talk therapy for depression—Augmented Depression Therapy (ADepT)—is showing promise. A recent pilot study by researchers at University of Exeter found that it may be more efficient and cost-effective compared with traditional cognitive behavioral therapy (CBT). *We asked psychologist Barney D. Dunn, PhD, who led the development of ADepT, how it works...*

There are two sides to the depression coin—experiencing heightened negative emotions such as sadness and fear...and experiencing reduced positive emotions such as happiness. Classic CBT does a good job of reducing negative emotions but doesn't do much to build positive emotions. We know that reduced positivity predicts that people will stay depressed for longer and are more likely to become depressed again in the future.

ADepT is an enhanced talk therapy for depression that simultaneously reduces negativity and builds positivity. It was developed by following a co-design process with clinicians and people suffering from depression, integrating elements from effective existing therapies, and determining and then targeting psychological mechanisms driving negative and positive emotions in depression.

How ADepT works: During therapy, the patient establishes what's important to him/her in work, relationships, hobbies and self-care...sets behavioral goals consistent with these values...and breaks these goals down into action steps. He also develops a well-being plan to continue to move toward positive recovery. The intention is for patients to consolidate skills they have learned and build a habit of maintaining and tracking progress toward their valued goals.

Study details: Participants in the pilot study received 15 weekly ADepT sessions followed by five booster sessions flexibly scheduled during the year after treatment to help them keep making well-being gains and troubleshoot any difficulties. ADepT did well treating anhedonia (loss of interest and pleasure), a hallmark feature of depression for many.

Result: While ADepT costs the same as CBT, it led to bigger quality-of-life gains by helping people reconnect to valued and pleasurable activities and identify and act opposite to behavior that can stop these activities.

Next steps: ADepT has been designed so that CBT therapists will require minimal additional training, and an ADepT treatment manual is currently being written. It is not yet available in the U.S., but a few academic therapy centers are interested in evaluating it.

Depression Doesn't Affect All Aspects of Life

Meta-analysis of four studies of 1,710 adults by researchers at University of London, UK, published in *Journal of Affective Disorders.*

People suffering from major depression often remain satisfied with certain parts of their lives, according to recent research, contrary to the widely held belief that they feel deeply negative about everything. Depressed people are particularly likely to feel satisfied with their relationships, including relationships with close friends, family members, and other housemates. Many also feel satisfied with their accommodations and their sense of personal safety. They're much less likely to feel satisfied with their financial situation and mental health.

The Disease of Loneliness

Charles B. Inlander, a consumer advocate and health-care consultant based in Fogelsville, Pennsylvania. He was the founding president of the nonprofit People's Medical Society.

You have probably never thought of loneliness as a disease, but, more and more, loneliness is being viewed as a serious health malady. In fact, studies have linked prolonged loneliness to mental health conditions such as depression and debilitating anxiety as well as contributing to heart disease and other physical conditions.

Loneliness is a worldwide problem. It is so serious that both the United Kingdom and Japan have Ministers of Loneliness as high-level appointees in their respective governments. Their role is to confront the degree of loneliness and isolation within their populations and develop programs and strategies to help people who suffer to find relief.

Obviously, the COVID-19 pandemic exacerbated the loneliness problem. People were forced to the confines of their own homes, with limited access to other people. Social gatherings became nonevents. Traditional meeting places, such as churches, recreation centers, entertainment venues, and even neighborly get-togethers became virtually nonexistent.

Older people are hit especially hard with loneliness. Seniors living alone or those with serious illnesses that limit their mobility and ability to perform daily functions such as cooking, showering, or grocery shopping report high rates of depression and anxiety directly linked to isolation and loneliness.

Even if you are housebound, there are many ways to combat loneliness. Here are some strategies you can employ for yourself or a loved one.

•**Stay engaged.** The most important thing you can do to combat loneliness is to be engaged with other people. Whenever possible, attend gatherings of friends or colleagues. If possible, regularly participate in your religious congregation and volunteer for things that need to be done.

If you are housebound, let your minister or rabbi know, and they can arrange for other congregants to come visit you on a regular basis. If you need assistance with meals, contact your local Meals on Wheels program. Check to see what programs are sponsored by local charities that bring people together.

•**Go low tech.** The good-old telephone is a wonderful way to keep in touch. Throughout the pandemic, I called a wide range of family and friends every day, just to chat and reminisce. It aways made me smile when I got off the phone.

If you have a smartphone, you can do video calls with friends and family. Seeing and talking to a grandchild is a spirit booster. And don't forget your legs. In my grandfather's later years, he would take a daily walk to a nearby park, where he and a few of his old buddies would sit and schmooze for hours.

•**High tech works as well.** During the pandemic, I did two Zoom calls a week with two different groups of old friends. We have continued to do so, and it is a wonderful way to combat loneliness. If you have Internet access, you can easily do these video calls. Ask one of your grandchildren or another kid from the neighborhood to help you set it up. You can be linked all over the world with this technology. And be on the lookout for new ways to engage through the emerging technology of artificial intelligence.

Loneliness can be deadly, especially over a long period of time. The most important strategy is to work hard at staying engaged and not give up.

When Your Fear Is Actually a Phobia…and What to Do About It

Michael Tompkins, PhD, codirector of the San Francisco Bay Area Center for Cognitive Therapy, Oakland, California. SFBACCT.com

If you're like most people, there's probably at least one thing that gives you the heebie-jeebies. Maybe it's snakes or heights or needles or clowns. And you may wonder if your fear is ordinary…or does it rise to the level of a phobia? Michael Tompkins, PhD, codirector of the San Francisco Bay Area Center for Cognitive Therapy, explains how to distinguish a phobia from an everyday fear and what to do if, in fact, you do suffer from a phobia…

Defining Phobias

Psychologists consider phobias to be anxiety disorders. When someone fears one object or setting, they call it a specific phobia. Specific phobias differ from ordinary fears if they meet three essential criteria…

•**Excessive distress.** If you cringe when you encounter a spider on your bathroom floor and call your partner to come dispatch it, you probably don't suffer from arachnophobia. People with arachnophobia would struggle just to finish reading this paragraph…or they might be unable to ever bring themselves to touch a book that contains photos of spiders.

•**Disproportionate emotional response.** People with a specific phobia won't quietly suffer when confronted with the object that causes their terror.

Example: Imagine two people on the ground floor of a skyscraper—one with a fear of elevators and the other with a diagnosed specific phobia of elevators. The person who is fearful of elevators will uneasily step into the elevator and ride up to the 25th floor, perhaps while clenching his/her teeth and sweating. But if the person with the specific phobia is somehow forced onto the elevator, he/she would grow wild with panic.

- **Disruption of day-to-day life.** Specific phobias cause people to change their behaviors. In recent years, the popular press has bandied about the term nomophobia—fear of being out of cell-phone range. If you asked 100 people whether they feel anxious when they have no bars on their phones or are physically separated from their devices, plenty would answer "yes." But compare that with someone who won't travel abroad until his/her partner produces coverage maps proving that they'll always have full bars on their phones…or a student who fails his SATs because he had to leave his cell phone at the classroom door and couldn't focus on the questions. Those are examples of how true phobias disrupt everyday life.

How Phobias Form

Phobias don't materialize spontaneously—they're learned, and there are three main ways this happens…

- **Traumatic conditioning.** Someone who has been viciously attacked by a dog could develop a phobia of all dogs (cynophobia). In the instant of the attack, at the height of his fear response, his psyche learned the lesson, "Dogs are dangerous."
- **Vicarious learning.** A similar thing can happen by watching someone else experience trauma. Being in the presence of someone getting mauled by a dog could trigger the same kind of phobia as undergoing the attack yourself, provided that you were in a heightened fear state as you watched what happened.
- **Social learning.** Someone raised in a household where one or both parents had an intense fear of dogs could develop cynophobia by hearing stories about how dangerous dogs are.
- **Risk factors and protective factors.** Of course, not everyone who gets attacked by a dog…or sees someone else get attacked by a dog…or is raised by dog-fearing parents is going to develop cynophobia. Our genetics, experiences and environments can tip the scale toward or away from the development of a phobia.

Example: A person who has always had dogs as pets has decades of "safe learning" from which he has established that dogs are generally harmless. If he is then attacked, this safe learning can act as a buffer against developing a phobia.

Uncommon Phobias

The list of possible phobias is infinite—you can develop a phobia around just about anything, and the phobic object need not be inherently dangerous.

Example: The actor Billy Bob Thornton has confessed to having a phobia of antique furniture. But there are certain objects or situations that humans are genetically predisposed to be afraid of. We call these primed fears because it has been advantageous, from an evolutionary perspective, to fear certain things. Prehistoric humans who lacked a healthy fear of heights might wander too close to a cliff's edge and die before passing on their genes…the same goes for those who weren't wary around snakes or enclosed places.

But that doesn't mean every modern human is walking around with acrophobia (fear of heights), ophidiophobia (snakes) or claustrophobia (enclosed places), although it probably does explain why such rational fears so commonly develop into specific phobias. Specific phobias fall into three main groups…

- **Animal-object phobias.** Birds (ornithophobia)…cats (ailurophobia)…trains (siderodromo-phobia)…men (androphobia)…water (hydrophobia).
- **Situational-environmental phobias.** Darkness (nyctophobia)…being watched or looked at (sociophobia)…the color yellow (xanthophobia)…bathing (ablutophobia).
- **Blood-injection-injury phobias.** Needles (trypanophobia)…having the eyes touched (ommeta-phobia)…blood (hemophobia)…surgery (tomophobia).

Emotional Rescue

If You Have a Phobia

Most people simply arrange their lives to avoid phobic objects. But some phobias—especially the blood-injection-injury type—can be dangerously disruptive. Someone who avoids health care because of a phobia is in a very precarious position.

Good news: Most phobias are extremely treatable and typically with just a few hours of work. All that's required is a skilled therapist and a motivated patient. The best method—exposure therapy—is really the only thing that works. The therapist will design a series of engineered experiences in which the patient repeatedly learns, step by step, that the fear of the phobic object is misplaced.

Example: Someone with arachnophobia may start by simply thinking about a spider or reading a script about encountering one. Perhaps she will be asked to view a photograph of a spider. Next, she will touch the photograph…then look at a closed container with a spider inside…then touch the closed container. In that escalating fashion, as the patient is ready, the therapist will guide her toward remission of the phobia.

To find a therapist skilled in treating phobias: Visit the website of the Association for Behavioral and Cognitive Therapies at ABCT.org.

Success Secrets from a 78-Year-Old Ironman World Champion

Cherie Gruenfeld, 78-year-old Ironman veteran and USA Triathlon-certified coach, who recently became the oldest female competitor to complete the coveted VinFast Ironman World Championship in Kona, Hawaii. Gruenfeld is a member of the USA Triathlon Hall of Fame. CherieGruenfeld.com

Ironman events are among the toughest single-day endurance events in the world, consisting of a 2.4-mile swim, a 112-mile bike ride and a 26.2-mile run.

To Combat Your Mind's Negative Chatter…

Zoom out—thinking of your situation from a broad or historical perspective can help you see that others have found solutions. Use the second person—referring to yourself as "you" preserves a certain distance from your woes, allowing you to advise yourself as you would a friend. *Reframe* your experience as a challenge. "You can do this" makes you feel like less of a victim. *Make your bed*—restoring order to your physical environment can give you a sense of control. *Experience awe*—the night sky, a work of art or a piece of music can pull you out of your narrow focus and readjust your perspective.

Ethan Kross, PhD, professor of psychology, College of Literature, Science, and the Arts, University of Michigan, Ann Arbor. LSA.UMich.edu

---

Cherie Gruenfeld raced her first Ironman at age 48, just six years after she began running. Now at 78, she has won 14 Ironman World Championship Age Group awards. Cherie shares some of her top strategies for success, not only for athletes, but also for anyone looking to make a midlife change.

SECRET #1: View everything as a new opportunity. One Sunday morning in 1986, my husband and I were lounging in bed, enjoying coffee and watching the first Los Angeles Marathon on TV. I was 42, working in the high-tech industry and, aside from playing tennis and skiing, wasn't athletically active. But when I saw those runners pounding the pavement, I thought, I want to try that. The next day, I bought a pair of running shoes and a book called *How to Run Your First Marathon*. My first run lasted just 10 minutes, but six months later, I completed the Run Through the Redwoods marathon in Northern California in 3:26, a finishing time that qualified me for the Boston Marathon. Within just a few years, I was competing in Ironman.

Many folks tend to stay in their comfort zones, so they don't see things like a marathon on TV, a magazine article about starting your own business or a restructuring at work as the possibility it might be. If something nags at your gut or makes you feel a bit scared but also a little bit exhilarated, give it a serious look.

SECRET #2: Setbacks and mistakes happen—it's okay. When you start something new, you probably won't get things right the first time—maybe not the second time either. That's not failure—that's learning, and it's all part of the process.

Eight years after I began Ironman racing, I started the nonprofit foundation Exceeding Expectations, a program that works with at-risk kids. We use the sport of triathlon to help redirect lives, with the ultimate goal of each member getting a college education. These kids live in seriously disadvantaged circumstances, and every day I learn more and get better at helping them.

In the beginning, I selected 12 kids at an elementary school. I told the teacher, "We'll write a note to the parents, explaining to them that their child has been selected for our program and asking permission for them to train with us on weekends." She looked at me like I was crazy and said, "These parents usually are not around or involved. You'll need to physically go into each home and try to find a parent to speak with and earn trust that way." It was the first of several mistakes I made, but it informed my actions and mindset moving forward.

Being hit with an unexpected setback requires the same kind of determined learning process. In 2019, while training for the Ironman World Championship, I was diagnosed with two unrelated cancers. After spending several days in denial, I accepted my situation and chose to focus on becoming cancer-free while still working out. Except for the day of my surgery and one recovery day, I kept up my regular training schedule, even throughout radiation treatments.

SECRET #3: Work smarter, not harder. One of the advantages to making a big change in your life when you're older is that you have decades of experience and gained wisdom, much of it coming from mistakes and setbacks. As Will Rogers put it, "Good judgment comes from experience, and a lot of that comes from bad judgment."

Push yourself, yes, but keep your expectations reasonable and set attainable goals. Ask yourself, What do I need to do to get that promotion, to move cross-country to a new city, to start getting more fit? Be honest about the answer to those questions.

Hire a coach or expert in the field if that would work for you. Write down your goals and put them where you'll see them often. I stick notes with my long-term goals on the bathroom mirror. Every time I look at them, I recommit myself to accomplishing those goals.

Keep in mind—part of working smarter is making sure you're enjoying what you're doing. If not, you'll lose your drive and won't stick with it. A few years back, while training for a full Ironman in the grueling Palm Springs desert heat, I realized that training was no longer as enjoyable as it used to be. So I made the strategic choice to temporarily shift my focus to Ironman 70.3s, which are half of the Ironman distance (70.3 miles instead of 140.6 miles). I was much happier, and it showed in my performance.

SECRET #4: Find your support system. When you're venturing into unknown areas, support is absolutely critical. You need someone who believes in you. After I'd been a marathoner for a few years, I read a *Competitor* magazine dedicated to the Ironman World Championship event in Kona, Hawaii. This was interesting to me, but it never occurred to me that I could do such a thing. My husband, Lee, who believes I can do anything, read the magazine, and said, "I know you can do this. I think you can be good at it." He gave me the push I needed, and the rest is history.

Not every loved one will do this. Some may say it's not practical to apply to graduate school at age 50, too hard to write and self-publish a book, too risky to start an Etsy shop selling your hand-poured candles. Don't listen to them. Change can feel risky. Surround yourself with people who believe in you and will support you.

To-Do Items Can Be Threats for People with Task Paralysis

Ellen Hendriksen, PhD, clinical psychologist, clinical assistant professor, Center for Anxiety and Related Disorders (CARD), Boston University, and author of *How to Be Yourself: Quiet Your Inner Critic and Rise Above Social Anxiety.* EllenHendriksen.com

People facing many things that must get done, especially perfectionists, tend to freeze when the to-do list is long or an item is major. For those struggling with task paralysis or fear of failure or of letting others down can make it hard to do anything at all.

Self-defense: Use whatever stress-reduction technique helps you. Then, if facing a huge task, break it down into the tiniest possible steps and take any first step that you can do without feeling internal resistance. If faced with numerous tasks all at once, devise and follow a strategy—for instance, do the most important or most timely task first, or do the most enjoyable one to generate feelings of accomplishment.

Breath Work Improves Mood and Reduces Anxiety

Study of 114 volunteers by researchers at Stanford University, Stanford, California, published in *Cell Reports Medicine.*

Performing *cyclic sighing,* a type of controlled breathwork that emphasizes prolonging exhalation, for five minutes a day improved mood more than mindfulness meditation in recent study participants. It also worked better than box breathing (equal duration of inhaling, breath retention and exhaling)...and cyclic hyperventilation (longer inhalation and shorter exhalation). Search for "cyclic sighing" at YouTube.com.

How to Beat Medical-Test Anxiety

Justin Gillis, MSW, LICSW, clinical therapist, McLean Hospital, Belmont, Massachusetts, McLeanHospital.org... Suzanne Salamon, MD, associate chief of gastroenterology, Beth Israel Deaconess Medical Center, Brookline, Massachusetts. BIDMC.org

Whether you're scared of needles, worried about the effects of radiation or contrast dye, claustrophobic, or concerned about the health problems a test could reveal, there are ways to manage your anxiety. *Shift your mindset*—skipping out on a test won't make hidden health problems disappear, and getting a diagnosis offers your best fighting chance. *Tell your providers* so they can numb an injection site, prescribe a tranquilizer, or

Crying Is Good for You

The ancient Greeks believed that crying released "ill humor" and cleared the mind. Now science shows that they may have been onto something. Crying releases the hormone prolactin, which has a calming effect and helps manage the stress response. Studies also show that crying balances the brain and body and helps with cognition. Don't hold those tears inside! (Remind the men in your life, who cry about half as often as women.)

Caroline Leaf, PhD, cognitive neuroscientist and mental health researcher based in Dallas-Fort Worth and author of *Switch on Your Brain,* quoted at Lifehacker.com.

modify a test to make it easier for you. *Bring a buddy* for distraction and support. *Try relaxation exercises,* especially ones that focus on controlled breathing. Look away—not focusing on a needle helps you ignore the pain. *Focus on something fun*—a reward you can look forward to.

Recovering Your Mental Health After a Medical Emergency

Lawson Wulsin, MD, professor emeritus of psychiatry and behavioral neuroscience at University of Cincinnati Medical School and author of *Toxic Stress: How Stress Is Making Us Ill and What We Can Do About It*. LawsonWulsin.com

Medical trauma is a pattern of lingering psychological distress extending beyond the normal healing period of a medical event.

Example: For most surgery patients, the wounds heal and the psychological distress recedes. But a few people will continue to have psychological repercussions in a way that impairs their functioning. In that regard, medical trauma can be thought of as a form of post-traumatic stress disorder (PTSD). But medical trauma is not "just" PTSD. It's often more complex and difficult to diagnose than other forms of PTSD because it is wrapped up in the medical issue itself. If you're in an awful car accident but walk away unscathed, you could develop PTSD, but it is purely psychological, requiring no physical recovery. Medical trauma can become a snake eating its own tail—the psychological trauma interferes with physical healing and, since trauma often manifests in physical ways, may cause a confusing pile-up of medical issues.

Symptoms: One of the tricky things about diagnosing trauma is that humans can repress traumatic experiences for months, years, even decades. That can make it difficult to connect the trauma to medical events

---

What Not to Do When You're Stressed Out

Stress Makes You More Vulnerable to Online Scams

A recent study found that people are significantly more likely to fall for a "phishing" e-mail scam when they are experiencing a high level of stress—in particular, feeling overwhelmed by challenges that they are unable to handle.

Self-defense: When possible, postpone opening e-mails and texts until you're calm and have your responsibilities under control. If you must open e-mails and texts while stressed, remind yourself to be especially cautious about clicking links.

Study of 153 employees by researchers at U.S. Department of Energy's Pacific Northwest National Laboratory, Richland, Washington, published in *Journal of Information Warfare*.

Don't Lift Heavy Stuff When You're Stressed

According to a recent study, when you are dealing with psychological stress, your body moves in ways that increase the pressure on the neck and lower spine when lifting or lowering heavy objects, increasing risk for injury.

Study by researchers at The Ohio State University, Columbus, and University of Michigan, Ann Arbor, published in *Ergonomics*.

---

from the relatively distant past. *Trauma manifests in two opposing ways…*

Hyperarousal is an emotional overreaction consisting of flashbacks, nightmares and reliving the trauma either through explicit memories or the re-experiencing of a sensation associated with the traumatic event.

Psychic numbing is a coping mechanism marked by a flattening of emotions and withdrawal from other people.

The same patient can experience both sets of symptoms or may lean more one way than the other. Psychological numbing is harder than hyperarousal to recognize in oneself or a loved one.

Who is susceptible? We know surprisingly little about who develops medical trauma and why. But we do know that somewhere between 20 and 30 percent of people exposed to the same event will develop a traumatic psychological reaction. That's in line with other forms of PTSD.

We also know that trauma thrives on surprise. The less prepared we are for a situation, the more likely we are to later experience trauma.

Example: Imagine a passive patient who ignores her doctor and signs a consent form without understanding what it says, then awakens from surgery to find her left foot gone. Besides the normal psychological burden of such an event, she may feel shock, betrayal, anger, and injustice, making the situation even harder to process.

People with any kind of psychiatric history, including depression, anxiety, and addiction, are more likely than others to develop medical trauma. We also know that people who have experienced prior traumas are more susceptible. That runs counter to the popular notion that we get tougher the more we endure. Instead, our bodies and minds "keep score" and eventually reach a breaking point. Given trauma's strange incubation period, it can sometimes be difficult to sort out which of a series of shocking events has triggered the PTSD.

Common causes: Just about any surprising or painful medical event—emergency bypass, colostomy, chronic infection, miscarriage—can produce medical trauma.

Prevention: Unfortunately, there's no way to guarantee that you or someone you love won't ever experience medical trauma. But we can take what little we know about trauma's causes and use it to reduce our risk.

Given that medical trauma appears more often in people with psychiatric histories and those who have experienced trauma in the past, medical professionals should ask screening questions before undertaking procedures that could trigger a trauma response. But since few doctors do this, you should report any personal history and voice any concerns about developing trauma. Also speak up if you've experienced intraoperative awareness (waking up during surgery) or delirium.

Because surprise tends to exacerbate the trauma response, enter medical situations with your eyes wide open. Taking control of the situation, being your own advocate, asking questions, making lists, calling specialists—anything proactive you do to make yourself more informed and more in control will provide a psychological buffer against trauma.

Treatment: Trauma is treatable, but since we can't erase the past and we can't cure trauma—we can only manage it. The gold standard for managing trauma is a branch of cognitive behavioral therapy called cognitive processing therapy (CPT). Over the course of weeks and months, the therapist helps the patient identify situations that trigger trauma. She learns alternative ways of thinking about the situation that triggered the reactions. By recording thoughts and story-building, the patient begins to construct a narrative about the events that gives her control over her emotional life and physical reactions to her feelings. Ultimately, the patient will be able to think about the traumatic event without re-experiencing the old emotions and feelings of threat. Some patients will need medication to help this process along.

Reminiscence Therapy Benefits Older Adults

Study by researchers at Hospital General Universitario Gregorio Marañón, Madrid, Spain, published in *Journal of the American Geriatrics Society*.

Being hospitalized for any injury or illness often is associated with depression and anxiety.

Recent finding: With reminiscence therapy (RT), a patient accesses his/her past through conversation, photos, mementoes, music, and art. Among older patients who participated in RT during their hospitalizations for illnesses unrelated to mental health, only 13 percent had moderate-to-severe anxiety at discharge and 20 percent had depression—versus 32 percent and 49 percent, respectively, for similar patients who did not participate in RT.

Hyperbaric Oxygen for Opioid Addiction

Two studies of 39 adults by researchers at Washington State University, Pullman, published in *Journal of Addictions Nursing and Pain Management Nursing*.

Hyperbaric oxygen therapy—breathing pure oxygen in a pressurized environment—helped reduce pain and withdrawal symptoms for people being treated for opioid addiction. This therapy also may make it possible to lower doses of methadone (also an opiate drug but longer-acting than heroin)—patients who received the treatment were able to maintain a dose reduction of 4.3 milligrams (mg) three months after the study, versus a dose reduction of 0.25 mg for people who did not get hyperbaric oxygen therapy.

Cannabis-Use Disorder Is Linked to Schizophrenia Risk

Study involving nearly seven million adults ages 16 to 49 over 50 years led by researchers at National Institutes of Health, Bethesda, Maryland, published in *Psychological Medicine*.

People with cannabis-use disorder—who are unable to stop using marijuana despite its negative effects in their lives—are more likely to develop schizophrenia, according to recent research. The association is stronger for men than for women. Cannabis-use disorder is estimated to be associated with 15 percent of cases of schizophrenia among men and 4 percent among women—and the association is especially strong for young men. In fact, among young men in their 20s, up to 30 percent of preventable schizophrenia cases are related to cannabis-use disorder.

Forgotten Courtesies We All Need to Practice

Lifehacker.com.

Be on time—chronic lateness sends the message to others that their time is not important to you. Letting someone know that you're running late shows that you do care about them...and their time. *Let people finish what they're saying*—cutting someone off mid-sentence gives the impression that you don't care about what the other person is saying. *RSVP to events*—letting your host know if you're coming helps him/her plan how much food and drink to provide. *Park within the lines*—encroaching on another parking spot even for just a few minutes has a domino effect. *Put down your phone and interact with those around you*—not only is it polite, it can be rewarding.

Stress Really Does Make Your Hair Gray

Study led by researchers at Columbia University, New York City, published in *eLife*.

Scientists have developed a method of analyzing human hairs that is similar to studying the rings of a tree. Just as a tree's rings record the effect of outside stressors on the life of the tree, the new tool gives a picture of the recent history of stress on the body and how it affects the proteins and other molecules of human hair as it grows.

Results: For hair that was not about to turn gray due to the natural aging processes, periods of stress are linked with periods of the hair losing pigment—and when the stress was reduced, hairs that had grayed prematurely resumed normal pigmentation.

How to Benefit from Pet Therapy

Jamison Starbuck, ND, naturopathic physician in family practice in Missoula, Montana.

Humans have long healed ills by connecting with animals. In 1792, Quakers working in England recorded the benefits patients gained from interacting with poultry and rabbits. In the 1860s, Florence Nightingale spoke about the value of a "small, pet animal" for patients with chronic, long-term illness that kept them shut in and socially alone. In our time, research in the field of pet therapy is growing.

Benefits of Pet Therapy

Pet therapy is most useful at enlivening mental function and quieting emotional difficulties. Patients with depression, anxiety, post-traumatic stress disorder, poor self-esteem, phobias, autism, and attention-deficit disorder often respond well to pet therapy. Pet therapy can bring relief to people with dementia or Alzheimer's disease or who are isolated in a long-term care facility. Pets are used to give blind people more freedom and mobility.

My tiny Papillon dog, Pippin, comes to work with me daily. She often helps out by sitting next to children who are getting scary procedures, such as a blood draw or allergy testing.

Try It for Yourself

If you'd like to try pet therapy, follow these guidelines for the best experience…

•**Set specific goals.** Know what you want to achieve from the therapeutic animal interaction. Goals can be simply seeing your child smile for the first time in months, noting a depressed elderly person move from indifference about life to happy anticipation of a pet visit, or finding a new ability to speak about difficult emotions. Pet therapy can help with stress reduction, lowering blood pressure, or the development of empathy and regard for others.

•**Talk with your doctor.** Your provider may be able to refer you to a qualified pet therapy professional and can help you set specific timelines to evaluate the progress and benefits of your pet therapy.

•**Interview providers of your proposed pet therapy.** Find out where and when they trained. Ask about clinical experience with pet therapy and ask for details about the therapy animals. If the pet therapist has a facility, visit the site before agreeing to work with the provider.

•**Be realistic.** Pet therapy isn't going to cure severe mental illness or reverse the course of a terminal disease, but therapeutic interactions with animals can soften the edges of many harsh and scary conditions.

When my patient Debbie brought her daughter, Kaylee, to try animal therapy to deal with a traumatic family experiences, Kaylee was initially afraid to come out of the car. But after observing for a bit, she couldn't resist the opportunity to touch and brush a horse and climbed out of the car with a tentative smile. That tiny breakthrough of happiness set both mother and daughter on what became a successful road to recovery.

Food and Mood

Rachele Pojednic, PhD, EdM, associate professor and program director of exercise science in the Department of Health and Human Performance at Norwich University, Northfield, Vermont.

If you've ever felt hangry after going too long between meals, stress eaten a chocolate bar, or lost your appetite when anxious, you've experienced the food-mood connection firsthand.

A bidirectional highway exists between the brain and the gut that allows nutrients absorbed in the gut to impact mood. The route between your mouth and rectum is actually lined with hundredsof millions of neurons—yes, neurons, as in brain cells!—that make up what's now known as the enteric nervous system (ENS) or, more colloquially, "the second brain."

As you might expect, healthy, whole foods like fruits and vegetables, whole grains, and fatty fish have the most positive effect. In contrast, excess intake of processed foods high in sugar and refined carbohydrates can create inflammation linked with mood disorders such as anxiety and depression.

The following three nutrients are incredibly beneficial when it comes to mood support:

Complex Carbohydrates

Carbohydrates have been vilified by diet culture, but the truth is they're an essential component of a healthy diet.

The brain actually runs exclusively on glucose, a type of sugar (a.k.a. a carbohydrate). Regular consumption of complex carbs like oats, quinoa, brown rice, whole-wheat bread and pasta, legumes, and beans also stabilizes blood sugar levels. Without sufficient complex carbs (or if simple carbs like those found in candy and white bread are eaten in large quantities), blood sugar levels fluctuate, which can lead to mood swings. Ideally, you want 45 to 65 percent of your diet to come from complex carbs. When consumed in these quantities as part of an overall healthy diet, carbs don't cause weight gain.

Fiber

You've likely heard the term "microbiome" before—it's the massive ecosystem composed of trillions of bacteria residing in your gut that helps regulate several bodily processes, including digestion and immunity. These bacteria feast on the foods you eat, pulling out various nutrients and using them to create compounds that help your body hum with energy and health. One of their favorite things to eat? Fiber.

Fiber is a type of complex carbohydrate that the body cannot digest on its own. It needs help from the good-for-you bugs in your microbiome, most of which reside in the large intestine. When you eat beans, berries, whole grains, peas, nuts, seeds, and other high-fiber foods, the fiber passes through the small intestine without being digested. Once it hits the large intestine, those bacteria get to work, using special enzymes to break it down and ferment it. As this happens, compounds called short-chain fatty acids are produced. These fatty acids have a mood-based mission: They interact with neurons within the gut to create serotonin, a feel-good neurotransmitter intricately linked to mood. This serotonin works locally, strengthening the gut-brain axis and improving the gut's ability to communicate with the brain and other organs.

Ample amounts of fiber also help create a thick protective layer of mucus in the gut, which serves as a protective barrier, ensuring that compounds that are meant to stay in the gut, including partially digested food particles, do indeed stay there and don't escape into the bloodstream by sneaking through the gut lining. When that happens, it can lead to all manner of inflammatory symptoms, including diarrhea, headaches, joint pain, fatigue, and mood troubles.

The Institute of Medicine recommends that women ages 51 and older eat 21 grams of fiber daily. Men ages 51 and older should consume 30 grams daily.

Omega-3 Fatty Acids

Heart- and brain-healthy omega-3 fatty acids—found in fatty fish such as salmon, trout, and sardines; seeds like flax and chia seeds; and walnuts—enable the brain to carry out its daily to-do list, including emotional and mood regulation. They're called "essential fatty acids" because the body can't produce them itself—it's essential that you eat them.

Omega-3s are anti-inflammatory, which may protect against depression. Several studies have shown that combining an antidepressant medication such as *fluoxetine* (Prozac) with an omega-3 supplement boosts the efficacy of the medicine. These fatty acids help regulate levels of serotonin and dopamine (other mood-boosting neurotransmitters), which may explain their antidepressant effects.

Let Yourself Eat Cake!

While your diet can bump your mood up or down, that doesn't mean you need to eat oatmeal and salmon for every meal for the rest of your life. Food brings us joy, and it brings people together, which has its own list of mental health benefits. Fill your plate with nutrient-dense foods as often as possible, but don't deny yourself a slice of birthday cake. There's a balance between eating for your mood and cultivating a healthy relationship with food.

Colorful Environments Boost Mood

Study of 36 adults by researchers at University of Lille, Lille, France, published in *Frontiers in Virtual Reality*.

When study participants took virtual-reality tours of green environments (natural outdoor settings), their pace slowed, their gaze lingered and their heart rates increased—indicating they were more alert and experiencing pleasure—versus when they took tours of gray urban settings with sidewalks and buildings. A stroll through environments with a spectrum of colorful objects is better for us than making our way through the grays and blacks of a city. To boost your mood, walk in places that offer a robust color palette.

Chapter 6

FOOD, DIET, AND FITNESS

Finding the Best Weight-Loss Program for You

Which weight-loss program will work for you? The one you'll follow at this moment, says obesity medicine specialist Holly F. Lofton, MD. As long as the plan creates a calorie deficit—you expend more calories than you take in—you'll lose weight if you stick with it. And surprisingly, the same diet may not work for you at different stages of your life.

Any diet plan you're considering should have the following elements...

•**Maintenance plan**—a way to bridge to the "forever" stage.

•**Foods that work with your tastes.**

•**Strategies for improving lifestyle habits.**

•**Tailored recommendations** delivered via a platform you're comfortable with.

•**Credentialed administrators**—therapists and coaches who stress the psychology of weight loss or, for a medication-based program, a medical director and doctors.

App-Based Programs: A Cheerleader in Your Phone

Apps can reinforce your meetings with coaches and therapists and counter the "obesogenic environment" we live in, which is not conducive to weight loss. We know what to eat to lose weight, but we are bombarded with messages that distract us. App reminders act as your cheerleader for reaching daily goals. Since costs vary, take advantage of any free trial period to see if you like an app before you pay.

Reminder: Spending more doesn't guarantee success—you get out what you put in. Look for these key features...

•**Ability to track food intake.** The app should tally calories and offer nutrition information to help you make better choices. Calorie counts should come from reliable sources such as the USDA or the nutrition labels of packaged foods.

•**Goal setting and motivational help,** including affirmations, stress-management tools, and cognitive-behavioral strategies. Higher level interactive apps should offer

---

Holly F. Lofton, MD, obesity medicine specialist, clinical associate professor at NYU Grossman School of Medicine, director of the NYU Medical Weight Management Program, and a weight-loss clinical researcher, New York City. Med.NYU.edu

Food, Diet, and Fitness

coaches for guidance and accountability with feedback via text messages, video calls, and/or phone calls.

•**Syncing with other apps and devices.** Connectivity with an Apple Watch or Fitbit and a wireless scale let you track other important components such as physical activity and pounds lost.

App-based programs to consider...

•**LoseIt! Premium.** Track your meals and workouts, and set goals. Enter the amount of weight you want to lose and your time frame, and the app creates your daily calorie limit. If you can't find a brand-name food in the database, you can scan the barcode and the information will be added. You can tap into wellness articles and recipes under the "Discover" tab and access the user community for nutrition- and weight-loss–related forum discussions. $40 per year...lifetime membership, $150. LoseIt.com

•**Noom** focuses on the psychology of weight loss with interactive lessons to help you make behavioral changes. It offers ways to manage emotional eating. Features include virtual coaches, food and activity tracking, and recipes. A stress-management program called Noom Mood is available for an additional fee. $59 per month...$199 per year. Noom.com

•**Train With Kickoff.** After an online questionnaire consultation, you will be matched with a coach for customized workouts and personalized nutrition advice. There's daily support and guidance to improve lifestyle habits, learn easy food swaps, access live workouts, and get feedback about your form. Coaches include certified personal trainers and registered dietitians. $95 per month...live workouts start at $13 per session. TrainWithKickoff.com

•**MyBodyTutor** offers personal coaching to help you change your eating habits and your mindset around food along with a customized diet and exercise program. This program is good for those who want daily accountability, but it's expensive—$299 per month...$599 for a daily scheduled phone call. MyBodyTutor.com

Online Medical Programs

The effectiveness of doctor-prescribed glucagon-like peptide-1 (GLP-1) medications for weight loss, including Wegovy and Ozempic, has led to an explosion of online programs offering these drugs. They can be worthwhile, but you still must do your due diligence. Look up the credentials of a program's medical director and the doctor or other providers who will be supervising you. Bona fide programs will require an initial, possibly virtual, doctor visit plus blood tests to check for any underlying medical conditions. They will prescribe GLP-1 medications only to those who qualify according to FDA guidelines—people with a body mass index (BMI) of 27 or more and a medical condition related to being overweight...or with a BMI of 30 or over who do not have a risk for medullary thyroid cancer or a history of pancreatitis, among other contraindications.

Important: Most GLP-1s are injectables that you'll need to give yourself. Other things to consider...

•**GLP-1 medications don't work for everyone**—about 13 percent of participants had no response to the medications.

•**You may experience side effects**, such as headache and nausea.

•**The required blood tests and drugs can be very expensive** and aren't always covered by insurance. The cost of joining a program itself, without the medications, is expensive, too.

•**Beware of any company that prescribes alternate versions of GLP-1 drugs.** These formulas have not been sufficiently tested and are not FDA-approved.

One important benefit of reputable online programs: They are accessible if you don't have a local board-certified obesity specialist or have shied away from the medical community after not being treated respectfully or being made to feel uncomfortable because of your weight. Look for programs that offer personalization and remote patient monitoring, including weigh-ins via Bluetooth. Some prescribe less expensive generic drugs, such as metformin, as an alternative to GLP-1s.

Medical programs to consider (note that the costs below do not include lab tests or the medications)...

• **Noom Med.** This Noom program makes GLP-1 medications available to existing members who qualify. You'll start with a health evaluation by a board-certified physician or a physician-supervised nurse practitioner and get necessary lab work, followed by an individualized program. $49 per month plus basic Noom membership ($59 per month or $199 per year). Noom.com/med

• **Calibrate** includes an initial virtual visit with a board-certified doctor and one-to-one video coaching with a credentialed and Calibrate-trained "accountability coach" who will help you set goals and make lifestyle changes and monitor your progress. It requires $199 per month, with an initial three-month commitment. JoinCalibrate.com

• **Found** offers less expensive medications for those who can't afford or take GLP-1s. Its doctors are board-certified and specially trained in weight management. You'll get a one-to-one consultation to customize a plan for you and have access to a library of recipes and health articles curated by registered dietitians. $149 per month...less with a longer commitment. JoinFound.com

To Find a Weight-Loss Specialist

If you're looking for a medically supervised program, consider working with a doctor certified by the American Board of Obesity Medicine. These specialists were initially board-certified in an area of medicine by the American Board of Medical Specialties (or the osteopathic medicine equivalent) and then trained and certified in treating obesity. Search at ABOM.org by clicking on "Find A Physician."

Another source of weight-loss specialists is ObesityCareProviders.com, a service of the national nonprofit Obesity Action Coalition (ObesityAction.org).

Dieters Beware

Some in-person and online medical weight-loss programs now offer extensive DNA testing on blood, saliva and hair to supposedly identify unique biomarkers that will determine the best diet for you.

But: There's no scientific evidence that designing a diet and fitness plan according to your genes makes any difference.

What has been proven is that you need a caloric deficit to produce weight loss, even if the diet itself is a healthy way of eating.

Examples: The DASH diet is great for hypertension and the Mediterranean Diet is great for heart and brain health, but you won't lose weight on either one unless you eat fewer calories. Also, look at the quality of the diet being recommended. A low-calorie diet is not necessarily bad, but it is unhealthy if all you're eating is cabbage soup.

Reminder: Avoid programs with unrealistic guarantees. One chain in the Northeast promises "up to 40 pounds lost in 40 days." If you weigh 200 pounds, that equals a 20 percent reduction in body weight—a loss that would take about six months even with medication.

10 Tips for MediterAsian Eating

William W. Li, MD, president and medical director of the Angiogenesis Foundation, is the author of *Eat to Beat Your Diet: Burn Fat, Heal Your Metabolism, and Live Longer* and *Eat to Beat Disease: The New Science of How Your Body Can Heal Itself.* His TED Talk, *Can We Eat to Starve Cancer?* has garnered more than 11 million views. DrWilliamLi.com

The MediterAsian approach to eating dates back 2,000 years, and its origins are rooted in the exchange of foods by ancient traders who traveled the Silk Road, a series of routes that connected China to the Mediterranean Sea. Long before anyone coined the term fusion in relation to cuisine, these travelers were exchanging and combining fresh, dried, and fermented ingredients along this trading route. They intermingled and swapped spices like turmeric, ginger, pepper, saffron, and cinnamon, which are now common to the cooking of China, India, Central Asia, and the Mediterranean countries of Italy, Greece, Spain, and the south of France.

Fresh vegetables, fruits, herbs, spices, and dried and fermented foods, all now recognized as being important for gut health and immunity, were a cultural currency for ingredient exchange.

1. Eat with intention. Choose your food wisely. You have only so many meals in your lifetime, so make each one count. Cut down or cut out the foods that harm your health and focus on the ones that bring you joy and improve your health.

2. Skip a meal (or two). If you can't find anything healthy you want to eat, feel free to miss a meal. Skipping a meal improves your metabolism, burns body fat, and activates your health defenses. Just be careful not to overeat at your next meal.

3. Go for fresh. Fresh foods are the backbone of MediterAsian eating. They contain the bioactive compounds that you want to activate your health. Avoid ultra-processed foods whenever you can.

4. Personalize your food choices. It's all about you: your preferences, your tastes, your circumstances, and your health concerns. Choose what you enjoy that is healthy and available and have it your way. Don't settle for less.

5. Respect tradition. Respect traditional recipes and methods of preparation. This means buying the right ingredients, preparing them from scratch, and making sure to develop full flavors in your meals. Take advantage of the wisdom of centuries. When it comes to healthy food, new inventions are rarely better.

6. Eat in moderation. Eat for enjoyment, but do not overload your body. Portion control is key.

7. Drink the trinity. Three beverages have uncontested health benefits: water, tea, and coffee. Drink them before, during, or after a meal or any time of the day.

8. Eat together. It's better for your health to eat with family and friends. Social bonds lower your stress, and you tend to eat more slowly in company. Sharing food makes it easier to appreciate what's on your plate.

9. Open your mind and explore. Be adventurous and try new foods. Variety helps you become healthier. Take the opportunity to discover your next favorite dish.

10. Live to eat. Give yourself permission to enjoy the pleasure of food.

If you follow these basic MediterAsian principles, you will find yourself loving your food and loving your health at the same time. With so many countries and cultures in the mix, almost everyone can find something they love to eat on a Mediterranean or Asian menu.

---

5 Percent Weight Loss Improves Health

If you're overweight, losing just 5 percent of your body weight has significant health benefits, but not all weight loss methods are the same. After examining data on more than 20,000 people, researchers reported that improving your diet and getting more exercise can help you lose weight and reduce heart disease risk, but skipping meals and taking diet pills doesn't appear to be effective.

Ohio State University.

To Maintain Weight Loss, Sleep Matters

Study of 195 adults led by researchers at University of Copenhagen, Denmark, published in *Sleep*.

Among study participants with obesity who lost weight—29 pounds, on average—during an eight-week low-calorie diet program, those who slept less than six hours per night gained back nearly 12 pounds during the following year...compared with those who regularly slept more than six hours nightly and maintained their new lower weight.

Worse: Reduction of percentage of body fat was also less for those who regularly slept less than six hours a night.

Artificial Sweeteners Are Fattening

University of Minnesota Medical School.

After conducting a 20-year-long study, researchers from the University of Minnesota have reported that long-term consumption of aspartame, saccharin, and diet beverages is linked to increased fat stores in the abdomen and within muscle. The relationship persisted even after accounting for other factors, including how much a person eats or the quality of their diet. They found no such relationship with sucralose.

The USDA's MyPlate Should Not Be Your Plate

Marion Nestle, PhD, Paulette Goddard Professor of Nutrition, Food Studies, and Public Health, Emerita, at New York University, New York City. She is author of *Slow Cooked: An Unexpected Life in Food Politics*. FoodPolitics.com

It has been more than a decade since the US Department of Agriculture (USDA) toppled its well-known "Food Guide Pyramid" dietary guidelines in favor of the "MyPlate" program. But despite the millions of tax dollars spent promoting MyPlate, most Americans don't know what it is, and fewer still follow its advice. It turns out, they're not missing much.

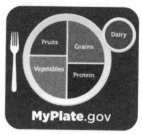

Like the Food Guide Pyramid, MyPlate is meant to distill dietary guidance down to an easy-to-understand visual image—but it doesn't do that very well. The MyPlate graphic (shown above) features a circular plate divided up into four quadrants labeled "fruits," "vegetables," "grains," and "protein"...plus a smaller second circle labeled "dairy," no doubt meant to represent a glass of milk consumed with the meal on the plate.

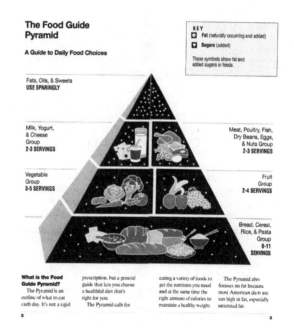

While the Food Guide Pyramid (shown above) made it obvious which categories should form the core of a healthy diet—grains and fruits/vegetables were the largest layers at the pyramid's base—the relative sizes of the MyPlate categories are tricky to compare. *Among MyPlate's other shortcomings...*

•**Protein problem.** The quadrant of the MyPlate graphic that represents meats, poultry, seafood, eggs, meat substitutes, and so forth is labeled "protein." Chefs use the term "proteins" to refer to these foods, but nutritionists don't because it creates the impression that these are the only sources of protein. In fact, a range of foods contain protein, including grains, fruits and vegetables, and dairy foods.

• **Dairy dodge.** The circle labeled "dairy" creates the impression that dairy is a necessary component of a healthy meal—which it isn't.

• **Fruit flub.** Fruits are given their own quadrant on the MyPlate plate. Fruit certainly has a place in a diet, but shoehorning it into this dinner plate graphic creates the impression that healthy sit-down meals must include fruit. In fact, people usually consume fruit as a snack.

What to do: If you want nutrition guidance, ignore MyPlate and stick with the original Food Guide Pyramid, which was based on years of nutrition research.

Secret Superfoods

Sharon Palmer, RDN, a registered dietitian nutritionist based in Ojai, California. She is author of several books, including her latest, *The Plant-Powered Plan to Beat Diabetes: A Guide for Prevention and Management—100 Vegan Recipes Cookbook.* SharonPalmer.com

You don't have to add kale and blueberries to your plate to get a superfood in every meal. Nor do you have to splurge for exotic ingredients like açai berries or maqui berries. These have rightfully been dubbed "superfoods" because they deliver exceptional nutritional value, but they're far from the only foods that do so. In fact, there are plenty of ultra-healthful, antioxidant-rich foods out there, many of them widely available and extremely affordable, says registered dietitian nutritionist Sharon Palmer.

Check out these humble foods that are some of the world's best superfoods in disguise...

• **Black pepper** often is an afterthought, typically just shaken or ground onto prepared meals to add a bit more flavor. But black pepper is much more than just a flavoring. Numerous studies have found that piperine, the alkaloid in black pepper that gives its distinctive bite, has anti-inflammatory, antioxidant, antihypertensive, antiarthritic, and neuroprotective properties.

Even better: When combined with other spices, piperine has a synergistic effect.

Example: The spice turmeric, commonly used in Asian and Indian foods, contains the antioxidant and anti-inflammatory compound curcumin—and when turmeric and black pepper are consumed together, the piperine improves the body's absorption of the curcumin by 2,000 percent, according to a study by researchers in India.

• **Canned tomatoes** have greater antioxidant activity than fresh tomatoes—that's surprising since typically fresh ingredients are most healthful. The cooking process for canned tomatoes significantly increases the bioavailability of the antioxidant *lycopene*—in other words, it increases how much lycopene is absorbed by the body. Lycopene reduces risk for cancer and cardiovascular disease. Tomatoes are versatile, too—stir them into pasta dishes, casseroles, soups, stews, and more—and they are a great source of potassium and fiber.

Note: Cooking tomatoes does somewhat reduce the amount of vitamin C they deliver but not dramatically so. You could buy fresh tomatoes and cook them yourself, but canned tomatoes generally are less expensive than fresh tomatoes when they are out of season and can be stored for months.

• **Peas** might not be glamorous, but they're excellent sources of vitamins, minerals, fiber, protein, and "slow-digesting carbs"—the body takes a significant amount of time to break down these carbs. This results in a slow-and-steady release of glucose into the bloodstream that is linked to lower rates of obesity, type 2 diabetes, heart disease, and other health problems. A recent study by researchers at Toronto's

St. Michael's Hospital found a strong link between the consumption of peas and other legumes with lower risk for cardiovascular disease. Frozen peas are as nutritious as fresh peas, and—like canned tomatoes—they're inexpensive, last for months, and are easy to add to many different meals.

•**Onions** contain antioxidant and anti-inflammatory compounds. Onions have been linked to better heart health, improved immune system function, and reduced rates of some cancers. One review of dozens of previous studies by Italian researchers at the Mario Negri Institute for Pharmacological Research concluded that people who regularly eat lots of vegetables of the genus Allium, including onions and garlic, are 22 percent less likely to get stomach cancer than people who rarely eat onions. They often are used like a spice because of their bold flavor, but they actually are vegetables and are a particularly good source of potassium and vitamin C.

Similar: Garlic has the same anti-inflammatory and antioxidant properties as onions. Numerous studies suggest that garlic protects against heart disease and lowers cholesterol and blood pressure. It also is an excellent source of the minerals manganese and selenium. Garlic powder even can serve as a heart-healthy substitute for salt in many dishes, and it contains the active ingredients found in fresh garlic.

•**Medjool dates** are the rare food that can deliver health benefits while satisfying a sweet tooth. They are rich in fiber and several important minerals, such as potassium, selenium, and magnesium. They're also a good source of heart-healthy antioxidants, according to several studies, including one by Algerian researchers. You can eat dates on their own as a snack, or grind them up and use them to sweeten desserts.

•**Sunflower seeds** are among the best sources of cholesterol-lowering phytosterols, according to numerous studies. They're also rich in heart-healthy polyunsaturated fats, fiber, the antioxidant vitamin E, and minerals including manganese and magnesium. And they are an excellent plant-based protein source. The seeds can be roasted or turned into sunflower butter, which can be used in place of peanut butter.

Similar: Hemp seeds offer many of the same benefits as sunflower seeds, plus they're rich in omega-3 fatty acids, which are great for heart and brain health. Hemp seeds tend to be a bit pricier and harder to find than sunflower seeds. Sesame seeds are rich in fiber and healthy fats and a great source of important minerals, including copper, manganese, calcium, iron, magnesium, and zinc. They provide lignans, which research suggests could reduce risk for heart disease and certain cancers…and cholesterol-controlling phytosterols. Tahini, made largely from sesame seeds, is a tasty and versatile dressing and sauce.

•**Beans** are a healthful, low-fat source of protein, especially when compared with red meat, the most common protein source in the U.S.

One big health plus: Beans provide antioxidants. The amount and type of antioxidant vary depending on the bean variety, but black and other dark-colored beans are great choices—the compound that provides their dark pigmentation, anthocyanin, is an antioxidant linked to lower rates of heart disease, type 2 diabetes, and certain types of cancer. Beans also are fiber-rich and satiating relative to the number of calories they contain, so we tend to feel full after eating them. That helps explain why eating beans regularly tends to reduce body fat and waist size, according to a study by Brigham Young University researchers…and reduces risk for type 2 diabetes, according to a study by researchers at Australia's University of Sydney.

•**Celery** is loaded with fiber, potassium, folate, and vitamins K and C. It also contains coumarin compounds that appear to lower cancer risk…and phthalides that reduce high blood pressure. A study by Indonesian researchers confirmed that drinking celery juice regularly significantly reduces both systolic and diastolic blood pressure among people who have hypertension. Just chop up a celery stick and toss it into a sauté or soup, and you've added an unobtrusive serving of a very healthful vegetable.

•**Bell peppers** are rich in vitamins A and C. They're also great sources of antioxidant carotenoids such as lycopene and beta-carotene, which are associated with lower risk for cancer, cardiovascular disease, and type 2 diabetes. Different-colored bell peppers have different antioxidants, so including several varieties in a meal broadens its health benefits.

Foods You Should Refrigerate

Academy of Nutrition and Dietetics, Chicago. Eat Right.org

Tortillas—they will last much longer. *Pecan and pumpkin pies*—they quickly attract bacteria and are safe to eat at room temperature for only an hour or so after they come out of the oven. *Maple syrup*—refrigeration will significantly increase its lifespan. *Citrus fruits* can last more than a month if kept cold. *Uncooked corn on the cob*—it loses sugar content and taste quickly at room temperature. *Peanut butter*—refrigeration keeps it fresh and prevents separated oil in natural peanut butter from becoming rancid. *Eggs* can be prone to salmonella bacteria at room temperature. *Ketchup* retains freshness and flavor better when kept cold.

Low-Calorie Sugar Substitute Danger

Tod Cooperman, MD, president and editor in chief of ConsumerLab.com, White Plains, New York, commenting on a study of 4,000 adults published in *Nature Medicine*.

Among study participants at high cardiovascular risk, those who had the highest blood levels of the sugar alcohol erythritol, a popular sugar substitute, had twice the risk for heart attack or stroke and increased risk for death within three years. Erythritol appears to stimulate clotting.

Self-defense: Avoid or limit products that list erythritol among the first ingredients, especially if you have cardiac disease or diabetes.

Safer sugar alternatives: 100 percent monk fruit or stevia.

Skip the Banana to Boost Flavanols

University of California, Davis.

Adding a banana to your smoothie appears to decrease the absorption of flavanols, bioactive compounds that are good for your heart and mind. Researchers used smoothies to test how various levels of the enzyme polyphenol oxidase (PPO) affect the absorption of flavanols. PPO is the enzyme that causes apples and bananas to turn brown when exposed to air. One group of study participants drank smoothies made with banana, which has naturally high PPO activity, and another group drank smoothies made with mixed berries, which have naturally low PPO activity. Blood and urine samples showed that people who drank the banana smoothie had 84 percent lower levels of flavanols in their body compared with the control group.

To boost flavanol absorption, consider preparing smoothies by combining flavanol-rich fruits like berries with other ingredients that also have a low PPO activity, like pineapple, oranges, mango, or yogurt.

Almonds Keep Your Gut Healthy

Alice Creedon, PhD, a researcher at King's College London's Department of Nutritional Sciences and lead author of a study published in *The American Journal of Clinical Nutrition*.

Gut bacteria of people who consumed two ounces of whole or ground almonds per day produced significantly more butyrate, the primary fatty acid fuel source for colon cells. Increased butyrate levels can optimize nutrient absorption and reduce gut wall inflammation. Butyrate also has been linked to heart and immune system benefits. If you're not a fan of almonds, other high-fiber nuts, fruits, and vegetables likely provide a butyrate boost as well.

Fiber Makes You Fuller, Especially This One

National Public Radio.

The new anti-obesity medications Ozempic and Wegovy mimic a natural hormone called GLP-1 that suppresses appetite. You can increase levels of this hormone naturally—though not to the same extent—by eating more fiber.

First, consider what happens when you eat a low-fiber meal. Digested food moves into the small intestine, which releases hormones, including GLP-1, that tell your body to start absorption and to suppress hunger signals. GLP-1's actions are extremely fast, so the hunger signals are not suppressed for long and you are hungry again quickly.

But if you add high-fiber foods to a meal, you have an additional opportunity for your intestine to release GLP-1. Fiber moves through the small intestines largely unchanged and takes about four to 10 hours to reach the colon.

Once there, it can finally be broken down by molecules that release GLP-1 and another appetite-suppressing hormone called PYY. Since this extra boost of GLP-1 and PYY occurs hours after you eat, it can decrease cravings between meals and even the overall desire to eat the next meal.

But not all fiber is equal: To get this extra boost of satiation hormones, you need to eat fermentable fiber, such as beta-glucan, which is found in barley, oats, and rye. Human studies have found that beta-glu-

Kidney Beans Caution

All legumes contain proteins called lectins. But red kidney beans and white kidney beans (cannellini) contain a lectin called *phytohaemagglutinin* (PHA) in high enough quantities to cause vomiting, diarrhea, and other gastrointestinal illness. Unless properly prepared, as few as four beans can cause sickness. Slow cookers do not reach high enough heat to remove PHA from beans that are put dry into the cooker.

To remove PHA: Soak dried beans for at least five hours, preferably overnight... drain the soaked beans, place in a large pot, and add enough fresh water to cover them by two inches...bring to a boil, and boil the beans for 30 minutes. Then it is safe to drain the beans and use them in any slow-cooker recipe. Canned kidney and cannellini beans have already been soaked and cooked and can be used as is in slow-cooker recipes... and are healthful and inexpensive ways to add protein, fiber, and iron to meals.

EatingWell.com

can fiber may improve insulin sensitivity, lower blood pressure, and increase satiety between meals. Other fermentable fibers include dextrin in wheat, oligosaccharides in beans, peas, and lentils, and pectin in apples, pears, and green bananas.

Most Eco-Friendly Straws Contain Toxic Chemicals

Food Additives and Contaminants.

Close to 70 percent of eco-friendly straws contain low levels of the forever chemicals poly- and perfluoroalkyl substances (PFAS), researchers have found. In a study of 39 straw brands, PFAS, which are used to make products resistant to water, heat, and stains, were detected in 90 percent of paper straws, 80 percent of bamboo straws, 75 percent of plastic straws, and 40 percent of glass straws. None were detected in steel straws. PFAS can remain in the body for many years, so concentrations can build up over time. PFAS have been associated with thyroid disease, increased cholesterol levels, liver damage, kidney cancer, and testicular cancer.

Revisiting Dairy

Amy Goodson, MS, RD, CSSD, LD, a registered dietitian in the Dallas-Fort Worth area and a certified specialist in sports dietetics who has worked with the Dallas Cowboys and Texas Rangers. She is the author of *The Sports Nutrition Playbook* and co-author of *Swim, Bike, Run, Eat, a Sports Nutrition Book for Triathletes.* AmyGoodsonRD.com

You may think that dairy foods—milk, yogurt, and cheese—are a bad choice for health. After all, the components in dairy can seem like a who's who of nutritional villains. But there's another side to the dairy story. We spoke with Amy Goodson, MS, RD, CSSD, LD, to learn more.

Decades of research—including many recent studies—show that many people who consume more dairy are likely to be *healthier*. In these studies, dairy intake is linked to *lower* rates of chronic diseases —including cardiovascular disease and type 2 diabetes. And the preponderance of evidence also shows that dairy does not increase the risk for cancer. Let's take a closer look at the scientific evidence.

Inflammation

One of the most common misconceptions about dairy products is that they cause chronic low-grade inflammation—a risk factor linked to many chronic conditions and diseases. But research suggests that dairy is either neutral or lowers inflammation.

A study published in *Advances in Nutrition* analyzed data from 16 studies on dairy intake and signs of inflammation. The consumption of dairy products did not show a proinflammatory effect in healthy people or in people who had type 2 diabetes, were overweight or obese, or had metabolic syndrome (a complex of conditions including high blood pressure, high blood sugar, and abdominal obesity). In fact, most of the studies showed an anti-inflammatory effect from milk.

Yogurt may be particularly anti-inflammatory, according to the Framingham Offspring study. Researchers reported in 2021 in the journal *Nutrients* that the effects may be due to yogurt's probiotics, which could help alleviate inflammation by modulating gut microbiota.

What to do: Eat a cup of low-fat, unsweetened yogurt before eating an inflammatory meal.

Cardiovascular Disease

Cardiovascular disease (CVD)—most commonly, the buildup of plaque in the arteries, triggering a heart attack or stroke—is the leading cause of death in America. Full-fat dairy is often cited as a cause of CVD because of its saturated fat. But in a 16-year study, a team of researchers looked at more than 4,000 60-year-olds and found that those with the highest blood levels of fatty acids, considered biomarkers of dairy fat, had the lowest risk of CVD.

The researchers then analyzed the results from 18 studies on dairy fat and cardiovascular disease and found that two biomarkers of dairy fat consumption were linked to lower levels of CVD. The study was published in *PLOS Medicine*.

"Our study suggests that cutting down on dairy fat or avoiding dairy altogether might not be the best choice for heart health," said Kathy Trieu, PhD, the lead author of the study. "Although dairy foods can be rich in saturated fat, they are also rich in many other nutrients and can be part of a healthy diet."

Dairy fat has more than 400 fatty acids—the building blocks of fat—including a good mix of monounsaturated, polyunsaturated, and saturated fats. A complex substance like dairy fat has many potentially healthful components that science is just starting to reveal. For example, research shows that the membrane or outer surface of milk fat globules are uniquely bioactive, reducing inflammation, including the neuroinflammation that plays a role in memory loss and dementia, according to a study in the *International Journal of Obesity* in 2021.

What to do: If your doctor has advised you to eat a low-fat diet, choose no-fat or low-fat diary. Otherwise, feel free to enjoy two to three servings a day of full-fat dairy foods.

Type 2 Diabetes

A large international study, published in the medical journal *BMJ* on May 18, 2020, linked two daily servings of dairy to a lower risk of type 2 diabetes—with the lowest risk for those eating full-fat dairy products.

> ### Dairy Is Not for Everyone
> While dairy isn't an unhealthy food, it can cause problems for some people. Those with lactose intolerance, for example, can experience gastrointestinal issues from eating or drinking certain dairy products, and dairy may exacerbate symptoms of various health conditions among sensitive people. If dairy doesn't agree with you, you can find milk, yogurt, cheese, and more products made from nondairy alternatives, like oats, soy, peas, and coconut.

What to do: If you want to prevent blood sugar problems, or you have prediabetes or type 2 diabetes, enjoy three servings of dairy daily.

Cancer

In an ongoing review, the American Institute for Cancer Research concluded that consumption of dairy products probably protects against colorectal cancer and decreases the risk of pre- and postmenopausal breast cancer. A study in the journal *Nutrients* found that dairy consumption is not associated or is neutral when it comes to cancer-related mortality.

What to do: If you're concerned about cancer, there's no need to be concerned about dairy. If you have a family history of colorectal cancer, eat two to three servings of dairy a day.

Common Beverages Contain Toxic Metals

Tulane University.

After testing 60 beverages, researchers at Tulane University found that mixed-fruit juices and plant-based milks had higher levels of toxic metals than other drinks.

The researchers suggested that heavy metals likely enter the products through contaminated soil or water used during the growing or manufacturing process. Five out of 60 beverages tested had levels that exceeded Environmental Protection Agency recommendations. While the health risks are likely low for adults, parents should be cautious about giving these drinks to infants and young children.

Should You Go Gluten-Free?

Chris Iliades, MD, a retired surgeon and regular contributor to Bottom Line Health.

According to Harvard Medical School's *Harvard Health Letter,* about 20 to 30 percent of Americans are following a gluten-free diet. Gluten is a protein found in grains, including wheat, barley, rye, and oat. People with celiac disease or a wheat allergy need to avoid gluten, but only about one to two percent of people have these conditions, so why are all the other people avoiding gluten?

Most people on a gluten-free diet either claim to have gluten sensitivity or think that a gluten-free diet is healthier for them. Surveys show that most people go gluten-free because they believe that gluten-free foods are a healthier option for digestive health. Gluten sensitivity was first recognized about 30 years ago. Symptoms may include crampy pain, bloating, gas, brain fog, diarrhea, nausea, headache, or fatigue. Because gluten sensitivity does not cause any changes that can be measured with diagnostic testing, doctors have been slow to accept it as a real condition.

Today, to be diagnosed with gluten sensitivity, or non-celiac gluten intolerance, you need to go to a doctor to rule out celiac disease and wheat allergy with a blood test or skin testing. You would then go on a gluten-free diet for several weeks to see if your symptoms go away, and then reintroduce gluten to see if they come back. Not surprisingly, most people who say they are gluten sensitive or gluten-intolerant are self-diagnosed.

A recent commentary in the journal *Digestive Diseases and Sciences* notes that when tested under research conditions, few people with gluten sensitivity symptoms test positive for non-celiac gluten intolerance. Available studies suggest that only about six percent of the 20 to 30 percent of Americans going gluten free need to avoid gluten.

What's Causing the Symptoms?

When people with symptoms of gluten intolerance are given a placebo instead of actual gluten under double-blinded study conditions (neither the subjects nor the researchers know who is getting real gluten or fake gluten), as many people given the placebo as the gluten may have sensitivity symptoms. These people may be experiencing what is called the nocebo effect. Nocebo is a well-documented response in clinical studies. When people expect to get certain symptoms or side effects, they are more likely to get them.

Undoubtedly, there are people without celiac disease or wheat allergy who really do react to foods that contain gluten, but evidence is growing that gluten may not be the main culprit. Most researchers now believe that these symptoms are caused by FODMAP foods, not gluten. These are sugars in foods, including wheat and other grains, that are rapidly fermented in the intestines and create gasses that cause pain, bloating, and diarrhea.

FODMAP is an acronym for fermentable oligosaccharides, disaccharides, monosaccharides, and polyols. For some people, these sugars are hard to digest and are poorly absorbed in the small intestine. People with FODMAP intolerance can have the same symptoms as gluten intolerance. Treatment of FODMAP intolerance requires a very restrictive elimination diet to find out what foods you need to avoid. This diet should be supervised by a dietitian. Along with grains, FODMAP foods may include dairy, beans, specific vegetables, and some fruits. People react differently to different foods.

Is Gluten Bad or Good for You?

According to the Harvard School of Public Health, gluten-free foods are a rapidly growing food industry worth about $12 billion in 2015 and much more today. Media campaigns have spawned gluten-free cookbooks, restaurants, food aisles, and celebrities. The vast majority of people supporting this industry do not have celiac disease or wheat allergy. They may not even have any intolerance symptoms. The gluten-free food industry claims that the gluten-free lifestyle is healthier and, without any evidence, blames gluten for everything from autism and heart disease to acne.

The Harvard School of Public Health notes that many studies consistently show people who include more whole grains in their diet (and more gluten) have less heart disease than people who eat less grains. Harvard also warns that gluten-free foods tend to be highly processed with lots of sugar, salt, calories, and saturated fats. Gluten-free foods are low in fiber, vitamins (especially B vitamins), nutrients, and iron. In fact, people with celiac disease, who need to avoid gluten, have an increased risk of obesity, high blood pressure, and diabetes. Gluten-free foods are also more expensive than most whole foods.

Bottom Line on Gluten-Free

If gluten foods do not cause any symptoms, like cramps, gas, or bloating, you don't need to go gluten-free. There is no advantage to avoiding gluten for you. In fact, it may be unhealthy. If you do have symptoms after eating gluten, you should check in with your doctor. Even if going gluten free makes you feel better, don't diagnose yourself with gluten sensitivity.

Anyone on a gluten-free diet should be on a diet that is also low in fat and high in fiber, and should get regular blood testing to check for anemia, iron deficiency, vitamin B deficiency, high cholesterol, and high blood sugar. If you really are sensitive to gluten, you should work with your doctor and a dietitian to make sure you are getting as much nutrition and fiber from your diet as possible.

Another reason to get checked is that you may have another condition that needs treatment. Your symptoms could be due to celiac disease, wheat allergy, other food allergies, irritable bowel syndrome, inflammatory bowel disease, lactose intolerance, or FODMAP intolerance. A FODMAP elimination diet is more complicated than just avoiding gluten, and many people who have celiac disease do not know they have it. All these conditions require the right diagnosis and treatment. So, don't self-diagnose, and don't be fooled by the benefits of a gluten-free lifestyle.

Most Healthful Deli Meat Options

Danielle Crumble Smith, registered dietitian nutritionist, Eat Well Live Well, LLC, Mableton, Georgia. EatWellLiveWellRD.com

Turkey, chicken, and roast beef are the best choices—preferably sliced at the deli counter, because the meats there usually are freshest and contain the fewest ingredients. Salami, bologna, pepperoni, and pastrami have more sodium and usually are more processed—and some may come from mixed meat sources.

If prepackaged deli meats are your only option: Look for ones with fewer than five ingredients, preferably listed as nitrate-free and free of artificial colors.

Truffles Are Worth a Try

Environmental Nutrition. UniversityHealthNews.com

The fruits of underground fungi, truffles' musky, nuttiness is intense and aromatic enough that they are used only in small amounts. They also are expensive. Truffles contain calcium, potassium, magnesium, and digestible protein. Some research has found that they have antioxidant and anti-inflammatory compounds… and may have anticancer properties and antimicrobial properties that fight *E. coli, staphylococcus* and *salmonella*. Just a tiny piece provides 12 percent of recommended dietary fiber. Available fresh, frozen, as oil, salt, butter, and cheese. You can grate, slice, or dust truffles raw—cooking reduces flavor—into soups, sauces, and entrées.

The Health Benefits of Eating Insects

University of Colorado.

Chitin, a type of fiber, and healthy fats from insects appear to contribute to healthy gut microbiota and are strong sources of protein and nutrients. "These components may provide unique benefits for the gut by encouraging healthy gut microbiota and reducing intestinal inflammation," notes researcher Tiffany Weir, PhD. Edible insects are unusual in the American diet, but they are common in many traditional cuisines.

Easy Egg Substitutes

Reader's Digest. RD.com

To replace one large egg: In baked goods, three tablespoons aquafaba, made from chickpea liquid, plus one tablespoon cornstarch…or one-quarter cup of unsweetened applesauce…or one-quarter cup of mashed ripe bananas. In meatloaf, use one tablespoon ground flax or chia seeds plus three tablespoons water. In baked goods and casseroles, one-quarter cup silken tofu. For fluffy baked goods, one-quarter cup carbonated water. In baked goods and sauces, one tablespoon arrowroot powder plus two tablespoons water.

Should Your Oil Be Cold-Pressed or Refined?

Karin Evans, PhD, RD, CHES, adjunct faculty member at Winthrop University in Rock Hill, South Carolina, certified health education specialist, and a registered dietitian focusing on wellness, women's health, and eating disorders. She can be reached at TopNutritionCoaching.com.

The cost of cooking oils, as well as their individual nutrient profiles, are often related to the processing method used to make them. Oils labeled "cold-pressed" or "expeller-pressed" were extracted without heat or chemicals and are more expensive. Oils labeled "refined" were extracted using heat and solvents and then bleached (to remove the solvents) and deodorized. Refining enables manufacturers to get the most oil possible from the plant source, enabling them to sell it more cheaply, but some nutrients will be lost in the process.

You might decide to spend more money on higher-quality oils that you value for their taste, such as olive oil for your vinaigrette, and less on oils you use in bulk, say canola for occasional deep frying.

But resist becoming obsessed over all the nuances between oils: You're already making a huge stride toward better health by replacing saturated fats with unsaturated ones. Take a big-picture view when it comes to the guiding principles of nutrition, such as following the Mediterranean diet, enjoying the act of cooking, and engaging with friends and family. Everything can fit into your lifestyle, even occasional French fries, as long as you learn to listen when your body says, "I've had enough."

Note: To keep oils fresh, store them in a cool cabinet, away from the heat of your oven or, for very delicate oils, in the fridge.

Don't Throw Out Overripe Avocados

The Penny Hoarder. ThePennyHoarder.com

Avocados are expensive—there is no need to toss them just because they're past their prime. Scrape away the brown spots, and use the remaining green flesh in dressings, sauces, appetizers, egg salad, baked goods, puddings, smoothies…even as a face mask.

Recipes: Check https://tinyurl.com/mrxtmuj8.

Choose Your Chocolate Carefully

Tod Cooperman, MD, president of the independent testing group ConsumerLab.com, White Plains, New York.

Recent testing has revealed that some dark chocolates and cocoa powders contain troubling levels of dangerous heavy metals including…

•**Cadmium.** Dark chocolate is a leading source of dietary cadmium—the tree that produces cocoa beans sucks up cadmium from the surrounding soil. Cadmium—a carcinogen—can cause kidney damage and weakened bones. If consumed only occasionally, the cadmium in most dark chocolate and cocoa powders isn't a major concern, but cadmium levels vary dramatically from product to product.

•**Lead** can be found in dark chocolate and cocoa powder but usually in concentrations too low to cause problems for most adults, though it could be a consideration for children and pregnant women.

•**Don't throw out your chocolate yet.** Multiple studies have identified a link between the antioxidant flavanols found in cocoa beans and improved cardiovascular and cognitive health. In fact, the U.S. Food and Drug Administration announced earlier this year that it will allow high-flavanol cocoa-powder makers to cite these cardio benefits on packaging and in advertising.

Caution: Concentrations of flavanols in dark chocolate and cocoa powders vary dramatically from product to product. To select a dark chocolate or cocoa powder with high flavanol content…

•**Avoid products featuring the terms "alkalized," "Dutched," and/or "Dutch processed" on the packaging.** The process to reduce bitterness also dramatically reduces flavanol content.

•**Choose 72 percent or higher cocoa/cacao content.** Products with cocoa percentages below this level almost inevita-

---

The World's Most Nutritious Vegetable

Watercress is the only vegetable with a score of 100 for nutritional density on the CDC's scale of 0 to 100. This peppery-flavored, nutrient-dense leafy green vegetable has more vitamin C than an orange and is high in vitamin A and potassium. Use young shoots in salads or as toppings…cook more mature leaves in stir-fries or savory broths. Avoid overcooking, which depletes the nutrients. Watercress can be hard to find—it usually is available only in specialty supermarkets such as Whole Foods.

Delish.com

Food, Diet, and Fitness

bly have a low flavanol content...though a high percentage does not guarantee high flavanol content.

The following products provide especially high levels of flavanols but very low levels of heavy metals...

•*Sweetened dark chocolate:* Ghirardelli Intense Dark 72% Cocoa Dark Chocolate.

•*Unsweetened dark chocolate:* Montezuma's Dark Chocolate Absolute Black 100% Cocoa.

•*Cocoa powder:* Target's Good & Gather Unsweetened Cocoa Powder 100% Cocoa.

•*Cocoa powder supplement:* CocoaVia Cardio Health Powder—this contains by far the highest flavanol content among the 40 products tested.

Products best avoided include: Alter Eco Deep Dark Blackout, a dark chocolate found to have high levels of cadmium...and Hershey Cocoa Special Dark, which had high cadmium levels and hardly any flavanols.

The Best Rx: Take a Walk

Joyce Shulman, cofounder and CEO of the virtual walking challenge 99 Walks, Bridgehampton, New York. She is CrossFit Level 1 certified, hosts *The Weekly Walk* podcast, and is author of *Walk Your Way to Better: 99 Walks That Will Change Your Life* and *Why Walk: The Transformative Power of an Intentional Walking Practice.* 99Walks.fit

Hippocrates is known for commanding, "Do no harm." But the ancient Greek physician also wisely proclaimed, "Walking is man's best medicine." Perhaps he recognized that walking can improve our health and decrease risk for heart disease, dementia, depression, cancer, and early death in general. This low-impact exercise promotes nourishing blood flow throughout the body...strengthens the heart...is easy on our joints...can be tailored to any fitness level...and is free.

There is more than one way to walk, says expert Joyce Shulman—and by switching up your pace, adding in special equipment and/or changing your environment, you can address some significant health concerns. Here's how...

•**Regulate blood sugar.** Your grandmother was onto something when she used to tell you to go for a walk after eating. Also called *post-prandial walking,* strolling after meals helps mitigate post-meal blood sugar spikes by moving glucose out of the bloodstream and into muscles. Over time, blood sugar spikes are bad news for heart health, can make it harder to maintain a healthy weight and can foreshadow type 2 diabetes.

Studies from George Washington University Medical Center and other institutions indicate that a 15-minute walk after each meal is ideal, but a *Sports Medicine* meta-analysis of seven studies found that walking for as little as two to five minutes after a meal is enough to help regulate blood sugar levels. These walks don't have to be vigorous—the reviewed studies involved "light-intensity" walking, described as easy and comfortable and/or slower than two miles per hour. But they need to be frequent—these findings apply when a two-to-five-minute walk is done every 20 to 30 minutes over the course of a full day.

Anyone who wants to help reduce their diabetes risk can try post-meal walking... and Michigan State University research has shown that moderately paced 15-minute walks after meals help regulate blood sugar in people with prediabetes.

•**For mild depression.** Adults who are active experience lower rates of depression, in part because they have lower levels of the stress hormone cortisol and increased levels of the feel-good chemicals serotonin, dopamine, and endorphins. Walking is ideal for older adults, in particular, because it gets the heart rate up high enough to kick-start these important mood-boosting chemical changes and can be tailored to all fitness levels.

Walking in the great outdoors bumps things up a notch. Spending time surrounded by the green and blue of nature is linked with increased happiness and decreased stress.

Most of us think of walking in nature as hiking, but that can feel intimidating due to its physical intensity. Here's where soft hiking comes in—walking off-road in areas where you can enjoy the sights and sounds of Mother Nature. You don't need to traverse streams or scramble over boulders—meandering through woods, strolling along a river, or walking on the beach all count.

Even better: In addition to the antidepressant benefits, you'll get a dose of mood-enhancing vitamin D from the sunlight.

Note: If you have moderate-to-severe depression, you'll likely also need therapy and/or medication.

•**For better sleep.** Our bodies and brains are governed by our circadian rhythm, a built-in body clock that keeps nearly every system, from metabolism to mental health to sleep, on a 24-hour cycle. This clock uses the sun's ultraviolet rays to determine when the body should release different hormones. The early morning sun's blue rays are particularly important for regulating your sleep-wake cycle—they enter your eyes and signal your circadian rhythm to halt melatonin production… increase production of cortisol and other energizing hormones…and raise your

---

Best Types of Walking Shoes

For foot pain: Built-in arch support will help if you suffer from flat feet…or your foot rolls too far inward toward the arch, called overpronation…or if you have plantar fasciitis.

Consider: Aetrex Carly Arch Support Sneakers for women, $129.95, or for men, $149.95. Aetrex.com

For toe pain: If you have bunions or arthritis of the big toe, a thick-soled sneaker with a rocker-bottom style will reduce range of motion through the toe joint.

Consider: Hoka Bondi 8 for women, $165, or for men, $165. Hoka.com

For swelling or sensitivity: A stretchy, wide toe box and smooth interior reduces risk for swelling or irritation. Also consider a tieless lacing system and a heel strap, so you can loosen or tighten areas of the shoe.

Consider: Orthofeet Verve Tie-Less sneaker for women, $140, or Orthofeet Sprint Tie-Less sneaker for men, $140. Orthofeet.com

For arthritis in your hands or if you have difficulty bending over: Tieless slip-on sneakers with crushable heels allow you to step into your shoes hands-free.

Consider: Kizik Women's Madrid Eco-Knit sneaker for women, $99, or Kizik Lima Graphite sneaker for men, $109. Kizik.com

For sweaty feet: Breathable sneakers keep feet cool and prevent blisters. Merino wool is breathable, as are mesh uppers.

Consider: Allbirds Women's Wool Runners, $110, or Allbirds Men's Wool Runners, $110. Allbirds.com

To strengthen foot muscles and/or optimize foot health: If you're free from podiatric problems, look for a lightweight sneaker with minimal cushioning and ultra-flexible soles that promote flexing.

Consider: Xero HFS Lightweight Road Running Shoes for women, $119.99, or for men, $119.99. Xeroshoes.com. *Note:* People with flat feet or a history of plantar fasciitis should avoid minimalist shoes.

Emily Splichal, DPM, MS, CES, Center for Functional & Regenerative Podiatric Medicine, Chandler, Arizona. DrEmilySplichal.com

Food, Diet, and Fitness

> **When You Exercise Affects Weight Loss**
>
> People who exercised moderately to vigorously between 7 a.m. and 9 a.m. had an average body mass index (BMI) of 27.5...versus an average BMI of 28.3 among those who exercised at midday or in the evening.
>
> Study of more than 5,200 adults by researchers at Hong Kong Polytechnic University, China, published in *Obesity*.

body temperature in preparation for the day to come.

As we get older, we tend to spend less time outside, depriving our circadian rhythm of the sun. This reduced light exposure is one reason that residents of senior living centers and nursing homes often have disrupted sleep and insomnia.

• **For your bones.** If you have poor posture or want to slow age-related bone loss, try rucking—walking with weight on your back, typically in a backpack. This low-impact exercise is based on military training workouts. *Not only does rucking increase calorie burn, improve endurance, and improve balance, it can...*

• Slow bone loss. Wearing a lightly weighted backpack or vest places an increased load on your skeleton. Bones respond to this load by growing stronger at the cellular level—the weight stimulates bone-building cells called *osteoblasts*.

• Improve posture. If you spend hours a day in front of a computer or driving, your posture may have defaulted to an unhealthy "C" shape instead of a natural "S" curve. Wearing a lightly weighted backpack or vest can correct posture by pulling your shoulders back. It also naturally activates your core, strengthening the muscles in your abdomen and back.

When choosing a vest or backpack: Start with a few pounds, and see how it feels. You can work your way up to 5 percent or 10 percent of your weight, but don't exceed 10 percent.

Example: If you weigh 150 pounds, don't wear anything more than 15 pounds. The vest or backpack should fit your body closely—if it's loose, the weight could throw off your balance.

Warning: Don't simply add a small weight to a backpack you already own—the weight will sink to the bottom of the bag, changing your center of gravity.

Consider: Jetti Pack (JettiFit.com, $88), a backpack that distributes weight evenly, and has padded shoulder straps, a chest strap and ventilation to allow heat from your back to escape. (*Note:* Joyce Shulman is CEO of Jetti Fitness and receives financial compensation from the company.) Or try the Aduro Sport Weighted Vest Workout Equipment (AduroSport.com, $49.99 for a four-pound vest).

Caution: People with hyperkyphosis—an excessive rounding of the upper back caused by osteoporosis—should not wear weighted backpacks. And always check with your doctor before starting a new workout routine or incorporating new equipment into your walks.

Water Workout

Melissa Layne, MEd, assistant professor of kinesiology at University of North Georgia, Dahlonega, and triple-certified by the Aquatic Exercise Association, SCW Fitness Education and the American Council on Exercise. She is author of *Water Exercise, a Comprehensive Guide to Water Workouts*. UNG.edu

Love being in a pool? Then what better way to get your exercise than by working out in a pool! Water exercise is a non-impact way to stay—or get—in shape. It's also excellent for rehab after an injury or a joint replacement because the water cushions and supports you as you build muscle strength. In water that reaches only up to your navel, the impact on your joints is reduced by 50 percent...at mid-chest (the level at which most people feel comfortable, especially if they're not strong swimmers), by 75 per-

Food, Diet, and Fitness

cent...at the collar bone, by 90 percent, and your core muscles will get a great workout because this depth makes keeping your balance more difficult. To remove all the impact, try exercising in the deep end where your feet can't touch the bottom.

Water is a great equalizer. Compared with many other fitness environments (such as classes at a health club), the pool is a much more inclusive place mentally, socially, and physically, and the typical excuses to avoid exercise fall away...

I feel uncomfortable in gym clothes. Being in water eliminates the friction of fabric against skin that many people find irritating.

I feel self-conscious. No one can see you under the water. Wear a robe to the pool, and drop it right before getting in. Instead of a swimsuit, try a bodysuit made for water or even shorts and a T-shirt.

I can't swim. Stay near the side of the pool...and you don't have to put your head in the water.

The basics: To find a pool, look beyond the obvious choices, such as neighborhood pools, YMCAs, aquatic or recreation centers, and health clubs. There may be a local hotel with a pool willing to give you a monthly nonguest rate.

Add-ons: In the shallow end, you can use a $1 pool noodle to increase resistance, especially for arm and shoulder exercises. Wearing webbed gloves also will give you more of an upper-body workout.

If you want to work out in the deep end or have more stability in the water, consider bringing a flotation device such as a belt (if you carry extra weight in the front, put the buckle in the front and vice versa).

On your own or with a group: Most people can follow exercise descriptions and work out on their own. But if you have any physical limitations or want the social experience of taking a class, look for a group instructor who is water-certified by the Aquatic Exercise Association or SCW Fitness Education. "Land-based" teachers don't have the training to understand the differences between buoyancy in the water and gravity on land.

Getting Started

Warm-up and cooldown. Begin your water workout by walking back and forth across the pool from one side to the other for five to 10 minutes. At the end of each exercise session, return to water walking at a slow, relaxing pace, followed by stretches that target your quads, calves, and arms.

If you're new to exercise, start with just two or three repetitions of each of the following exercises for a total of 10 minutes every other day. As you progress, increase the reps to 12 and work out daily if you like.

Note: Many exercises begin with a bounce, also called rebounding—step down onto one or both feet as directed, slightly bend at the knee, and push off the bottom, letting buoyancy comfortably lift the body.

Exercises

• **Basic Jumping Jack.**

Focus: Inner and outer thighs, and elevating heart rate. Face the pool wall, feet together and flat on the pool bottom, hands gently holding the edge. With a small bounce or rebound, jump with both feet at the same time, and land with your feet hip-width apart. With another small bounce, 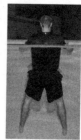 jump with both feet and land with your feet back together in the beginning position. Be sure that your heels reach all the way to the pool bottom on every landing.

To increase the difficulty: Move to the center of the pool, and let your arms rise at your sides, stopping just short of the water level. Keep your arms in the water at all times to avoid stress on the shoulder joints.

131

Food, Diet, and Fitness

- **Criss-Cross Jumping Jacks.**

Focus: Muscles surrounding the shoulder joints. Stand in the middle of the pool, feet together. With your legs remaining straight, give a bounce off the pool bottom and land with your feet shoulder-width apart, arms extended straight out from the sides at a 45-degree angle with shoulders relaxed (keep arms just below the water's surface). 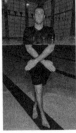 As you jump to bring your feet back together, let one foot cross behind the other as your arms come down in front of your body and cross at the wrists or forearms. Push off again, and return to the shoulder-width stance with arms extended out to the sides. Jump again, and bring your feet back together, but this time, cross the other foot behind and cross your arms in front with the other arm on top.

- **Cross-Country Skiing.**

Focus: Shoulder, leg, and core muscles, and elevating heart rate. Stand sideways by the pool wall, and place your right foot in front of the left with your feet hip-width apart. Extend your arms with your right hand in front, touching the pool wall if needed for balance, and the left hand behind you (opposite to the position of your feet). 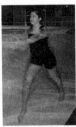 Make a small bounce to push off the pool bottom with both feet, and reverse your leg and arm positions while off the bottom. Land on the toes of both feet at the same time, and roll down onto your heels. Repeat, reversing your leg and arm positions again, to return to start.

To increase the difficulty: Let go of the wall while moving your arms and legs in opposition, keeping your core stable and upright.

- **Water Running.**

Focus: Balance and the cardiovascular system. Run back and forth from one side of pool to the other. Your feet stay close to the bottom of the pool as the leg in back passes by the leg that was in the front. 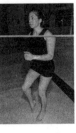 The faster the pace, the less time you'll have to lift your knees (whenever you increase the pace of an exercise, the moves decrease in size).

For more of a challenge: Try serpentine running—stand in chest-deep water, and run across the pool in a zigzag pattern as though weaving through an obstacle course of cones. Turn around and repeat.

- **Rocking Horse.**

Focus: Entire body. Stand in the middle of the pool. Rebound forward onto your right foot, landing with a soft knee as you simultaneously bring your arms in front of you (as though hugging a tree), and lift your left back heel toward your glutes. With a small rebound, transfer your weight to your back foot as you open your arms to stretch 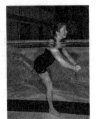 your chest and your front right knee lifts to hip level (if possible). Rebound forward to your front leg, and repeat. Make sure your heels roll completely to the pool bottom on every rocking horse repetition.

If the arm movements are too difficult: Bend your elbows as you rock forward, and do a biceps curl. As you rock backward, straighten your elbow joints.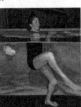

- **Twisting Mogul.**

Focus: Leg and core muscles. Stand in the middle of the pool with your feet together. As you bend your knees to push off with your feet, rotate your body to the right side, and land with both feet together at a 45-degree angle. Always land on the balls of your feet, and roll all the way down 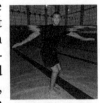 onto your heels. Next, push off both feet and rotate your body to the left side, and land with both feet together at a 45-degree angle.

To increase the difficulty: Pull your knees up into a tucked position after each push-off, then straighten them as you land facing the opposite side.

• **Deep Water Seated Core.**

Focus: Core, hips and triceps muscles. Hold a noodle curved around your waist, and assume a seated position with your legs extended straight out in front of you. Engage the muscles in your core and hips to maintain a right angle at your hip joints. Straighten your arms to push the noodle down into the water. Hold briefly, then relax the arms to return to start.

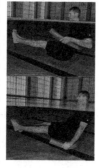

If keeping your legs straight causes any lower back discomfort: Bend at the knee joints so that your body position resembles sitting in a straight-backed chair.

Simple Exercises for Strength and Energy... In Just 6 Minutes

Jonathan Su, DPT, CSCS, C-IAYT, physical therapist, yoga therapist, and former U.S. Army officer based in the San Francisco Bay area. He is author of *6-Minute Fitness at 60+* and *6-Minute Core Strength*. SixMinuteFitness.com

You can squeeze a surprising amount of productivity into just six minutes. You can make and enjoy the first few sips of a cup of coffee...complete a guided meditation...unsubscribe from annoying e-newsletters...even declutter your car.

Guess what else you can accomplish in six minutes twice a day? You can counter the effects of age-related muscle loss while also improving heart health and aerobic endurance...easing chronic pain... boosting mood...protecting cognition... regulating blood sugar levels...and reducing your risk of falling. So says former U.S. Army officer Jonathan Su, DPT, CSCS, C-IAYT, now a physical therapist and yoga therapist.

When you exercise strategically, targeting key muscle groups with movements that alternate between high- and low-intensity, you can generate impressive strength and balance results in a fraction of the time. The magic lies in interspersing shorter workouts with quick bouts of higher-intensity exercise. High-intensity interval training (HIIT) involves pushing yourself harder than you're used to for small bursts of time (say, 30 seconds), then catching your breath while you move through a minute or so of lower-intensity exercise before repeating the sequence.

Several shorter (less than 10 minutes) bouts of higher-intensity exercise spread throughout the day are just as effective as a single daily 30-minute session. This is likely due, at least in part, to the fact that you can maintain a higher intensity during each shorter session.

Keep in mind: High intensity doesn't mean high impact. In fact, lower-impact moves spare joints from unnecessary stress. High intensity simply means that you're exerting more effort than usual. To reap the benefits, you need to challenge yourself more than you're used to—to push until you feel tired...then push just a little bit more. Exercise scientists refer to this effect as the overload principle.

The following routine takes six minutes and should be done twice a day. It targets key muscle groups you need to stay active, mobile and independent—namely, the muscles in the hips and legs. A strong, healthy lower body lets you stand and walk safely and confidently, even on uneven or slippery surfaces. If you do fall, strong hips and legs help guard against major injury. Working the quadriceps (thighs) and glutes (buttocks) will enhance your ability to walk longer and navigate stairs, inclines, and uneven surfaces.

Food, Diet, and Fitness

Strong calves also can prevent or reduce swelling in the feet...discourage the formation of blood clots...help propel your body forward while walking...and let you elevate on your tiptoes. HIIT moves that target leg and hip muscles also boost production of testosterone in men and human growth hormone, both of which preserve muscle but decline with age.

HIIT improves cardiovascular endurance and builds muscle, and it is safe for adults with heart or lung disease, diabetes, obesity, and cancer. A Mayo Clinic study found that regular HIIT workouts have the power to slow aging at the cellular level in people over age 65.

Below is Dr. Su's six-minute plan to help you become more fit!

The Big Three Workout

Perform the following routine twice a day, every day for two weeks. After that, you can drop to once a day, five, or six days a week. The routine consists of the Big Three—three simple exercises to do at home that work the hips and legs, performed at a pace that taxes muscles in a good way. These moves are designed for individuals who have no difficulty standing but lack the strength or energy needed to walk for at least six minutes at a vigorous pace or navigate stairs easily.

Space your sessions at least three hours apart. Perform 15 repetitions of each exercise without resting before moving onto the next exercise. Each time you complete all three exercises is one round. Your goal is to complete as many rounds as possible in six minutes—aim for four to five rounds. Performing moves continuously qualifies as HIIT. You can rest for 30 seconds after a round if you feel you need it.

A note on safety: Check with your doctor to see if there's any reason you should avoid this workout. If you have untreated cardiovascular disease or significant balance issues, your health-care provider may want you to go a bit easier.

MOVE #1: Chair Squat.
Muscles worked: Quadriceps and glutes. You'll need two sturdy chairs for this move—one should be backed up against a wall to keep it from moving. Begin by sitting on the front half of this chair, feet flat on the ground (hip-width apart, feet under knees, knees at a 90-degree angle). If the seat is too low for the 90-degree angle, place a pillow on the seat and sit on that. Place another sturdy chair directly in front of you with the back of the chair facing you. Use this chair for support if you need it. With your arms crossed over your chest, lean forward at the waist to bring your nose over your toes as you stand up by pushing your legs into the ground.

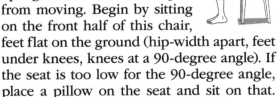

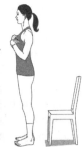

Lower yourself down to the starting position with control, bending at the waist to bring your nose back over your toes and reaching your hips back toward the seat. Repeat this at a moderate pace 15 times.

Why it works: Older adults with weaker legs tend to use their arms to push themselves out of chairs, sofas, or beds. This keeps their legs weak. Crossing your arms ensures that your lower body does the work.

If it's too difficult at first: Place your hands on your knees to help push yourself up to standing position. This is different than pushing off the chair because your legs still do all of the work.

For an extra challenge: Increase the resistance by wearing a sturdy backpack loaded with heavy items like books or soup cans...or consider purchasing a weighted vest.

MOVE #2: Heel Lift.
Muscles worked: Calves. Using the same two chairs as you did for the Chair Squat, stand in front of the chair that's backed up against the wall, with your back facing

the chair. This chair is for safety, to catch you if you stumble. Place your hands on top of the chairback in front of you for balance.

With your feet hip-width apart, toes pointing forward, lift your heels off the floor. Keep your knees straight, and resist the urge to lean forward. (Bending your knees will take the pressure off your calves, but you want to work your calves.) Hold the elevated position for just one-half second before slowly lowering your heels to the floor. Repeat at a moderate pace 15 times. You can rest your hands lightly on the chairback in front of you for support.

If it's too difficult to lift your heels all the way up: Lift them as high as you can. This will improve quickly as your calves strengthen.

For an extra challenge: Wear a heavy backpack or a weighted vest...or let go of the chairback.

MOVE #3: High Knees Marching.

Muscles worked: Quads and hip flexors. Using the same two chairs as you did for the Chair Squat and Heel Lift, begin in the same hip-width stance. (Put a few extra inches between you and the front chair so you have room to lift your knees.) With hands lightly balanced on the chairback, lift your left leg so your thigh is parallel to the ground, left knee bent 90 degrees.

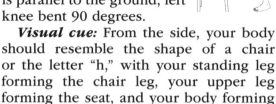

Visual cue: From the side, your body should resemble the shape of a chair or the letter "h," with your standing leg forming the chair leg, your upper leg forming the seat, and your body forming the backrest.

Hold your left leg up for a quick beat before lowering the left foot back down to the ground, then lift the right leg. Continue marching for 15 left-right alterations.

If it's too difficult to lift your leg all the way up: Lift it as high as you can. You'll improve quickly as your hip flexors strengthen.

For an extra challenge: Wear ankle weights or challenge your balancing abilities by hovering your hands over the chairback rather than grasping it.

Why hip flexors matter: Positioned on the fronts of the hips, your hip flexors allow you to lift your knees up toward your chest. Strengthening these makes your legs feel lighter and helps you avoid the stereotypical "senior shuffle" (dragging your feet while walking, which increases fall risk).

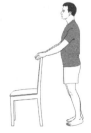

Exercise illustrations: Jonathan Su, DPT, CSCS, C-IAYT

11 Minutes of Activity to Lower Disease Risk

University of Cambridge.

Just 11 daily minutes of moderate physical activity can lower the risk of heart disease, stroke, and cancer. That comes out to 75 minutes per week, enough to reduce the risk of developing cardiovascular disease by 17 percent and cancer by 7 percent. "Moderate activity doesn't have to involve what we normally think of exercise, such as sports or running," said Dr. Leandro Garcia from Queen's University Belfast. "Sometimes, replacing some habits is all that is needed. For example, try to walk or cycle to your work or study place instead of using a car, or engage in active play with your kids or grandkids. Doing activities that you enjoy and that are easy to include in your weekly routine is an excellent way to become more active."

Food, Diet, and Fitness

8,000 Is the New 10,000...Steps, That Is

Piedmont Healthcare, private not-for-profit organization, Atlanta. Piedmont.org

New research suggests 8,000 steps once or twice a week may be just as effective as 10,000 steps. The study, by researchers at Kyoto University in Japan, and University of California, Los Angeles, published in *JAMA Network Open,* found that 8,000 steps leads to a lower risk of dying from heart disease or any cause, for that matter. Adults who walked a minimum of 8,000 steps—about four miles—one or two days a week were 14.9 percent less likely to die within a decade versus adults who walked less. Walking at least 8,000 steps a day for three to seven days a week reduced mortality rates by 16.5 percent. Even 6,000 steps once or twice a week was shown to be advantageous.

Exercises to Improve Your Balance

Grace T. DeSimone, ACSM-CPT, ACSM-GEI, editor of the *American College of Sports Medicine's Resources for the Group Fitness Instructor Manual (LWW 2011)* and associate editor of its *Health & Fitness Journal,* a past IDEA Health & Fitness Association Program Director of the Year, and the current Wellness and Group Fitness Director of the Wyckoff Family YMCA in New Jersey. GraceDeSimone.com

Balance training isn't just for preventing falls later in life—good balance is essential for everyone, and it helps reduce the severity of an injury when you take a spill at any age. Even if you think you have great balance now, you'll benefit from adding balance-enhancing exercises to your day. Don't wait until a problem occurs—these exercises can help you avoid one.

Why balance matters: Balance is an integral part of everyday activities. Technically speaking, it is the ability to control your body when you're upright whether you are moving or standing still. Every time you step from one foot to the other, that's a balancing act!

Balance also helps with proprioception, or body awareness—the ability to know where you are in space at any given time.

Examples of proprioception: Typing without having to look at the keyboard... walking in the dark without losing your balance.

Better balance builds confidence and prepares your body for any sport. Even people who do cardio and strength training should include balance and stability exercises in their routines.

Don't assume that just because you can walk easily, you're doing enough to promote balance. There's always benefit to balance work, but the younger and stronger you are when you start, the better you'll be for it later in life.

Do It Right

For most of us, the American College of Sports Medicine recommends doing balance exercises at least two to three times a week. For older adults at risk of falling, the recommendation is three or more times per week and possibly a structured fall-prevention program. The National Council on Aging offers a list of evidence-based programs at NCOA.org/article/evidence-based-falls-prevention-programs, and many communities offer free or modestly priced programs.

Best: Regardless of your age, incorporate a few minutes of balance exercises into every day. To ensure you are doing these exercises safely...

•***Be sure you have support***—a doorway, counter, wall, or sturdy chair that you can hold with both hands, especially when you first start doing the exercises. As you gain confidence, decrease your level of support—use one hand instead of two or just your fingertips, and eventually no support (but keep your source of support handy just in case).

Suggestion: Do these exercises in the kitchen while you're waiting for your morning coffee to brew or stirring a pot of stew... or combine them with an existing habit such as brushing your teeth.

• **Make sure your posture is correct.** If your head is jutting forward, that's 20 pounds (the weight of your head plus the force it exerts on your neck) throwing you off balance. Your posture should maintain the three natural curves of your spine—at your neck, mid-back and low back. Your head should be above your shoulders, and the tops of your shoulders should be over your hips.

• **Work with a partner** to boost motivation and be accountable to each other. Or you might prefer the camaraderie of a class and working with a qualified professional who can help you fine-tune your technique.

Building Up Your Balance

There are two types of balance—static (standing still) and dynamic (when you are moving, such as walking). It's important to exercise both.

• **Static Exercises.** Each of the following exercises can be repeated three to five times.

Wide Stance: Stand with your feet slightly wider than hip-width apart. Imagine you're on a moving boat or train and have nothing to hold onto. Bend at the knees, and press your feet into the floor to steady yourself. Hold for 30 seconds.

Narrow Stance: Stand with feet together, centered in line with your belly button. Your toes should face forward, not inward or outward. Hold for 30 seconds.

Inline Stance: Looking straight ahead, stand with one foot immediately behind the other foot so that the back foot's toes touch the front heel. Hold for 30 seconds. Reverse stance and repeat.

Stork Stance: Stand on one foot, raising the nonweighted foot mid knee height (or as high as you deem comfortable). Balance for up to 30 seconds. Switch feet and repeat.

Standing March: March in place slowly for 20 to 30 seconds, lifting the moving leg until the thigh is parallel with the floor and bringing it down completely before reversing legs.

Chair Rises: Sit toward the front of a sturdy chair. Shift your weight to the front of your feet, and slowly stand up by contracting your core, leg and butt muscles. The goal is to rise without using your hands. When you're able, increase the difficulty by crossing your arms over your chest.

As you gain confidence, challenge yourself by activating your vestibular system—located in the inner ear—and visual system. These two sensory systems provide your brain with information that helps your body adjust as needed. Add one of these elements at a time (always bring your head and eyes back to center between repetitions)...

• **Look down and up.**

• **Look over at different objects in the room.**

• **Move your head from side to side.**

• **Extend one arm in front of you.** Raise your index finger. Using only your eyes, follow your index finger as you move your arm from side to side.

• **Close your eyes.** Once that feels comfortable, move your head from left to right, then right to left.

Another option: Do these exercises on a balance pad (a rectangular piece of specialty foam) or a BOSU balance trainer, a rubber dome set on a rigid platform. Both are designed to create an unstable surface for greater balance training.

• **Sideways Walking.** Step to the left side with your left foot, then bring your right foot to meet it. Continue across the room. Reverse directions, stepping to the right with your right foot.

• **Heel-to-Toe Inline Walking.** Start in the Inline Stance (mentioned in previous column), and walk forward by placing one foot directly in front of the other, as though you were on a tightrope. Keep your head up, eyes open and looking forward. Walk this way for the length of the room (or counter if you need support), turn around and return to your starting point.

• **Backward Walking.** Once you're comfortable with Heel-to-Toe Inline Walking, try going backward to return to your starting point. You'll be challenged to develop greater focus and coordination because you can't see behind you. With each step you take backward, place your toes on the ground before your heel (the opposite of forward walking). Keep an even and smooth stride.

Caution: Dehydration, fatigue, certain medications, and chronic conditions all can impact your balance. If you have any of these concerns, check with your doctor.

Get the Most from a Standing Desk

Linda Miller, occupational therapy doctor (OTD), certified professional ergonomist (CPE), CEO and senior ergonomist at the occupational ergonomics company EWIWorks, Edmonton, Alberta, Canada, EWIWorks.com.

Alan Hedge, PhD, CPE, professor emeritus of ergonomics, Cornell University, Ithaca, New York. Human.Cornell.edu.

Position your computer screen an arm's length away and two inches below eye level. The desk should be elbow height so your arms are at a 90-degree angle. Stand with your feet shoulder-width apart, preferably on a mat. If using a laptop, get a separate keyboard and external mouse, and position the mouse so you don't have to reach forward…also elevate the laptop so you don't have to bend your neck.

Best: Alternate between sitting, standing, and moving around.

Offset Sitting with Just a Little Exercise

Study titled "Device-Measured Physical Activity, Sedentary Time, and Risk of All-Cause Mortality: An Individual Participant Data Analysis of Four Prospective Cohort Studies," led by researchers at Arctic University of Norway, Tromsø, published in the *British Journal of Sports Medicine.*

Most of us sit in front of computers for extended stretches of time to work and play. That's dangerous. Over the past several years, many studies have found that sitting for long periods, called sedentary time, is associated with harmful conditions such as obesity, high cholesterol, and high blood sugar. One recent review of several of these studies found that sitting for more than eight hours a day without physical activity is as bad for you as being obese or smoking. And since the average adult in developed countries spends nine to 10 hours in an office chair, many have tried to solve the sitting problem with standing desks or treadmill walking while on the phone. Or the sitters set timers to indicate when to stand and move about.

But all that can be a hassle.

Good News for Long-Term Sitters

A new study from a collaboration of researchers in Norway, Sweden, and the United States finds that you can safely sit down if you average more than 22 minutes of moderate-to-vigorous physical activity (MVPA) per day. That amount of MVPA was found to eliminate the health risk of sedentary time. That amount of MVPA corresponds to the lower level of MVPA recommended by the World Health Organization, 150 to 300 minutes of moderate-intensity exercise per week.

The new study, which is published in the *British Journal of Sports Medicine,* analyzed data from four previous studies involving close to 12,000 adults age 50 and over. All study participants had a minimum of four days that included 10 daily hours monitored for activity for at least two years. To measure sedentary and MVPA times, the studies reviewed used a type of fitness tracker worn on the belt called a hip accelerometer. This device measures the force of forward movement (acceleration).

The researchers wanted to find out how both sedentary time and MVPA were associated with mortality. Acceleration data can be used to measure MVPA, but for people without the data, moderate exercise can be defined as exercise that increases breathing rate without causing shortness of breath, works up a mild sweat in about 10 minutes, and does not affect talking. Vigorous exercise makes you a bit short of breath, works up a quicker sweat, and makes it hard to talk normally.

22 Minutes Makes a Big Difference

During the study period, 805 people died (about 7 percent). After adjusting for other mortality risk factors such as sex, obesity, smoking, cardiovascular disease, cancer, and diabetes, these were the key findings of the study...

• **Getting less than 22 minutes of MVPA per day,** along with more than 12 hours of sedentary time, was associated with a 38 percent higher risk of death compared to eight hours of sedentary time.

• **Getting more than 22 minutes of MVPA** was associated with a lower risk of death no matter the sedentary time.

• **Ten more minutes of MPVA per day** was associated with a 15 percent decreased risk of death in people with less than 10.5 hours of sedentary time and a 35 percent lower risk in people with more than 10.5 hours of sedentary time.

• **Long sedentary time may be a risk factor for death** because it allows large muscles and heart muscles to become weak, called deconditioning. When we're deconditioned, it becomes harder to exercise and stay fit. Deconditioning has also been associated with poor mental health, injuries, and poor sleep.

But you can reduce your risk. The research team concludes that even small amounts of MVPA may be an effective strategy for reducing the health risks of sedentary time.

Women Need Less Exercise Than Men

Study titled "Sex Differences in Association of Physical Activity With All-Cause and Cardiovascular Mortality," by researchers at Cedars-Sinai Medical Center, Los Angeles, published in the *Journal of the American College of Cardiology*.

For once, women do not have to work harder to get the same good results procured by men. A new study from Cedars-Sinai Medical Center in Los Angeles has uncovered the good news: Women may be able to get the same benefits from exercise as men with about half the time and effort. Since women can get more for less, the researchers hope this will encourage inactive women to start exercising.

For example, for men to reach their maximum survival benefits from moderate to vigorous physical activity they must exercise for five hours per week. Women reached the same survival benefit at just two-and-a-half hours per week.

Large Survey Confirms Benefits from Exercise

The research team from the Cedars-Sinai Department of Preventive Cardiology analyzed data from over 400,000 U.S. adults who responded to the National Health Interview Survey between 1997 and 2019, of which 55 percent were women. This survey was conducted by the Centers for Disease Control and Prevention (CDC) and the National Center for Health Statistics in all 50 states.

Survey data included all types of leisure-time physical activities including frequency, duration, and intensity of the activity. The age of the adults averaged about 44 and ranged between 27 and 61 at the start of the study. Adults included in the study did not have a history of cardiovascular disease or other long-term conditions that would limit physical activity. The study is published in the *Journal of the American College of Cardiology*. These were some of the key findings...

During the study period, there were about 40,000 deaths, of which about 12,000 were heart related.

For all the adults (men and women), those who reported regular physical activities had a lower risk of death from any cause and a lower risk of death from cardiovascular disease than adults who reported being physically inactive.

Men reached their maximal survival benefit, which was a 15 percent reduced risk of death, from 300 minutes of moderate-to-vigorous physical activity per week.

Woman reached the same benefit as men at 140 minutes per week but had a 24 percent reduced risk of death if they reached 300 minutes per week.

For muscle strengthening activities, men reached their peak benefit at about three sessions per week. Women required just one weekly session to get similar benefits.

Adults Need to Get Exercising

Less than 25 percent of adults meet the minimum physical activity guidelines for physical activity from the CDC and American Heart association, which is 150 minutes per week of moderate physical activity or 75 minutes per week of vigorous activity, along with at least two days of muscle strengthening activity.

Moderate aerobic activities include brisk walking. Vigorous physical activity includes jogging or tennis. Muscle strengthening activities are the use of weights or resistance training to increase muscle strength of the legs, hips, back, abdomen, chest, shoulders, and arms.

Why Women Fare Better with Exercise

Although there are several explanations for the exercise gap, part of the difference is that men have larger hearts, bigger lung capacity, and larger muscle fibers, so it takes more exercise to supply the energy needed to stimulate growth and stamina. Women have less muscle mass, and they also have better blood flow during exercise than men.

It's well documented that women usually exercise less often than men do and engage in less physical activity. The conclusions of this study are that women get greater benefits for survival and reduction of cardiovascular risk than men for the same amount of activity. The researchers hope that these finding will encourage more women to take advantage of these benefits and close the gender gap in leisure-time physical activity.

Difficulty Walking Predicts Higher Fracture Risk

Garvan Institute of Medical Research.

Trouble walking even short distances is associated with a higher fracture risk over five years. Researchers discovered that women who said they were limited "a lot" had a 60 percent higher fracture risk than women with no limitation. For men, the increased risk was more than 100 percent. This suggests a direct relationship between low walking ability and weaker bones.

Running Doesn't Harm Your Knees— It Protects Them

Study of 2,637 adults, average age 64, led by researchers at Baylor College of Medicine, Houston, published in *Arthritis Care Research*.

Common medical wisdom holds that running can lead to knee problems later in life.

Recent finding: Current and former runners had had less knee pain and fewer symptoms and less radiographic evidence of osteoarthritis than non-runners.

Possible reason: Runners may have lower body weights on average, which puts less stress on knee joints over time.

GET THE BEST MEDICAL CARE

Depersonalized Health Care

The delivery of medicine has changed dramatically over the past 50 years. While you still go to a doctor for most of your medical needs, chances are your doctor does not own his own practice. In fact, unlike 50 years ago, the majority of American physicians are employees of either hospital-owned medical practices or large group practices owned by for-profit companies.

Changing Relationships

This change in ownership has had a major impact on the doctor/patient relationship. Unlike in the past, physicians and other health-care professionals are obligated to look out for the best interests of their employer and are forced to do so by their employment contracts. This easily leads to depersonalization between doctors and patients.

Studies have found that depersonalization leads to a higher likelihood of medical errors being made. The doctor simply confuses you with another patient, possibly ordering the wrong medication or being unaware of an underlying condition you may have. I recently spoke with an oncologist who sold his practice to a hospital and is required, by his contract, to see at least three patients an hour. He said he hardly gets to know his patients.

Fragmented Services

My wife recently went to a large group practice for cataract surgery. There were eight doctors associated with the practice, each one having a different ophthalmic specialty (such as cataracts, dry eye, retina, post-surgical education). When my wife had a postoperative question about a pain in one eye, her cataract surgeon had her see the practice's retina specialist. In other words, another visit, another bill, and another opinion. And by the way, the waiting room on every visit had at least 20 other patients waiting and a half-dozen clerks checking people in and out. This is the new reality of medical care delivery. The old personal touch of the doctor/patient relationship is a relic of the past. Even your primary care doctor may sim-

---

Charles B. Inlander, a consumer advocate and health-care consultant based in Fogelsville, Pennsylvania. He was the founding president of the People's Medical Society.

ply be a gatekeeper to other parts of the health system and, if she is a member of a large practice with several different office locations, she may be shuffled from office to office, forcing you to follow her around or else see another doctor in the practice.

What to Do About It

Here are some steps you can take to make sure your relationship with your doctors is as personal as possible.

•**Come prepared.** No matter how well you think your doctor may know you, come armed with your basic medical information to each visit. Not only should you bring your list of medications, but also bring a list of conditions you may have or had, surgeries you have had, and what other primary care or specialists you have seen. Bring a list of questions you may have, and make sure the doctor answers each one.

•**Don't get passed off** to a physician's assistant or nurse practitioner until the doctor has explained everything in detail. The more you interact, the more personal your relationship will be.

•**Get second opinions.** Depersonalized medicine underscores the need to seek out second opinions when a major diagnosis or treatment plan is raised. Second opinions mean another set of eyes are looking at your needs.

•**Monitor your medical records.** You have the right to copies of your medical records, both physician and hospital. Check them out regularly to make sure all your test results, visit summaries and prescribed treatments are listed. If you see a gap or a mistake, call your practitioner to have it corrected. Remember, your medical record is the way most doctors know you. Its accuracy is vital.

Shop Around for Care

If you feel like you are being shortchanged, seek out another practice. You can set up what is called an interview appointment in which you simply talk to a prospective doctor about becoming a patient in that practice. You may have to pay out of pocket for this visit, but it is worth it.

—Charles Inlander

Medical Gaslighting: Don't Let Your Doctor Dismiss Your Symptoms

Karen Lufey Spencer, PhD, professor of health and behavioral sciences who studies medical decision-making at University of Colorado, Denver. CLAS.UC Denver.edu

Shortly after tennis champion Serena Williams gave birth, she started having trouble breathing. She worried it might be a pulmonary embolism, a blood clot in her lungs—a problem she had suffered in the past. She asked for a CT scan and a blood thinner. A nurse told Williams that the pain medication she was taking was making her "talk crazy." But a subsequent CT scan did reveal a clot in her lungs.

If you've ever had a health-care provider dismiss your symptoms...say you were "just stressed"...or blame your concerns on psychological factors...you're not alone. Patients around the country are complaining about a phenomenon known as *medical gaslighting,* a term derived from the 1944 Ingrid Bergman film *Gaslight,* in which a husband manipulates his wife into questioning her perceptions of reality and her sanity.

Most doctors aren't intentionally trying to gaslight their patients, nor do they even realize they're doing it, says behavioral health-care expert Karen Lutfey Spencer, PhD. But there can be grave consequences when real symptoms are brushed aside—it may delay a correct diagnosis, force you to endure unnecessary or ineffective treatments, and cause you to second-guess your symptoms and conditions in the future.

We asked Dr. Spencer to explain why medical gaslighting is so prevalent now, as well as suggest strategies for spotting it and preventing it from compromising your medical care...

Why It Happens

Health-care practices today are heavily influenced by what insurance companies are willing to cover and pay for. That has forced doctors to make medical care as efficient as possible, and it shows. A study of 21 million patient visits to primary-care medical practices around the country found that the average visit lasted just 18 minutes...and 22 percent of primary-care physicians spend only nine to 12 minutes with patients. When doctors are rushed or distracted, they tend to fall back on preconceived notions about patients, which can lead to oversights and diagnosis errors. *Examples...*

•**Age bias.** An elderly man consults his doctor because he is having a hard time coordinating his hands when he plays golf. The doctor assumes the cause is arthritis and recommends a nonsteroidal anti-inflammatory medication without exploring whether it's a more serious neurological condition.

•**Gender bias.** Women's ailments often are not taken as seriously as men's.

Recent findings: Women waited in hospital ERs an average of 12 minutes longer to be evaluated and treated than men. Heart problems often are misdiagnosed in women because they may not experience the typical symptoms such as chest pressure or pain that men do. Researchers have attributed these disparities to bias among health-care workers.

Are You Being Gaslighted?

Gaslighting can be hard to spot. Just because a doctor offers a different interpretation of your symptoms or declines to recommend a test that you requested doesn't mean that he/she is disregarding your concerns. But there are telltale signs that should put you on alert. *Take notice if your health-care provider...*

•**Immediately blames your symptoms on general lifestyle causes,** such as your weight, stress or work overload, rather than asking further questions or exploring other medical possibilities.

•**Is condescending and unhelpful if you challenge the diagnosis.**

•**Uses phrases that minimize your concern,** such as, "It's all in your head"..."You've got to expect this as you get older"..."Your pain is manageable."

•**Interrupts you repeatedly.** One study found that clinicians interrupted patients just 11 seconds, on average, into their conversation. This makes it difficult to present a full picture of your concerns.

How to Advocate for Yourself

Many patients are intimidated by physicians. After all, they're the experts, right? And you don't want to appear dramatic or foolish or paranoid in front of your health-care providers.

But remember—you are the foremost expert on your body, and that means your input is not only valuable but essential. You need to collaborate with your health-care provider and make shared decisions on a realistic and sustainable treatment plan. *Steps to take...*

Before your doctor visit...

•**Keep a symptom diary.** Record details about your condition including dates and times when symptoms occur...when you first noticed symptoms...what triggers them...whether they come and go or are constant...what makes them better or worse. It's particularly important to track your pain. And because pain is subjective, it is easy for doctors to downplay it. Record the intensity of your pain on a scale of 1 to 10...how long it lasts...its quality (a sharp stabbing sensation, a dull ache)...and how it specifically is affecting your life ("My lower back aches when I drive for more than 30 minutes").

Helpful resource: Use Symple (Symple App.com), a symptom-tracker and health-diary app.

Cost: Free to monitor up to five symptoms…additional features for $9.99 per month.

•**Schedule your appointment for first thing in the morning.** Studies show that patients get better care early in the day, rather than later, when physicians may suffer mental fatigue that could compromise their decision making.

During your visit…

•**Tell the doctor's assistant you would prefer to explain your problems to the doctor while you are still dressed.** Only change into that skimpy hospital gown for the physical checkup. Reducing the obvious power differential means your initial complaints and input may be taken more seriously.

•**Set the agenda.** Tell the doctor your main priority for the visit so he spends the majority of time on that problem, not lesser concerns you have. Many patients are reluctant to self-diagnose or worry that their Internet research about their symptoms won't be seen as legitimate, so they let the doctor decide what to focus on.

•**Ask permission to record your appointment.** Not only does a recording make the doctor more accountable, it's easier for you to remember what he says.

•**Bring along a friend or family member,** especially someone who has been with you when you've had your symptoms. In addition to taking notes and providing emotional support, that person can validate and reiterate your concerns if the doctor is dismissive.

•**Pin down the next steps before you leave.** Ideally, you should leave your appointment with a best guess as to what is causing your symptoms…a plan for diagnosing or ruling out different possibilities…and potential treatment options depending on what is found.

After your visit…

•**Find an ally/liaison in the doctor's office.** This might be a physician's assistant or a nurse administrator. They often are easier to reach and less intimidating.

•**If your visit didn't have the outcome you hoped for,** strategize with this liaison about what to do. If you decide to get a second opinion or see a specialist, your liaison can help you get an in-network referral.

•**If you are in the hospital, contact the patient-advocacy office.** Patients who are critically ill are particularly susceptible to medical gaslighting. Studies show that patients who have someone advocating for them at their hospital bedside have much better outcomes. If your hospital doesn't have an in-house patient advocate, find one near you at the website of the National Association of Healthcare Advocacy (NAHAC.com/directory-of-advocates).

When to Go to the Emergency Room

Jay Itzkowitz, MD, chair of emergency services at Mount Sinai Hospital South Nassau in Oceanside, New York. Dr. Itzkowitz is a 2023 Castle Connolly top doctor for emergency medicine.

When you have an unexpected illness or injury, you have a variety of options: your doctor's office, a walk-in medical clinic, an urgent care center, an emergency room (ER) or calling 911. The choice you make could be the difference between a long and short wait, a big or small bill, and in some cases, life or death.

What Are Emergency Services?

The ER is a lot more than just a room. It is the center for a hospital service called emergency medicine, which is a medical department and specialty, just like the departments of surgery or internal medicine. If someone is having any type of life-threatening emergency or any condition that can cause significant disability, the emergency department is the place to go. *The American Board of Emergency Medicine describes the following conditions as emergencies...*

• **Chest pain, trouble breathing, or stroke symptoms** like sudden confusion, weakness, loss of speech, extreme headache, or loss of vision

• **Choking or passing out that requires CPR** because the person does not have a pulse or is unable to breathe

• **A severe injury,** such as a fall or motor vehicle accident

• **Injury or illness that causes you to be too weak or unsteady to drive.**

Other reasons to use the ER may include a head injury with loss of consciousness or confusion, a severe burn, a seizure, possible poisoning or overdose, vomiting or diarrhea that won't stop, heavy bleeding from any cause, high fever with stiff neck, any serious injury that causes loss of movement, or very severe pain.

Doctors who specialize in emergency medicine are trained to make immediate decisions and take actions needed to prevent death or disability. They head a team of nurses, medical technicians, and other health-care providers who are available 24 hours a day. Emergency medicine doctors are certified by the American Board of Emergency Medicine. Before certification, a doctor must have at least three years of training in emergency medicine.

If you are not sure if your condition is an emergency, your insurance company may have a nurse hotline that can help you decide if you need to go to an emergency department or to an urgent care center. You can also call your primary care provider. If your provider is not available, there should be an on-call doctor to help you decide.

Even though the ER is supposed to be for emergencies, many people use it for less serious medical problems or injuries.

If you are not in a life-threatening situation, you may have to wait. Generally, concerns like colds, earaches, rashes that aren't affecting your breathing, and other discomforts that are not life-threatening are better treated in an urgent care facility, retail health clinic, or doctor's office.

What to Expect at the ER

When you arrive at the ER, you may see a waiting room full of patients. Unlike at a doctor's office, ERs are not first-come, first-served. Instead, people are triaged: A trained health-care provider, usually a nurse, will assess you and decide how quickly you need to be seen and, importantly, how urgent your needs are compared with other people who are waiting.

If there are more serious emergencies in front of you, you may need to wait, and that can mean a long wait at a busy ER—even if you arrive by ambulance. *Becker's Hospital Review* reports that the average wait time is as little as 104 minutes in North Dakota and as long as 228 minutes in Maryland. Even if the waiting room looks empty, the treatment area may be filled with patients.

It's a good idea to bring something to read and your phone (and a charger), so you can keep in contact with your family. Having someone to stay with you and help you through the process is helpful for support and for another set of ears. Having your primary physician call the emergency department to give them a heads-up for what is coming in can be a good idea, as the physician can give the ER providers additional information that you might not be aware of, but it won't affect your wait time.

If you have a chronic illness, keep an updated file containing any physician reports, test results, allergies, and medications, and take it to the ER. It could save valuable time.

While the wait can be frustrating, know that health-care providers are seeing people as quickly as they can. Yelling at the front-desk staff won't get you seen any faster. On the other hand, if you're condition worsens while you're waiting (for example, you begin to have difficulty breathing) let the triage nurse know so they can ensure that you're in the right place in line.

After you leave the waiting room, you'll go to a bed to wait for a doctor. What happens next depends on your condition and diagnosis.

It could include immediate treatment or diagnostic tests. The visit may result in treatment and discharge with instructions for home and follow-up care, admission to the hospital for treatment, or transfer to another facility that may be better suited to treat your condition. After you're stabilized, you may still have to wait a while to be discharged.

When Can You Use Urgent Care?

If your problem is not life-threatening or a risk for disability, you can save time and money by going to an urgent care center or even a retail health clinic. Even if you have insurance, your copays for urgent care are likely to be less than for an ER visit or ambulance trip.

Some examples of urgent care problems include common infections, colds, flu, earache, sore throat, nosebleed, nausea, vomiting, diarrhea, stomachache, fevers, rash, sprains, pains, minor burns, cuts, and bruises. In most cases these illnesses and injuries are problems you are familiar with, but you can't wait for a doctor's appointment.

Not all urgent cares have the same types of providers. Some may have physician assistants or nurse practitioners. Some urgent care centers have physicians working, but not all the physicians are emergency medicine trained. In any case, most of these centers can manage most nonemergency problems, or get you to the next level of care.

Making the right decision about emergency or urgent care is important. If in doubt about urgent care, call your doctor or health-insurance advice hotline. If you or a loved one are having signs of a heart attack, stroke, or difficulty breathing, go immediately to the ER. If in doubt about a possibly life-threatening situation, call 911. *To prepare for these situations make sure you have contact information easily available that includes...*

- **Your health-care provider.**
- **Your closest ER contact and location**
- **Your insurance advice hotline and other hotlines like poison control.**
- **Your closest urgent care or walk-in clinic contact and location.**

Don't Drive Yourself to the ER

Driving or having someone drive you to the ER with any life-threatening condition is almost always a bad idea. You may lose valuable time, and driving may make you a danger to yourself and others. Surviving or avoiding disability from a stroke or a heart attack can depend on minutes saved. An ambulance gets you to the ER faster and safer, and treatment can start as soon as emergency responders arrive. If you have any life-threatening illness or any condition that could possibly lead to harm or disability, call 911.

Beware These Risks When You're in the Hospital

Peter Pronovost, MD, PhD, chief quality and transformation officer at University Hospitals Cleveland Medical Center and professor at Case Western University's School of Medicine. He is a member of the President's Council for Science and Technology Patient Safety Working Group and is coauthor of *Safe Patients, Smart Hospitals.* UHHospitals.org

Patients go to the hospital to get their health problems treated, but it's distressingly common for hospital stays to cause health problems instead. A 2022 report by the Department of Health and Human Services Office of Inspector General estimated that 25 percent of hospital patients experience "care-associated harm" during their stays. While that research relied on data from 2018, there's little reason to believe things have improved since then. If anything, the widespread resignations and retirements of experienced health-care workers during the pandemic probably made things worse.

We asked leading patient-safety expert Peter Pronovost, MD, PhD, what patients and their families can do to prevent the health risks caused by hospital stays...

•**Medication errors.** A large-scale study by researchers at Texas Tech University and UCLA found that more than 5 percent of hospital patients experience medication errors. Some of these errors are as straightforward as a nurse handing a patient the wrong pill, but medication mistakes also involve the interactions between drugs prescribed to a patient in the hospital and drugs the patient already is taking. Hospitals attempt to avoid this by compiling a list of all the drugs a patient is taking, a process called *medication reconciliation,* but oversights are common. *What to do...*

• Create and continually update a list of all the medications you're taking, both prescription and over-the-counter, and bring this list with you when you go to a hospital.

• If you have not recently updated such a list when a trip to the hospital becomes necessary, bring all of your medication bottles or instruct a loved one to do so. Use your list or bottles to confirm that the hospital has a complete record of all the drugs you're taking.

• When you're given a drug in the hospital, say something along the lines of, "I know you're working hard to provide me the best care, but could you help me understand what this drug does and how it interacts with the drugs I'm already taking?" Voicing confidence in the doctor or nurse's good intent before asking a question can deflate defensiveness.

•**Surgical errors.** Every week, surgeons in the U.S. accidentally leave sponges or other foreign objects inside patients nearly

> **Take Care at Urgent Care Centers**
>
> Urgent-care centers often are staffed by inexperienced non-physician practitioners. The corporations that own them pressure staff to see enormous volumes of patients, so exams may be cursory and serious conditions overlooked. At emergency departments, you are more likely to see a board-certified emergency physician, and non-physician practitioners may be more seasoned.
>
> *Also:* "Freestanding emergency departments" can look like urgent-care centers but charge emergency-room prices.
>
> Mitchell Li, MD, founder of Take Medicine Back PBLLC, a public benefit company opposed to corporate practice of medicine. TakeMedicineBack.org

40 times...they perform the wrong procedure around 20 times...and they operate on the wrong side of the body 20 times, according to Johns Hopkins researchers. These figures include only errors that result in malpractice claims, so the actual number of surgical errors is likely significantly higher. A separate study by University of Michigan researchers found that the overall postoperative complication rate—a useful though imperfect proxy for surgical errors—was 14.5 percent. *What to do...*

• Before settling on a doctor for a surgery, ask him/her, "How often do you do this procedure?" Numerous studies have found a very strong link between quantity and quality when it comes to surgery—doctors who do a particular procedure often are much less likely to make mistakes with that procedure.

If the doctor's answer is only a handful of times per year or less, strongly consider choosing a different doctor unless it's an extremely rare procedure that few doctors perform often. Also ask, "Does the hospital where you will perform this procedure on me handle this procedure often? Is this where you usually do this procedure?" The experience of the team that will be working with the surgeon during the operation and caring for you after the operation matters, too.

None of this should come as a surprise—practice might not make perfect, but we all know it makes better. Yet many patients never ask doctors about their experience with the procedure and end up trusting their lives to novices. A recent study by a Stanford University professor found that hundreds of patients in California receive cancer surgery at hospitals that perform only one or two of their type of procedure all year—even though a hospital that performs the operation much more frequently is located within 50 miles in more than two-thirds of these cases.

•**Infections, blood clots, and other medical complications.** A 2014 study by the Centers for Disease Control and Prevention (CDC) suggested that around 4 percent of hospitalized patients experience a hospital-acquired infection. This risk is substantially higher for intensive-care patients—a large-scale German study estimated that nearly 20 percent of ICU patients acquire one or more infections while in the hospital.

Thrombosis, also known as blood clots, are another common hospital complication—they're among the leading causes of hospital deaths. The National Blood Clot Alliance estimates that up to 40 percent of surgery patients—including up to 60 percent of patients who have major orthopedic surgery—will experience blood clots if proper preventive steps are not taken. *What to do...*

•If a hospital staff member is about to put a catheter into any part of your body, ask, "Do I really need that?" If the answer is yes, ask, "Do you follow a checklist procedure to reduce catheter infections?" Catheters are a very common source of hospital infections, but research has shown that this risk is dramatically reduced when hospital staff use a simple best-practices checklist.

•Ask every day if you still need the catheter. They are sometimes left in longer than necessary simply because no one bothers to take them out—and the longer a catheter is in, the greater the odds of infection.

•Brush and floss multiple times each day while you are in the hospital. Oral hygiene sometimes is overlooked by hospital patients who are coping with major medical issues, but neglecting this increases the odds that bacteria from the mouth will get into your lungs and lead to pneumonia.

•Sit up in your hospital bed as much as possible—the more hours spent lying flat, the greater the odds that fluid from the mouth will find its way into the lungs.

•Following surgery, ask, "Have I had deep vein thrombosis (DVT) screening?" and "What DVT treatment am I receiving?" The answer might include anticoagulants, intermittent pneumatic compression devices (IPCs) or other strategies. What is most important is that the staff is monitoring your DVT risk.

•Ask, "What should I do to reduce my risk for DVT?" Getting out of bed and walking in the days following the surgery can reduce the odds of clots. If an IPC is used to reduce the odds of clots in your legs, periodically confirm that it's still connected to the machine that inflates it—sometimes these become disconnected and/or are not reconnected after a patient gets out of bed.

•**Falls.** Walking around a bit is generally healthier for patients than lying in bed all day, but patients who are very ill or recovering from surgery can be unsteady on their feet, leading to dangerous falls. These falls often occur when patients ring for a nurse to help them to the bathroom, then attempt to make this trip on their own when a nurse doesn't arrive quickly. *What to do...*

•Don't wait until you're desperate to use the bathroom to call for a nurse—plan ahead so you can wait for assistance if the nurses are busy.

•Confirm that a bedpan and/or urinal is within reach of your bed for emergencies.

•**Hospital staffing and policies.** It pays to select a hospital that performs the specific procedure you require regularly. It also pays to seek out hospitals that use staff and practices that are associated with lower error rates. *What to do…*

• Choose a hospital with "intensivists" on staff if you or your loved one is going to be in the intensive care unit (ICU). These doctors specialize in treating critically ill patients. Having these specialists on staff is associated with an astonishing 30 percent reduction in hospital mortality, according to researchers at Johns Hopkins University.

To find out which hospitals in your area have intensivists on staff: Search local hospitals on Ratings.LeapfrogGroup.org, then click the "Guided Search" tab and choose "Critical Care" from the drop-down menu.

• Look for a hospital that has implemented "Enhanced Recovery After Surgery" protocols (ErasUSA.org). These protocols are associated with substantially reduced odds of post-operative complications, shorter hospital stays, and less pain despite lower use of painkillers. They ensure the patient is as healthy as possible through exercise and weight loss. Unfortunately, only a small number of U.S. hospitals have adopted them so far.

Private Equity Increases Adverse Events

Medscape.

Hospital-acquired adverse events or conditions are 25 percent higher in hospitals that have been acquired by private equity (PE) firms, according to a study of Medicare claims for more than 4.5 million hospitalizations. These events include falls, infections, pressure ulcers, foreign objects retained after surgery, air embolism, and blood incompatibility. Bloodstream infections accounted for 37.7 percent of the increase, and falls accounted for 27.3 percent. Surgical site infections increased from 10.8 per 10,000 hospitalizations before acquisition to 21.6 per 10,000 hospitalizations after acquisition, despite a reduction in surgical volume. The increase is likely due to staffing cuts, a common tactic that PE firms use to increase profitability.

Understand What Your Medical Specialist Does

Study of 204 adults by researchers at University of Minnesota, Minneapolis, published in *Journal of Hospital Medicine.*

Like other professions, medicine routinely uses jargon that is familiar to health-care providers but that patients may not understand.

Recent survey: 94 percent and 93 percent of people understood what dermatologists and cardiologists do, respectively… but for other medical specialists, far fewer people knew exactly what these health-care practitioners do—only 31 percent understood what a hospitalist does…internists, 21 percent…nephrologists, 20 percent…intensivists, 29 percent.

Best: When your doctor refers you to a specialist, ask what that health-care provider's specialty is—and be sure you understand why you're being referred and what that person's role is in your treatment plan.

Micro Hospitals— A Growing Trend

Charles B. Inlander, a consumer advocate and health-care consultant based in Fogelsville, Pennsylvania. He was the founding president of the nonprofit People's Medical Society.

The old saying "What goes around, comes around" is the best way to describe what is happening in the hospital industry. Starting in the 1970s, small hospitals, mainly in less populated areas, began closing as the cost of new technology and overall cost of care began to rise. By the 1990s, most smaller and rural communities were without a nearby hospital, forcing those needing emergency care or same-day surgery or treatment to travel many miles to reach a large regional medical center able to meet their needs.

But by 2015, the cost of patient care in these large regional medical centers had become exorbitant. Treating patients on an outpatient basis or patients needing just a night or two in a hospital bed became too costly for many large hospital systems. What was needed were smaller hospitals (to augment the big mega facilities), with between three and 25 beds and fewer doctors, nurses, and technicians capable of serving both emergency patients and same-day surgical patients. The beds would serve patients needing a day or two of inpatient care after a more routine surgery or those needing a bit longer observation.

Welcome to the micro hospital! Since 2017, micro hospitals have opened in at least 19 states, and the numbers are increasing every year. They are all affiliated with large regional hospital systems in conjunction with private companies that help them develop the structure and management of the smaller facilities. Most are in suburban or rural communities, where research has shown there are specific needs. For example, micro hospitals have been constructed in communities with large elderly populations or in areas attracting young people for economic reasons.

Here are some pros and cons you should consider before utilizing a micro hospital.

•**Pros.** Micro hospitals offer patients the convenience of nearby emergency care without the long waits often encountered at large hospital emergency rooms. They also provide access to same-day surgery or treatments but with back-up beds if follow-up treatment or observation is necessary. And because they are community based, they can be designed to meet the needs of the surrounding population.

Micro hospitals differ from stand-alone surgi-centers and outpatient/same-day surgery centers because they provide overnight or longer care. Unlike those other facilities, they are licensed as hospitals and must meet the same safety standards and staffing requirements as any other hospital. And because they are smaller and limited in the services they provide, they are cheaper to build and operate than large hospitals. That savings is passed along to insurers and patients alike.

•**Cons.** Because of micro hospital's size, with far less volume of patients, critics have noted that micro-hospital staff may have limited experience diagnosing serious but less common problems. Since these facilities are usually staffed by an emergency room physician and nurses, the availability of specialists may be restricted. Other concerns that have been raised include staff turnover, which in a small facility can be cause for alarm.

Check Them Out

It is important that you check out a micro hospital before you need it. Check out the facility, its capabilities, and the training of the doctors on staff. This should be available on the website.

What goes around has come around in the hospital world, with the recognition that, in many instances, smaller is better than larger when it comes to patient care and convenience.

Home Medical Essentials

Chris Iliades, MD, a retired ear, nose, throat, head, and neck surgeon and now dedicates his time to providing information that helps people stay well.

People with high blood pressure benefit from high blood pressure monitors, and people with diabetes use home blood sugar monitors. Should you add a pulse oximeter or a smartwatch to your wellness toolbox?

Pulse Oximeters

You may not recognize the name of this gadget, but if you have been to a doctor or a hospital in the past 30 years, you have used one. Medical office and hospital-based pulse oximeters are the clips placed on your finger to measure the amount of oxygen in your blood. This is such an easy, quick, and valuable test that it has been called the fifth vital sign. This device estimates the percent of oxygen saturation in your blood by passing a light through your fingertip.

Pulse oximeters used by doctors and hospitals are regulated by the U.S. Food and Drug Administration and are accurate within about three percentage points. If you have a known lung condition, such as COPD or asthma, your doctor may prescribe an FDA-approved oximeter for you.

Over-the-Counter Devices

Over-the-counter pulse oximeters are easy to use, but they are less accurate. OTC pulse oximeters have been around for several years, but they really took off during COVID-19 when people became aware that a drop in blood oxygen was a sign of a more serious COVID infection. They give your oxygen saturation as a percentage that you read off the device. A normal reading is 95 to 100 percent saturation. Below 92 percent is the danger zone, and you should contact your health-care provider. Below 88 is very dangerous and requires immediate medical attention.

FDA Warning

Due to the rapid increase in the use of these devices, the FDA issued a safety communication in September 2022. It warns that OTC pulse oximeters are not checked or regulated by the FDA, and that users should be aware of certain conditions that may reduce the accuracy of pulse oximetry. These conditions include poor circulation, dark or thick skin, smoking, cool skin temperature, dark fingernail polish, artificial nails, or dirty nails.

Both the FDA and the American Lung Association say that readings from a pulse oximeter alone are not sufficient to diagnose low blood oxygen levels. You should do a few readings to make sure the reading stays the same and check for other signs of low oxygen, like a blue tinge of the nail beds or lips (called cyanosis), shortness of breath, or air hunger (taking deep breaths without felling relieved).

If you already have a long-term lung condition, your normal pulse oximeter reading may be a little low, but normal for you. In that case, look for a drop of three or four percentage points from your normal reading as a warning.

If you decide to try an OTC pulse oximeter, check with your doctor to find out your normal oxygen saturation number, and have your OTC oximeter checked against an FDA-approved office model. Ask your doctor what saturation drop would require either a doctor call or an emergency evaluation.

Bottom line: As long as you know the limitations, you could consider having this device in your home, especially if you have someone at home who may be at risk for lung problems.

Smartwatch Heart Monitor

In 2018, an Apple Watch that can do a simplified electrocardiogram (ECG) became available. This watch claims it can detect atrial fibrillation (A-fib), the most common heart rhythm abnormality, called an arrhythmia. There are pros and cons to consider before you spend your money. Like the OTC pulse oximeter, this device is not regulated by the FDA.

Studies suggest that using a smartwatch ECG increases the number of people diagnosed with A-fib. A-fib can come and go, and many people with it have no symptoms, so they don't realize they are in danger of a stroke. Finding out you have A-fib is certainly a big benefit because your doctor can prescribe medications to control it and to reduce your risk of stroke. If you are young and healthy, without any heart condition, the Apple Watch is less likely to be beneficial. The risk of A-fib increases with age, affecting about 10 percent of people over age 75 and 20 percent of people over age 80.

Limitations of the Apple Watch

A large, recent study of the Apple Watch was published in the October 2022 edition of the *Canadian Journal of Cardiology*. In this study that included 734 patients, Apple Watch electrocardiograms (ECGs), which use one sensor, were compared to 12-lead ECGs and evaluated for accuracy by cardiologists.

The key results were that the Apple Watch ECGs correctly identified A-fib in about 80 percent of patients, compared with 97 percent for the 12-lead ECG. People who had common and innocent ECG changes due to premature heartbeats were three times more likely to be incorrectly diagnosed with A-fib by the Apple Watch. People who had more serious arrhythmias due to other heart conditions were not accurately diagnosed by the Apple Watch. The researchers concluded that "smartwatches are not yet smart enough."

If you have risk factors for A-fib, like older age, high blood pressure, obesity, sleep apnea, or diabetes, the benefits of an Apple Watch may be worthwhile for you. Your best bet is to talk to your doctor to find out. If you get one, let your doctor know about any Apple Watch warnings, but don't panic. A-fib is not a medical emergency, and the Apple Watch ECG could be a false alarm. Also, let your doctor know about other warning signs of A-fib like an irregular pulse, palpitations, lightheadedness, fatigue, shortness of breath, or chest pain.

Beware of Oxygen Machines Sold Online

Richard Casaburi, PhD, MD, associate chief for research in the pulmonary division at Harbor UCLA Medical Center, Torrance, California, and first author of a study published in *Respiratory Care*.

FDA-approved, physician-prescribed portable oxygen concentrators (POCs) are expensive and not always covered by insurance.

But: Cheaper versions available online are not a good alternative.

Recent study: Only one of three models tested increased lung oxygen levels usefully...and that one didn't perform as well as the prescription model.

Health Screening Tests

Charles B. Inlander, a consumer advocate and health-care consultant based in Fogelsville, Pennsylvania. He was the founding president of the nonprofit People's Medical Society.

Health screening tests are designed to identify serious medical conditions early. The earlier a condition is identified, the better the chances that the treatment will be successful. Studies show that screening tests such as mammograms, colonoscopies, and prostate-specific antigen (PSA) tests have saved or extended countless lives over the past decades.

Experts have produced guidelines about when routine screening should begin, and physicians usually follow those guidelines. But what we do not hear much about is at what age these screening tests can be ceased. The same experts who recommend starting ages for tests also give ages when many of these tests can be stopped or done less frequently. Their recommendations are based on studies that show that, after a certain age, specific treatments will be of little benefit or have risks that are greater than the risks of the condition.

Many physicians, however, continue to recommend testing to their patients even when the data show little usefulness. A recent study of 30,000 men over age 70 underscores this dilemma. The U.S. Preventive Services Task Force has long recommended that men ages 70 and above not have PSA tests done. They base their recommendations on data that show that men above age 70 will likely die of something other than prostate cancer. Thus, testing is of little benefit, and over-testing can lead to unnecessary treatments, many of which can have serious side effects. Yet the study found that over 50 percent of those men were being tested—including almost 40 percent of men over age 80. The study's authors found that elderly patients asking for these tests was a common issue, and few were advised of the guidelines. There are similar guidelines concerning mammograms and colonoscopies based on age and history of cancer.

Here are some tips to help you decide if you should continue to get routine screening.

• **Do your research.** No matter what the screening test you are considering, do your research. Do online searches about the test. Check what expert guidelines recommend for a person your age and your medical history. Also, check out the treatments that are likely if the testing finds something wrong. Are you willing to undergo those treatments? What are the potential side effects?

• **Speak with your doctor.** It's important that you have a serious discussion with your doctor about the value of a specific screening test. Ask your doctor if there is anything that can be done if something is found. If so, what are the potential side effects or longer-term effects of the treatment. In other words, is the treatment worse or riskier than the condition?

• **What's best for you.** Guidelines are simply that—guides for you and your doctor to take into consideration when deciding on the benefit of a particular screening test. The important consideration is what is most appropriate for you, regardless of your age, and taking into consideration your overall medical status.

Take Your Temperature with Your Phone

University of Washington.

A team led by researchers at the University of Washington has created an app that transforms smartphones into thermometers without adding new hardware. The app uses the phone's touchscreen and repurposes the existing battery temperature sensors to gather data that a machine learning model uses to estimate people's core body temperatures. When the researchers tested FeverPhone on 37 patients in an emergency department, the app estimated core body temperatures with accuracy comparable to some consumer thermometers.

Genetic Testing and Medication

Ann M. Moyer, MD, PhD, associate professor of laboratory medicine and pathology and an assistant professor of pharmacology, Mayo Clinic, Rochester, Minnesota.

Every person has a unique set of genes, and these genes can influence how their body processes and reacts to different drugs. Tiny genetic differences can mean the difference between a drug working as intended or being either too strong or too weak. They can affect how people experience side effects and even toxicity.

Drugs and Genes

Pharmacogenomics, the study of these interactions, can be applicable to many drugs, but some medications are more likely to be influenced by a person's genetic makeup than others.

- **Antidepressants.** Studies have identified genetic variants that can affect how a person responds to antidepressant medications. Genetic variants can affect the enzymes involved in drug metabolism, neurotransmitter transporters and receptors, and other molecular targets that affect how antidepressants work in the brain. Changes in the cytochrome P450 enzyme system can affect the rate at which a particular medication is broken down in the body.

- **Cancer drugs.** Not all patients with the same type of cancer respond to treatment in the same way. Some patients have genetic variations that affect how their bodies break down and eliminate chemotherapy drugs, which can impact the effectiveness and toxicity of treatment. By testing for these variations, doctors can adjust the dose or type of chemotherapy drug used to better match the patient's individual metabolic profile, potentially improving the chances of a positive treatment outcome while minimizing side effects. For example, a *UGT1A1* genotyping test identifies genetic variants that impact the activity of UGT1A1 enzyme, which metabolizes irinotecan, a chemotherapy drug used to treat colorectal cancer. Variations in this gene can increase the risk of severe side effects, such as neutropenia and diarrhea.

Pharmacogenomics can also be used to develop therapies that are designed to target specific molecular abnormalities in cancer cells. (While we use the term pharmacogenomics here, some people use the term pharmacogenomics only to refer to inherited genetic variations in all of a patient's cells, not just the variants that are acquired in only the tumor cells.) These drugs are often more effective and have fewer side effects than traditional chemotherapy, but they work only for patients whose cancer cells have the specific molecular target that the drug is designed to inhibit.

- **Pain medications.** Nonsteroidal anti-inflammatory drugs (NSAIDs), like *ibuprofen* and *diclofenac,* block the production of certain enzymes that cause pain and inflammation. Genetic variations in the *CYP2C9* gene can affect the metabolism of NSAIDs, leading to slower clearance of the drugs from the body. This can increase the risk of side effects such as gastrointestinal bleeding, especially in older patients.

- **Proton-pump inhibitors.** Genetic variations in the *CYP2C19* gene can affect the metabolism of PPIs such as omeprazole, esomeprazole, and lansoprazole. People with a reduced-function *CYP2C19* genotype may metabolize these drugs more slowly. The reduced-function *CYP2C19* genotype is more common in Asian and African populations than in European populations. On the other hand, individuals with a rapid metabolizer genotype may metabolize these drugs more quickly, leading to lower drug levels in the blood and potentially reduced efficacy.

- **Thiopurines.** An enzyme called thiopurine *S-methyltransferase* (TPMT) helps the body process drugs that are commonly used to treat conditions such as leukemia, inflammatory bowel disease, and autoimmune disorders. If a person who is deficient in TPMT takes a thiopurine medication, the drug can build up and cause bone marrow damage and other side effects. Depending on your ancestral background, you may be less likely to have a TPMT variant, but instead have a variant in NUDT15. In the mid-2010s, studies revealed that, in some populations in which TPMT variants are less common, NUDT15 variants are more common and have a similar impact with regard to thiopurines. But a genetic test can prevent these effects by alerting the prescribing physician before it's too late.

Limitations

As exciting as pharmacogenomics is, there are limitations. While scientists have identified many genes that influence drug metabolism and response, there are still many more genes and interactions to be discovered. As a result, there may be cases in which pharmacogenomic testing doesn't provide clear guidance for medication selection or dosage. Furthermore, while pharmacogenomics can help identify which medications are likely to be most effective for a particular patient, for a lot of drugs, scientists don't know what role genetics plays or what genes may be involved. They're more using a patient's genetics to rule a drug in or out, not to select the perfect drug. This can limit the practical applications of pharmacogenomics in some cases.

Finally, pharmacogenomics testing can be expensive, and insurance may not always cover the cost. If your doctors offers a test, make sure you investigate your coverage.

DIY Testing

Several companies offer pharmacogenomic tests directly to patients. If you try these companies' tests, be sure to discuss the results with your physician before stopping any medications.

- **Color** offers a pharmacogenomic test that provides information on how you may respond to antidepressants, antipsychotics, and pain medications.
- **Nebula Genomics'** test offers recommendations for mental health, pain management, and cardiovascular disease medications.
- **Invitae** looks at how your genes may interact with antidepressants, antipsychotics, and pain medications.

Your health-care provider may also offer you a test from an academic medical center, such as Mayo Clinic, or a for-profit company.

- **GeneSight or Genomind** assess how you may respond to psychiatric medications.
- **Myriad Genetics** provides guidance on chemotherapy treatments.
- **OneOme** provides recommendations for mental health, pain management, and cardiovascular disease medications.

> ### Genetic Testing and Your Current Drug Intake
>
> If you choose to undergo testing, it's important to discuss the results with your health-care provider before making any drug changes. For example, you may get a report that notes a specific SSRI you already take can be less effective in people with your genetic make-up. But if it's working for you—and your doctor has already worked with you to get the dosage just right—there's no need to make a change. If, however, you're having a lot of side effects from a drug you take, a genetic test could help your physician choose a better alternative. Either way, the science is more complex than the report you may receive, and it requires professional input to best interpret.

Is Your Medicine in Short Supply?

Jack E. Fincham, PhD, clinical pharmacy faculty affiliate in the Osher Lifelong Learning Institute, University of Arizona, Tucson.

If you've been turned away from the pharmacy because the medication you need is out of stock, you're not alone. Medication shortages are a growing problem in the United States. According to the American Society of Health-System Pharmacists (ASHP), at the end of the second quarter of 2023, there were 309 active drug shortages. Those in shortest supply include medications for attention deficit/hyperactivity disorder, electrolytes, antibiotics, cardiovascular drugs, hormone therapies, gastrointestinal drugs, and the most dangerous of all: chemotherapy drugs.

Shortages have significant effects on patients. They can decrease medication compliance by forcing patients to wait for a drug to be restocked, force patients to turn to more expensive or less effective drugs, or go without. In an ASHP poll, 32 percent of pharmacists said the shortages resulted in rationing, delaying, or canceling treatments or procedures.

Causes of Shortages

Most of the products that face shortages are generics, lower-cost drugs that are less profitable—or not profitable at all—for pharmaceutical companies to produce. In the past 25 years, many generic drug production lines in the U.S. have closed. In the past year, Akorn, which made 75 common generics, went bankrupt, closed, and recalled all of its medications, and Teva, which makes 3,600 medicines, announced that it will shift to brand-name drugs and "high-value generics." Several other generic manufacturers are facing financial troubles as well.

When a company stops making a generic drug, there isn't always someone to step in to replace them. If only one or two manufacturers make an active ingredient or final product, any disruption can be devastating to the supply. Those disruptions could come from a vast array of issues, from company closures due to poor quality or consolidation, unexpectedly high demand, natural disasters, worker shortages, or even political crises. Last summer, a tornado halted production at a Pfizer plant in North Carolina for three months, threatening the production of virtually the entire national supply of sterile injectables.

Quality Concerns

To win sales contracts with the middlemen who buy and then distribute generic drugs, generics manufacturers are forced to accept lower and lower prices. "Bargain-basement prices have pushed production overseas," which makes it difficult for the FDA to monitor quality, reports Kaiser Family Foundation.

More than three-quarters of active pharmaceutical ingredients are made outside the United States, but in 2022, the FDA inspected only an estimated 3 percent of foreign manufacturing sites. The consequences can be dire. In spring 2023, three people died and eight were blinded after using bacteria-tainted eyedrops that were made in a plant in India that had never been inspected.

Another Indian company, Intas Pharmaceuticals, stopped production of most of its drugs after the FDA uncovered a systematic effort to conceal quality problems in 2022, as well as inadequate efforts to prevent microbiological contamination.

The plant made close to half of the U.S. supply of two cancer drugs, cisplatin and carboplatin, which are now in severe shortages. In June 2024, the National Comprehensive Cancer Network reported that 93 percent of cancer centers are currently experiencing a shortage of carboplatin, and 70 percent have a similar lack of cisplatin. The FDA is allowing Intas to return to manufacturing certain critical oncology products under strict supervision. Other chemotherapy drugs are also in short supply, and patients nationwide are affected.

What Can You Do?

More than ever, it's important to know the status of any medications that you rely on. The FDA maintains a database of all drugs that have shortages. You can find it online at https://www.access data.fda.gov/scripts/drugshortages/default.cfm or download an app called Drug Shortages to your phone. For any medication that you are on, or that your doctor recommends, check the database to see if you may run into problems. *If your medication appears on the list, try these steps...*

• **Ask your doctor for a 90-day supply** so you have more medication on hand.

• **Refill your prescription before the medication runs out.** While your insurer determines how early you can refill, many pharmacies will refill a week early unless it's a controlled substance.

- **When you get a new prescription,** ask your doctor if there are alternatives in case you can't get a refill.
- **If your pharmacy is out of a medication,** call other pharmacies to check their supply. Try both chain and independent providers.
- **Don't ration your medication.** If you can't get enough to maintain the regimen your physician prescribes, call the doctor to talk about alternatives.
- **Don't be afraid to take expired medication,** if it's in tablet or capsule form, as a last resort. Most medications are given a yearlong expiration date when you fill them, but studies have shown that most drugs last much longer. However, the exception is liquid medications, such as eye drops. Do not use these after they expire. If you take something like a hypertension drug or antihistamine, it is safe to stockpile.

Beware Online Medications

If a drug that's in short supply seems to be magically available on the internet, watch out. Unless a pharmacy is vetted, approved, and listed in the National Association of Boards of Pharmacy's (NABP) database, you have no idea what you're buying. Visit https://safe.pharmacy/buy-safely/ to use their online search tool.

The vast majority of online pharmacies—even those that appear to be legitimate Canadian pharmacies—are risky. In fact, the official-sounding Canadian International Pharmacy Association (CIPA) website is itself questionable. The CIPA website claims to list "certified" Internet drug access sites; however, the pharmacies listed on that site have not been verified by independent and valid inspections. Many of the listed locations sell drugs that are sourced from unreliable countries and have never had to pass through Canada's equivalent of the FDA (Health Canada) regulatory process for assurance of safety and efficacy. The NABP notes that there are no Canadian online pharmacies that consistently dispense Health Canada-approved medicines to American customers: The drugs you buy from a Canadian pharmacy are not the same ones a Canadian is getting at the pharmacy counter.

The New Obesity Drugs: Is One Right for You?

Angela Fitch, MD, FACP, FOMA, president of the Obesity Medicine Association, assistant professor at Harvard Medical School, and former associate director of the Massachusetts General Hospital Weight Center. She is cofounder and chief medical officer of knownwell (knownwell.co), a weight-inclusive health-care company. Dr. Fitch is on the advisory boards for Novo Nordisk and Eli Lilly and Company.

Thanks to decades of research, we now know that diet, exercise, and other lifestyle modifications are essential for general wellness but don't move the needle much when it comes to managing obesity. And now that we are recognizing obesity as a disease, treating it with pharmaceuticals is gaining acceptance. The rise in popularity of newer anti-obesity medications (AOMs) such as semaglutide (Ozempic, Wegovy) has demonstrated their power—people with obesity can lose more than 20 percent of their body weight with these drugs, resulting in major health benefits.

Research shows that Wegovy reduces risk for heart attack, stroke and cardiovascular death by 20 percent in heart disease patients who are overweight or have obesity. Over the next decade, the drug's widespread use could prevent up to 1.5 million heart attacks and strokes and 43 million cases of obesity.

We asked Angela Fitch, MD, FACP, FOMA, president of the Obesity Medicine Association, and chief medical officer of the health-care company knownwell, to explain how these drugs work...

- ***Semaglutide* (Ozempic, Wegovy).** The hot new obesity drug is neither new nor designed as a weight-loss drug. Semaglutide branded as Ozempic was FDA-approved as a treatment for type 2 diabetes in 2017, thanks to its ability to boost insulin secretion and keep blood sugar levels stable. In 2021, the same drug, rebranded as Wegovy and at a slightly higher dose, was FDA-approved for people who have obesity or who are overweight and have health problems related to their excess weight.

Semaglutide is a glucagon-like peptide 1 (GLP-1) receptor agonist, a medication that mimics the naturally occurring gut hormone GLP-1 that makes people feel full after eating. Like the synthetic thyroid hormone taken by people with hypothyroidism, semaglutide provides GLP-1, reducing the drive to eat while triggering insulin release to combat or help reverse diabetes. Semaglutide also slows the rate at which the food you do eat passes through the stomach into the small intestine.

Result: Almost 40 percent of people taking semaglutide lose 20 percent or more of their body weight. By comparison, only 5 percent of people lose 20 percent or more of their weight using diet and exercise alone.

How it is taken: Weekly self-injections under the skin of the upper arm, abdomen, or thigh.

Common side effects: Nausea is quite common. Diarrhea, vomiting, constipation, and stomach pain also can occur, as can low blood sugar levels in people with diabetes who are taking other medications to manage their blood sugar.

On the horizon: Oral semaglutide, in a class of drugs called oral GLP-1 receptor agonists, now is available as a diabetes treatment under the brand name Rybelsus, but it is expected to be approved for weight loss at a higher dose and under a different name. Taken daily on an empty stomach, you must wait at least 30 minutes to eat, drink, or take any other oral drugs. You can swallow the pill with only a few sips of water—no more than four ounces.

•**Tirzepatide (Mounjaro)** is another GLP-1 receptor agonist to treat diabetes. But unlike semaglutide, it includes the hormone glucose-dependent insulinotropic polypeptide (GIP, formerly known as gastric inhibitory peptide) that further dampens appetite. In 2022, Mounjaro was approved by the Food and Drug Administration for type 2 diabetes. In November 2023, the FDA approved a new version of Mounjaro called Zepbound for chonic weight management.

Result: 60 percent of people taking tirzepatide lose 20 percent or more weight.

How it is taken: Weekly self-injections.

Common side effects: Nausea, diarrhea, vomiting, constipation, stomach pain.

On the Horizon

•*Retatrutide.* In trials, 80 percent of people with obesity lost 20 percent of their body weight on retatrutide, a number previously unheard of with AOMs. Retatrutide adds a third agonist—a *glucagon agonist*—along with a GLP-1 agonist and GIP agonist, earning it the nickname "Triple G." (Glucagon is a pancreatic hormone that regulates blood sugar levels.)

Bonus: Retatrutide is effective at helping people with obesity and non-alcoholic fatty liver disease (NAFLD), an often-silent condition affecting 10 to 20 percent of Americans. Being overweight or having high blood pressure, type 2 diabetes, prediabetes, or high cholesterol can cause fat to accumulate in the liver, which can lead to cirrhosis, permanent scarring, and hardening of the liver. Retatrutide reverses NAFLD in 90 percent of patients. It will be several years before this injectable receives FDA approval.

•*Orforglipron and danuglipron.* These AOMs are in a class of drugs called *oral small-molecule GLP-1 receptor agonists.* Unlike oral semaglutide, you needn't wait 30 minutes to eat after swallowing orforglipron or danuglipron. They also don't require refrigeration during transit (Ozempic and Wegovy do), making them easier and less expensive to mass produce.

Frequently Asked Questions

•**Who can take AOMs?** The best candidates have a body mass index (BMI) of 30 or greater...or a BMI of 27 or greater plus at least one weight-related health complication such as high blood pressure, type 2 diabetes, or sleep apnea.

•**Will I need to take the drugs forever?** AOMs must be taken indefinitely. In theory, some individuals may be able to take temporary breaks, holding weight gain at bay with large amounts of exercise and dietary diligence, but as the weight creeps back up, medication would need to be resumed. Your doctor will want to see you every four to six weeks for the first six to nine months to conduct blood work to assess your cholesterol levels, kidney issues, thyroid function, and diabetes status. If your AOM dulls your appetite so significantly that you're not getting sufficient nutrients, you may need to take a multivitamin. Once your weight loss stabilizes, you can have annual or biannual check-ups.

•**Will insurance cover the cost of the drugs?** With a diabetes diagnosis, insurance (including Medicare) will cover most GLP-1 receptor agonists. But coverage is trickier if you don't have diabetes. Between 30 percent and 50 percent of employers offer coverage for medications to treat obesity. The bipartisan Treat and Reduce Obesity Act, before Congress for over a decade, aims to guarantee AOM coverage, but until that act passes, most people will need to pay out of pocket—typically more than $1,000 per month.

•**What about the scarier-sounding side effects?** *There are a few that you may have heard about...*

•**Ozempic face and Ozempic butt**—the wrinkling, gauntness, and sagginess sometimes seen in the faces or glutes of people who've quickly lost substantial weight. These occur as the skin struggles to keep pace with a changing body.

•**Stomach paralysis.** A few cases of AOM-related gastroparesis and intestinal blockages have made headlines. Patients who experience vomiting of undigested food that was eaten several hours earlier, severe constipation, abdominal pain,

Compounded Obesity Drug Is a Bad Idea

Supply issues and high cost are putting *semaglutide* (Wegovy) out of reach for some patients...who may turn to compound pharmacies that make their own formulations for significantly less money.

But: There is no way to know exactly what is in the compounded mixtures...and the FDA does not verify their safety or effectiveness.

Best: If you have trouble filling a prescription, ask your doctor for a safe alternative.

Fatima Cody Stanford, MD, an obesity medicine physician scientist at Massachusetts General Hospital and Harvard Medical School, both in Boston. HMS.Harvard.edu

nausea, and heartburn should speak with their doctors—this probably isn't the right drug for them.

•**Cancer risks.** AOMs carry a black box warning for medullary thyroid cancer, but this risk has been observed only in animal studies. If you have a personal or family history of medullary thyroid cancer/multiple endocrine neoplasia type II, GLP-1 receptor agonist medications are not recommended.

•**Surgical complications.** Slowing transit time through the gastrointestinal tract means food remains in the stomach longer. When under anesthesia, this can cause the food to enter the lungs. If you are planning to have a surgical procedure, tell your doctor and anesthesiology team that you are taking an AOM.

Unsafe Supplements

Carrie Ali, editor, *Bottom Line Health*. BottomLineInc.com

Cannabidiol (CBD), the non-psychoactive component of cannabis, is an increasingly popular and legal supplement. That popularity is putting dollar signs in the eyes of unscrupulous people and, as a result, there's a dangerous array of unsafe products being sold all over the United States. It was reported recently that two people unwittingly purchased CBD gummies that were tainted with fentanyl and heroin. They both fortunately recovered from drug overdose.

Dietary supplements, from CBD to vitamin blends and everything in between, are not regulated by the U.S. Food and Drug Administration. Undeclared, unapproved, and potentially dangerous ingredients can go unnoticed until after a product is already in your home.

A study published in *JAMA Network Open* reported that there are three types of supplements that are most commonly tainted: those targeted for sexual enhancement, weight loss, and muscle building. But they also found tainted supplements that were marketed to treat joint and muscle pain, osteoporosis, bone cancer, sleep issues, gout, and prostate health. Studies have shown that, aside from adulteration, supplement labels can list incorrect doses and ingredients.

That doesn't mean supplements are a no-go, but it's imperative that you buy them from reputable sources. Buy supplements that are verified by an independent organization, such as U.S. Pharmacopeia, ConsumerLab.com, or NSF International, to ensure that the manufacturing process was safe, sanitary, controlled, and documented. For CBD products, visit the manufacturer's website and look for a certificate of analysis. This document is produced by independent laboratories to ensure that CBD products are safe and properly labeled. And always make sure your doctor and pharmacist know about any supplements you're taking so they can watch out for medication interactions.

Antibiotic Overuse Can Be Harmful

Stanford University, Intermountain Health.

Viral infections don't respond to antibiotics, but many doctors give in to adamant patients and write a prescription anyway. This antibiotic overuse is a significant problem. A study published in the *Journal of Internal Medicine* found that overprescribing of antibiotics is leading to antibiotic resistance and causing significant patient harm.

The study by researchers at Stanford University and Intermountain Health examined 51 million patient encounters over a 15-year-period and focused on upper respiratory infections, including sinusitis, pharyngitis, laryngitis, bronchitis, and the common cold. Researchers tracked whether patients received oral antibiotics and if they were later diagnosed with diarrhea, candidiasis, and/or Clostridium difficile infection. They found that 62.4 percent of people with upper respiratory infection filled a prescription for an antibiotic, and 26 percent of those patients had a follow-up outpatient visit within 14 days.

Adverse events following antibiotics were found in up to one in 300 prescriptions. The researchers noted that the chance of adverse events is likely much higher as the study recorded only follow-up visits where the adverse event was coded.

One medication, *cefdinir* was commonly prescribed even though it is rarely recommended by prescription guidelines as an appropriate treatment for simple upper respiratory infections and has a high risk of adverse events.

These findings point to the need for physicians to prescribe antibiotics only when necessary, said Harris Carmichael, MD, principal investigator of the study. For patients, it means understanding that antibiotics aren't always the right medication and that overusing them isn't just ineffective; it can be harmful.

The Dangers of Polypharmacy

John Horn, PharmD, professor of pharmacy, department of pharmacy, University of Washington. Dr. Horn is one of the founders of the Drug Interaction Foundation.

If you're taking a prescription drug, you're taking a risk. You take a drug to *solve* a health problem, but a drug can also *cause* a health problem. And chances are one in four that you'll experience what experts call a "drug-related problem" during your lifetime—resulting in physical harm, hospitalization, or even death.

Drug-Drug Interactions

One of the most common types of drug-related problems is a drug-drug interaction (DDI)—an adverse side effect caused by taking two or more drugs, with one drug changing the action of the other drug. Some studies show that every year, DDIs harm 7.8 million people—5 million in hospitals and 2.8 million at home. DDIs cause up to 220,000 emergency room visits every year.

Are You at Risk?

Your level of risk for a DDI is very straightforward: The more drugs you take, the higher your risk for a harmful DDI. And a lot of seniors—many with multiple chronic conditions, like high blood pressure, high LDL cholesterol, and high blood sugar—are taking a lot of drugs.

Among adults 60 or older, an estimated 50 percent are taking five or more drugs, a risky level of intake called polypharmacy.

Seniors are also more vulnerable to harmful DDIs because as we age, we are less able to deal with the biological challenges of a drug-drug interaction.

Overwhelmed Doctors

Another big problem: Physicians ignore 90 percent of the DDI alerts generated by the standardized DDI software used in hospitals and clinics. When this type of software was first introduced in the late 1970s and early 1980s, many health professionals expected the problem of DDIs would be solved: The computer program would identify potential DDIs and drug combinations could be tailored to avoid them. But that hasn't happened.

The sheer number of prescription medications on the market—more than 20,000 in the United States—causes these programs to bombard physicians with untold numbers of DDI alerts every day. For example, in a study of 1,000 patients, 48,000 DDI alerts were generated—or 48 alerts per patient! With that many alerts, doctors have realized that most alerts are not truly applicable to their patients and have stopped paying attention.

Furthermore, current programs consider only the interactions of two drugs, but they fail to evaluate how two drugs interact with a third drug or beyond.

Good news: In the same study, a new type of software that takes into account specific patient-based factors—like diseases, lab results, gender, and age—generated only 3.2 alerts per patient. That software—Seegnal eHealth—has recently become available for widespread use.

How to Prevent DDIs

Aside from what your doctor can do, there are several ways you can lower your risk of a drug-drug interaction...

•**Maintain a list of all the drugs you take.** Each one of your prescribers and health-care providers—your primary care physician, your specialists, your pharmacist—needs to know all of the drugs you're taking. If they don't, they'll never be able to help you avoid a DDI.

Keeping all your providers informed about your medications sounds relatively simple, but it isn't. Health care is "siloed"—meaning information isn't typically shared between practitioners. You may have a cardiologist who treats your heart disease, an endocrinologist who treats your diabetes, and a neurologist who treats neuropathy. And each of them may prescribe you one or more medications—without knowing (or asking) what other medications you're already taking. Similarly, your pharmacist may not have a record of all the drugs you're taking—and won't be able to warn you about potential DDIs with a new prescription.

The solution: Don't rely on health-care professionals to keep track of your drugs. Make a list of all the drugs you're taking, and bring it with you every time you visit a doctor or a pharmacist. On your list, include not only prescription medications but also over-the-counter medications and supplements, which can also trigger DDIs. By keeping track of your meds in this way, you make sure that all of your health-care providers and pharmacists know what you're taking and why—and then they can do their best to help you avoid DDIs.

•**When you're prescribed a new drug, ask your physician about possible DDIs.** The physician who is prescribing the drug should tell you the specific signs that the drug is working, when to take the drug (with or away from meals), the drug's possible side effects (particularly serious side effects), what to do if a side effect occurs, and whether or not the drug is likely to interact with your other medications.

For example, selective serotonin re-uptake inhibitors (SSRI), like *sertraline* (Zoloft) and *paroxetine* (Paxil), relieve depression and anxiety. Nonsteroidal anti-inflammatory drugs (NSAID), like *ibuprofen* and *naproxen*, control inflammation and pain. NSAIDs increase the risk of gastrointestinal bleeding—but that risk is increased 10-fold when you also take an SSRI. If you're taking an SSRI and an NSAID, you must know about this potential DDI to protect your health.

If you develop a DDI—talk to your physician ASAP. You may have to stop one of the two drugs that is causing the problem. The physician and the pharmacist need to consider what other drug might be effective for your health problem, and the new drug should help you avoid another DDI.

If there's not an alternative—and that may be the case with medications for cancer, for example—then the physician should consider lowering the dose of the drug or using a different treatment.

Diseases and DDIs

Recent research shows there are several diseases and conditions in which DDIs are more likely. Check with your doctor and pharmacist for possible DDIs if any of the following apply to you...

•**High blood pressure.** Nearly one in five people with high blood pressure (a problem that affects 68 million Americans) also take a medication that could be elevating their blood pressure, according

If You're Taking a Drug, Don't Take This Herb

St. John's Wort, an herb commonly used for depression, anxiety, and insomnia, interacts with more than 50 percent of all prescription drugs. Specifically, it increases their elimination, reducing their effectiveness. If you're taking a prescription drug, it's probably best not to take St. John's wort.

Two other natural products to watch out for if you're taking prescription meds...

•**Grapefruit juice,** which interferes with the metabolism of many drugs. Don't drink more than one glass a week.

•**Piperine,** a bioactive compound in black pepper that is also available in supplement form. Limit or eliminate your use of black pepper, and don't take a piperine supplement.

to a study presented at the 2021 American College of Cardiology 70th Annual Scientific Session. (Those medications are discussed in the sidebar at right, "What Triggers a Drug-Drug Interaction?")

•**Depression.** More than 200 commonly used prescription drugs list depression as a side effect, including blood pressure, heart, and antianxiety medications, as well as painkillers. A 2018 study in the *Journal of the American Medical Association*, from researchers at the University of Illinois Chicago, found that 15 percent of people who use three or more of these medications are depressed—compared with 9 percent taking two such drugs, 7 percent for one medication, and 5 percent for those not using any of the drugs.

•**Cancer.** In a 2022 study of 718 adults with stage 3 or 4 cancer, 70 percent were at risk of drug-drug interactions.

•**Frailty.** In the condition called "frailty," an older adult has a decline in physical and mental ability, and in the ability to function day to day. They're also more likely to be hospitalized and to die.

An 11-year study in the *Journal of the American Geriatrics Society* found that older adults who take five or more medications were 1.5 times more likely to become frail compared with people who took fewer than five medications. And those who took 10 medicines were twice as likely to become frail as those who took less than five.

•**Memory loss and cognitive decline.** In the last 10 years, the incidence of older people who take three or more drugs that affect the brain—such as opioids, antidepressants, tranquilizers, and antipsychotics—has more than doubled. Symptoms from multiple use could include poorer memory, confused thinking, and falls, according to a study in *JAMA Internal Medicine*.

What Triggers a Drug-Drug Interaction?

There are two types of mechanisms that can trigger a drug-drug interaction (DDI).

•**Pharmacokinetic.** This is when one drug (in technical terms, the "precipitant" drug) changes how the body uses the other drug (the "object" drug). These changes can be in absorption, metabolism, distribution, or elimination. And all and any of those changes can affect the blood level of a drug, reducing or increasing levels—potentially leading to an adverse reaction. For example, antacids can decrease the absorption of some antibiotics.

Another example: Diuretics can decrease the elimination of lithium (for bipolar disorder), leading to increased lithium concentrations, which are toxic.

•**Pharmacodynamic.** This is when the activity of the object drug is changed, but not its blood level. For example, you might take an antihypertensive medication to lower blood pressure while you're also taking a second drug that inadvertently increases blood pressure (like nonsteroidal anti-inflammatory drugs, corticosteroids, oral contraceptives, decongestants, antidepressants, and stimulants for attention deficit hyperactivity disorder).

—John Horn, PharmD

Some of Your Meds May Cause Hearing Loss

Chad Ruffin, MD, cochlear implant surgeon, Hearing Speech and Deaf Center, Seattle. ChadRuffinMD.com

Certain drugs—even ones sold over the counter (OTC)—are ototoxic, meaning they can cause temporary or even permanent hearing damage.

Important: If your hearing changes after starting a new drug or increasing a dosage, contact the prescribing doctor immediately and make an appointment with an ear, nose and throat (ENT) doctor. Say the words "sudden hearing loss," and the ENT doctor won't make you wait weeks for an appointment.

The most frequent offenders…

•**Certain antibiotics.** For severe infections, doctors may prescribe *aminoglycoside* antibiotics, which include *gentamicin, tobramycin,* and *streptomycin*. These often are administered intravenously in intensive care units. Physicians weigh the benefits of defeating the infection against the risk for hearing loss.

•**Certain chemo drugs.** One of the most frequently prescribed chemo medications—*cisplatin*—is among the most ototoxic. Doctors prescribe cisplatin only after discussing with the patient the risk for hearing loss. Your oncologist likely will put you in the care of an ENT doctor to monitor your hearing.

Other ototoxic chemotherapy agents: *Vincristine, carboplatin,* and *oxaliplatin*.

•**OTC painkillers.** Aspirin and nonsteroidal anti-inflammatory medications such as naproxen and ibuprofen should be used in moderation. Taking aspirin at high doses or too often is associated with diminished hearing and reversible tinnitus.

•**Loop diuretics.** Heart failure and kidney drugs Lasix and Bumex often cause tinnitus or temporary or even permanent hearing loss.

•**Hydroxychloroquine.** This lupus drug, made famous as an alleged coronavirus treatment, can cause hearing loss and tinnitus, which stop when the drug is discontinued.

New Safety Warnings on Opioid Pain Medicines

U.S. Food and Drug Administration (FDA). FDA.gov

Labels for both immediate-release (IR) and extended-release opioids (EX/LA) must now warn that higher doses raise risk for overdose…and that opioid medications can lead to *hyperalgesia*—opioid-induced increased sensitivity to pain. The boxed warning label also must mention the risk for respiratory depression (abnormal retention of carbon dioxide). IR labels should state that the medicines should not be used for extended periods unless alternatives are inadequate…and EX/LA opioids are approved for "severe and persistent pain" only when there is no effective alternative treatment option. Health-care professionals should discuss the impact of a patient's pain on quality of life…identify potential causes of the pain…and prescribe the lowest possible opioid dose for the shortest possible period of time.

High-Intensity Interval Training (HIIT) Before Surgery Can Speed Recovery

University of Otago.

HIIT training alternates between periods of aerobic activity at about 80 percent of maximum heart rate and periods of active recovery. Training for four to six weeks before surgery can improve cardiorespiratory fitness (how well the body takes in oxygen and delivers it to the muscles and organs); reduce the risk of developing a postoperative issue, like cardiac complications, pneumonia, and postoperative bowel issues, by 56 percent; and shorten a hospital stay by about three days.

For Hip Replacement, Pay Attention to the Surgeon's Level of Experience

Chad A. Krueger, MD, assistant professor of orthopedic surgery at Thomas Jefferson University, Philadelphia, commenting on a meta-analysis of 63 studies published in *JAMA Network Open*.

When it comes to hip replacement surgery, it matters what surgeon you use. Recent research shows that there is little difference in outcomes among the eight most common surgical approaches. The direct lateral approach, now waning in popularity, showed the smallest patient improvements—but that doesn't necessarily indicate flaws in the approach itself. More important is finding an experienced physician well-versed in whatever approach will be used…and who communicates about risks and expectations.

You Could Be Rejected by a Hospital or Surgeon

David Sherer, MD, author of *What Your Doctor Won't Tell You*. Now retired from his clinical anesthesiology practice in the suburbs of Washington, DC, he was a repeat winner of HealthTap's leading anesthesiologists award. DrDavidSherer.com

Surgeons and hospitals may opt not to perform procedures on patients who are very overweight or old, have preexisting health problems and/or complications that increase risk for poor surgical outcomes. *In addition to concern for the patient, providers worry that high-risk patients could endanger their bottom lines for several reasons…*

• **Insurers sometimes pay surgeons and hospitals a flat fee for a procedure.** Unhealthy patients are more likely to need long hospital stays, making them less profitable.

• **Medicare links reimbursement rates to providers' medical outcomes,** such as surgical success rates.

• **Patients and families sometimes sue when surgical procedures fail.**

The rejection typically is presented as concern for that patient's well-being—and that may well be true.

Note: A patient is unlikely to be turned away in an emergency situation—emergency rooms are not allowed to refuse patients.

• **If a surgeon declines to operate due to concerns about your health or fitness.** Ask whether there's anything you can do to bring that risk down.

• **If there is no way to become a less risky patient** and you are committed to getting the procedure, you'll have to find a surgeon or hospital willing to work with you. Your primary care doctor might be able to provide recommendations.

Doctor Dilemmas

Doctors Are Under Attack

Physicians and scientists are facing high rates of personal attacks and harassment on social media, according to a study of 359 physicians, scientists, and trainees. A total of 66 percent of respondents reported experiencing harassment, a significant increase since 2020.

Medscape.

Sick Doctors Still Go to Work

Health-care workplaces that foster a culture of duty make physicians and nurses feel obligated to work even when they are unwell… and stay home only when symptoms are so severe that they might alarm patients.

MedPage Today. MedPageToday.com

Get the Best Medical Care

Were Your Medical Records Stolen?

Analysis of Health and Human Services data by USA Today.

Medical records for more than 40 million Americans were stolen or exposed in 2022. Half through security breaches caused by hackers, and one-third because of health-care employee errors, such as lost computers or accidental disclosure. Thieves use the records to create scams targeting people with specific conditions…create fraudulent insurance claims…and traffic drugs. Federal law requires steps to protect sensitive data, but as providers shift records online, many legacy systems become vulnerable.

Information: Check *USA Today's* searchable database of health-care data breaches going back to 2009 at https://bit.ly/3FS1q9R to see if a health-care provider you use is on the list.

Watch Out for Medical Billing Scams

Better Business Bureau. BBB.org

Victims get a letter or phone call saying they owe money on a medical bill and must pay immediately. Contacting the sender/caller brings the victim to a phony billing department, where he/she is bullied into giving credit card or debit card information and often personal data that can be used for identity theft. Some scams invent phony bills and medical services—but some find out about real medical care that victims received and try to get money sent to phony billing companies.

Self-defense: Verify all claims…never pay without contacting the doctor's office or hospital using a number you find on your own. Do an Internet search for the phone number that called you or that appears on a demand letter—if it is not registered to an official, traceable medical business, it is phony. Do not give out personal information to anyone who calls unexpectedly.

Beware Special Financing for Health Care

April Kuehnhoff, senior attorney at National Consumer Law Center, Boston. NCLC.org

Medical credit cards often have outrageous interest rates, and other financing offered in health-care settings may be more expensive than anticipated. Never agree to financing when you're receiving emergency care and thus vulnerable.

Before borrowing: Make sure that claims are submitted to your insurer, and appeal denials if necessary. Ask if the facility offers charity care or financial assistance. Exhaust public-assistance options.

If you must borrow: Shop around and look into loans from credit unions and small banks.

Less Expensive Medical Care from Costco

MoneyTalksNews.com

The Costco warehouse chain has arranged with health-care company Sesame to offer its members virtual primary care for $29 per visit…virtual mental-health therapy for $79…health checkups (standard lab panel and virtual follow-up with a provider) for $72. Other services will be offered at a 10 percent discount, including in-person appointments. Health insurance is not accepted—Sesame aims to reach people who don't have insurance or who pay cash because they have a high-deductible insurance plan. Costco members need to create an account at SesameCare.com.

Get the Best Medical Care

10 Drugs Medicare Will Negotiate

Kiplinger Personal Finance. Kiplinger.com

As part of 2022's Inflation Reduction Act, Medicare plans to negotiate the price of certain drugs with pharmaceutical companies.

The first 10 drugs, which together cost Medicare about $50 billion in 2023: Eliquis (for blood clots)...Jardiance (diabetes and heart failure)...Xarelto (blood clots, coronary or peripheral artery disease)...Januvia (diabetes)...Farxiga (diabetes, heart failure, and chronic kidney disease)...Entresto (heart failure)...Enbrel (rheumatoid arthritis, psoriasis, and psoriatic arthritis)...Imbruvica (blood cancers)...Stelara (psoriasis, psoriatic arthritis, Crohn's disease, and ulcerative colitis)...Fiasp and NovoLog (diabetes).

Watch Out for the Sun If You Take These Drugs

Orli R. Etingin, MD, director, Iris Cantor Women's Health Center, Weill Cornell Medical College, New York City, and editor in chief, *Women's Health Advisor.* Womens-Health-Advisor.com

Certain medications can cause hypersensitivity to the sun's ultra-violet rays, including blood pressure drugs such as beta-blockers and thiazide diuretics (also called "water pills")...antibiotics, antihistamines, nonsteroidal anti-inflammatory drugs, antipsychotics, antidepressants, and diabetes meds.

Symptoms to watch for: Rashes, hives, itching, and severe sunburn. Check label warnings...and ask your pharmacist if sun sensitivity is a concern.

Are Steroid Drugs Safe?

Linda Russell, MD, rheumatologist, Hospital for Special Surgery, and assistant professor, Weill Cornell Medicine, New York City. HSS.edu

Recent research raises concerns about the risks of taking steroid drugs. There seems to be little risk with occasional use—such as to treat a bug bite, poison ivy, or a bout of bronchitis—but taking steroid drugs, especially high-potency doses, regularly, such as daily inhaled steroids to treat asthma, for more than two weeks can lead to sometimes serious side effects.

Side effects include: Weight gain, high blood pressure, bone fractures, cataracts, thinning skin, osteoporosis, depressed or anxious mood, fluid retention, headache, glaucoma, insomnia, type 2 diabetes, dizziness, and avascular necrosis (insufficient blood supply to the bones causing them to collapse).

If you are prescribed a steroid drug: Ask your doctor about nonsteroidal alternatives...start with the lowest dose that is effective.

Did You Take Zantac? What You Need to Know

Jack Fincham, PhD, clinical pharmacy faculty affiliate in the Osher Lifelong Learning Institute, University of Arizona, Tucson. OLLI.Arizona.edu

You've probably seen advertisements for lawsuits regarding cancers associated with the heartburn medication Zantac. *If you took Zantac before it was pulled from shelves in 2020, here's what you should know now...*

What happened: Zantac, whose active ingredient is *ranitidine,* made its debut in the 1970s as a prescription heartburn medication. In 2004, the FDA approved over-the-counter sales of Zantac, making it

> ### Lifestyle Changes for Heartburn
>
> Several lifestyle changes can help reduce heartburn:
>
> • **Avoid foods and drinks that cause heartburn for you.**
>
> • **Lose weight** if you are overweight.
>
> • **Avoid eating within a few hours before bedtime,** and don't lie down within two to three hours after eating.
>
> • **Sleep with the head of your bed elevated,** or on an extra pillow to prevent stomach acid from seeping up into your esophagus.
>
> • **Sleep on your left side,** which helps stomach contents leave your stomach.

available in supermarkets and pharmacies until 2020, when it was discovered that it was tainted with the probable human carcinogen *N-Nitrosodimethylamine* (NDMA). NDMA has been linked to cancers of the liver, lungs, esophagus, bladder, stomach, and rectum. The FDA allows miniscule amounts of NDMA in medications, but Zantac's levels were unacceptable, especially since the NDMA in ranitidine increases under normal storage conditions.

In 2021, drug company Sanofi launched the new formulation Zantac 360 using *famotidine,* the same active ingredient in Pepcid products. You also can purchase generic famotidine. Zantac 360 is considered safe and effective.

If you took Zantac prior to 2020: Let your health-care provider know how much you took and when. If you have no cancer diagnosis but are experiencing continuing or worsening gastric reflux symptoms, report them to your doctor. Ask that everything be documented in your medical records, which will be helpful in the event of a lawsuit.

For heavy Zantac users—individuals who took the medication for months or longer—it's reasonable to ask your doctor about cancer screening and for a referral to an oncologist for a consultation. If you've already been diagnosed with one of the cancers mentioned above, you're likely eligible to join a class-action lawsuit. For information, go to MarinBarrettLaw.com/zantac-lawsuit.

How Safe Are Proton Pump Inhibitors?

Daniel E. Freedberg, MD, MS, associate professor of medicine and epidemiology at Columbia University, New York City. He is a practicing gastroenterologist at Columbia University Medical Center and lead author of the paper "The Risks and Benefits of Long-term Use of Proton Pump Inhibitors: Expert Review and Best Practice Advice From the American Gastroenterological Association."

Have you stopped taking Prevacid, Prilosec, Nexium, and other proton pump inhibitors (PPIs) for your acid reflux because they have been linked to dementia, kidney and liver disease, heart disease, stroke, cancer, and other serious health conditions? That is certainly understandable—but you may not have to stop.

Despite the drumbeat of articles reporting these frightening findings, PPIs are generally safe, says gastroenterologist Daniel Freedberg, MD, lead author of a paper published in *Gastroenterology* analyzing the evidence.

His findings: The vast majority of those adverse effects are overstated, and the actual risk of taking PPIs, even long term, is probably so low that it is not a significant factor in the decision of whether or not to take them. Instead, the decision to use (or not use) PPIs should be based on the benefits they have for specific conditions.

That is good news for the nearly 10 percent of Americans who take these medications to calm the burning and pain caused by acid reflux. *We recently spoke with Dr.*

Freedberg to get the details and help you make the right decision...

Not as Risky as Studies Imply

Studies that link PPIs to significant health risks almost invariably compare the rates of a major health problem such as dementia or chronic kidney disease (CKD) among people who take PPIs to the rates among people who don't take them. While that sounds reasonable, there is a problem—PPIs may not actually cause those health problems.

Rather, some underlying health factor that increases PPI users' risk for the health problem also increases their risk for acid reflux. Being overweight, depressed, physically inactive, and/or smoking all increase the odds of acid reflux as well as the odds of many health issues linked with PPIs. While researchers who conduct PPI studies attempt to factor these things into their studies, it's almost impossible to do so completely.

When studies are conducted that randomly assign some participants PPIs and other participants placebos, the risk of PPIs almost always disappears. That strongly hints that whatever is causing PPI users to have elevated rates of a long list of health problems almost certainly is not the PPIs themselves.

Example: Published studies reviewed by AstraZeneca researchers revealed similar pneumonia rates among patients taking PPIs and those taking placebos, despite earlier research that suggested PPIs increase risk for pneumonia.

Even if you're not ready to completely dismiss the studies that find links between PPI use and increased risk for health problems, the risk typically is only modest—though the results of these studies sometimes are reported in a way that makes them seem significant.

Example: One study conducted in Taiwan that found a link between PPIs and CKD concluded that PPI users' risk for CKD increases by 10 percent to 20 percent annually. That sounds steep, but it doesn't mean that PPI users have a 10 percent to 20 percent chance of developing CKD each year—it means that a PPI user's odds of developing CKD are, theoretically, 10 percent to 20 percent higher than the risk of someone who does not use PPIs. Fortunately, only a very small percentage of the overall population develops CKD, so that 10 percent to 20 percent actually amounts to only an additional 0.1 percent to 0.3 percent risk even if PPIs do increase risk for CKD...which, as noted above, they probably do not.

Are There Health Concerns?

Of all the health risks that have been linked to PPI use, only one stands out as probably real—the risk for bacterial infection in the gut, such as Clostridium difficile (C. diff), Salmonella, or Campylobacter infection. The associations between PPI use and these bacterial infections are much stronger than those between PPIs and the other health issues. And it also makes sense that taking PPIs would increase risk for bacterial infection in the gut—PPIs combat acid reflux by reducing the stomach's acid levels, and stomach acid helps kill these and other potentially dangerous gut bacteria.

But even with this risk, that doesn't mean taking PPIs is necessarily a mistake. The bacterial gut infections people get in the U.S. tend to result in just a day or two of diarrhea and discomfort. All medications have risks and benefits. Many people who have serious acid

Time to Talk to Your Doctor

Always let your doctor know if:

• **You have heartburn for more than four weeks.**

• **Over-the-counter medication and lifestyle changes** do not relieve your symptoms or your symptoms return after a short course of over-the-counter medication.

• **You have difficulty swallowing.**

• **You regurgitate or throw up blood.**

reflux issues are willing to accept increased risk for occasional intestinal discomfort to greatly reduce their acid reflux symptoms.

Exceptions: Some gut infections such as C. diff can be serious. Also, if you live in the developing world where bacterial infections such as cholera are relatively common, this elevated risk might be a reason to avoid PPIs.

There is a second legitimate drawback to PPIs—if you take them daily for multiple months or longer, it can be difficult to quit. Long-term users who stop taking PPIs often experience rebound acid hypersecretion (RAHS) phenomenon—the cells in their stomachs have grown accustomed to the PPIs and produce increased levels of acid. When the PPIs are discontinued, the acid reflux resumes full speed—similar to having your feet on both the gas and brake pedals of your car…when you lift your foot off the brake, your car will move forward.

Result: PPI users often conclude that their acid reflux is as bad as ever and quickly start taking PPIs again, perhaps for the rest of their lives. But in reality, that often isn't necessary—even if they didn't resume taking the PPIs, the rebound effect would fade after one to three weeks or so of discomfort.

Helpful: One way to reduce the discomfort caused by this rebound effect is to use other acid-reflux treatment options during the weeks after discontinuing extended PPI use. Options include antacids (Tums, Alka-Seltzer, Gaviscon, Mylanta, etc.) and histamine 2-receptor antagonists (H2RAs), such as *famotidine* (Pepcid).

The Big Decision

PPIs are generally very safe—but it still is best not to take them if you don't need to. When PPIs are beneficial… If you have ulcer-related bleeding, especially when the ulcer is not due to the stomach bacteria H. pylori. If you have been diagnosed with Barrett's esophagus, a precancerous condition where the lining of the esophagus changes due to acid reflux.

If you have been diagnosed with "complicated" or "severe" reflux esophagitis—this kind of reflux is likely to recur without long-term PPIs.

Acid reflux sufferers who do not fall into any of these three categories should instead try taking an over-the-counter H2RA, more commonly known as an H2 blocker, such as *famotidine* (Pepcid). These often are sufficient to control acid reflux, and they are less likely to increase risk for a gut bacterial infection and will not have a rebound effect when discontinued.

If H2 blockers fail to control your acid reflux, then you can consider a PPI even if none of the three categories listed above apply—the acid-reduction benefits that PPIs provide can easily outweigh their drawbacks. Often a few days of a PPI is sufficient to control symptoms.

Helpful: The new acid reflux drug *vonoprazan* recently was approved for use in the U.S. It has been available in a number of other countries, including Japan, for some time. Vonoprazan may reduce stomach acid levels even more than PPIs, although there are no studies to date that show it is definitively superior to PPIs.

Bottom line: For typical heartburn symptoms, try an over-the-counter H2RA such as famotidine first. If Pepcid fails, next try two weeks of an over-the-counter PPI. If you still have heartburn or if you find that you are unable to stop taking PPIs, it's time to talk to a doctor.

How to Create Your Family Medical History

David Sherer, MD, author of *What Your Doctor Won't Tell You*. Now retired from his clinical anesthesiology practice, he is a repeat winner of HealthTap's leading anesthesiologists award. DrDavidSherer.com

It is common to have only a limited sense of relatives' medical problems. But it's also dangerous—many problems have a significant genetic component. Listing family members' problems in a "family medical history" could save your life...and save you money—if there's a problem in your family that requires expensive care, you can select an insurance product that helps cover the medical bills.

Collecting the Data

Ask as many family members as possible what medical problems they've experienced, then gather this info into a document. To create a family history...

•**Focus on health issues that have a genetic component,** including cancers, heart disease/hypertension, neurodegenerative conditions, and more. If you're not certain if a disease could be genetic, enter its name and the phrase "does it run in families" into a search engine and look for results from trustworthy sources, such as nonprofits associated with the disease or sites with addresses ending in ".gov."

•**Get details about each diagnosis.** What specific form of the disease did this relative have? How old was he/she when diagnosed? If relatives can't recall key details, urge them to ask their health-care providers to check their medical records... or ask if they recall which treatments they received—that could help pin down these diagnoses.

•**Ask if any lifestyle or employment factors contributed to the medical problem.**

Example: If a relative had lung cancer, it's worth noting if he smoked or worked with asbestos.

•**Frame this as a project that could protect every family member.** Some loved ones might consider their health problems private, but they may decide that younger relatives' health outweighs their privacy concerns.

•**Ask if they've taken genetic tests for potential health risks.** If so, ask them to share the results and include these in the family medical history.

•**Ask if they know anything about the medical history of now-deceased relatives.** Surviving relatives might know that grandma had cancer but not which form of cancer, for example. Add the info they do have to your document, but include caveats noting any uncertainty.

What Is Palliative Care?

Joe Rotella, MD, chief medical officer of the American Academy of Hospice and Palliative Medicine.

If you have a serious health condition, anything from cancer to congestive heart failure to dementia to Parkinson's disease, you already spend plenty of time with doctors and other health-care providers.

But you may not have a care team focused on what may matter most to you: living your best life while you manage that condition. That will mean different things to different people, but often includes managing not only physical symptoms, but the psychological stress, practical issues, and even the spiritual challenges that come with any serious illness. That's where palliative care comes in. *Here are six things you might not know about palliative care...*

1. Palliative care is for people at any stage of illness. You can sign up for palliative care immediately after a serious diagnosis or any time after that. The condition can be curable, chronic, or life-threatening. That's one way in which palliative care differs from hospice care, which is reserved for people expected to live six months or less. Palliative care is meant for anyone dealing with considerable discomfort, disability, or distress as a result of their health condition. Palliative care specialists are skilled in treating pain, nausea, poor appetite, shortness of breath, fatigue, constipation, poor sleep, anxiety, depression, and other common problems. But patients and their caregivers can call on palliative care providers for other kinds of support as well. That includes help coordinating your care, dealing with paperwork, planning for long-term care, or figuring out how to pay for care.

2. You don't have to give up any other treatment to get palliative care. You can get palliative care while continuing care aimed at treating or even curing your underlying condition. That includes, for example, the chemotherapy and radiation that you hope will cure your cancer or the dialysis that you need for your chronic kidney disease. Palliative care should give you new options, not take any away. Research shows that patients receiving timely palliative care along with standard treatments often live longer than those not getting that kind of support.

3. Palliative care is a team endeavor. Some doctors are palliative care specialists, but if you start palliative care, don't expect to see just one doctor. Your team may include your existing primary and specialist providers, along with palliative care specialists who may include doctors, nurses, social workers, psychologists, pharmacists, and, for those who desire them, spiritual advisors. These teams may work out of a specialized clinic within a hospital or health-care system or at other locations. Some will see patients and their caregivers in their homes or through video visits; others stick to in-office care.

In any case, patients and their caregivers are considered very much a part of the team. In fact, the patient is the captain.

When you start palliative care, you should expect the professionals on the team to conduct a comprehensive assessment of your needs—and to really listen to what you have to say about what would make your life better.

4. You can ask for palliative care. If you think you might benefit from palliative care, you don't have to wait for a health provider to offer it to you. You can ask for it. You might find that's all you need to get a referral to a palliative care team. Or you might find that your doctor doesn't know much about palliative care or doesn't agree that you would benefit. In that case, you might need to dig a little deeper. You could start by getting a second opinion from another doctor. You might also want to contact your insurance provider. In many cases, insurers offer case management services that might help you get access to palliative care. If you aren't sure about what services are available near you, look for palliative care organizations in your state that have that information. You also can check out provider directories offered by the National Hospice and Palliative Care Organization and the Center to Advance Palliative Care.

5. Palliative care is widely—but not universally—available. Palliative care is much more widely available than it was a couple of decades ago. A recent survey found that 72 percent of U.S. hospitals with 50 or more beds had a palliative care team in 2019, up from 7 percent in 2001. But the national picture hides huge geographic differences, with hospitals in the Southeast, for example, much less likely to offer palliative care than those in the Northeast. In general, big urban hospitals are most likely to offer palliative care and small rural hospitals are the least likely to. A growing number of hospice agencies have developed separate palliative care programs.

6. Insurers vary in what they pay for palliative care. This is another way in which palliative care differs from hospice care, which is covered as a comprehensive benefit by Medicare, Veterans Affairs, and some other insurers, including some state Medicaid systems. That means patients pay nothing for any of the care they get under the hospice umbrella. When it comes to palliative care, Medicare, Medicaid and many other insurers often will cover the medical portions—such as your visits with doctors and nurses and your medications, with any of your usual co-pays—but insurers may or may not cover additional services, such as meetings with chaplains and social workers.

Chapter 8

HEART AND STROKE HEALTH

Understanding and Preventing Heart Attacks

Even if you have a family history of heart problems, you can take steps to prevent a heart attack or stroke, says cardiologist Michael Ozner, MD. *Here is his plan to do that...*

What Causes Heart Attacks

The root cause of *atherosclerotic cardiovascular disease* (CVD) is excessive cholesterol- and triglyceride-carrying atherogenic lipoproteins in your bloodstream—the result of a flawed lifestyle and/or genetic risk factors. If there are too many of these toxic lipoproteins, they can enter artery walls and, over time, cause a buildup of atherosclerotic plaque—a collection of cholesterol, fats and inflammatory cells. In early stages, plaque is soft, but as you get older, it can harden or calcify. And if plaque becomes highly inflamed, it can rupture, causing a heart attack or stroke.

Even though there are techniques to open blocked coronary arteries and others to remove clots from arteries in the brain to treat stroke, CVD remains the leading cause of death for more than a half million Americans every year.

Problem: The medical community tends to wait until a heart attack happens and then spring into action. But for many people, their first symptom is their last...and for those who survive, life is never the same.

It's time to eliminate the cause of atherosclerotic heart disease, says Dr. Ozner. How? By decreasing levels of dangerous lipoproteins beyond what can be achieved with statin medications. Over the last decade, genetic engineering has paved the way for new medications that lead to much lower levels of harmful cholesterol and reverse or shrink dangerous plaque. But it's up to you to be an informed patient.

Dr. Ozner's Three-Step Plan

STEP #1: Get your house in order—meaning your lifestyle. The foundation of heart health is a healthy lifestyle—following the heart-healthy Mediterranean

---

Michael Ozner, MD, FACC, FAHA, board-certified cardiologist, medical director, Wellness and Prevention, Baptist Health South Florida, clinical assistant professor of medicine (cardiology) at University of Miami Miller School of Medicine, and author of *Heart Attacks Are Not Worth Dying For*. DrOzner.com

diet, getting regular exercise, lowering stress, maintaining a healthy weight, not smoking, and avoiding exposure to air pollution. Double down on your efforts to reach these goals.

STEP #2: Find out your plaque status. Visualizing plaques in your arteries and measuring specific components in your blood can provide information about your risk status and guide appropriate treatment.

•*Apolipoprotein B-100 (ApoB)* is a protein that attaches to potentially harmful lipoproteins, such as LDL. A blood test that measures these particles is a better predictor of heart attack risk than measuring LDL cholesterol alone. A normal level is under 100 mg/dL.

•*Lipoprotein(a) (Lp(a))* is an LDL particle with a different protein attached (it resembles a little tail). It is more dangerous than run-of-the-mill LDL because it's linked to increased risk for heart attack, stroke and blood clots. High Lp(a) is a genetic, or inherited, condition and affects up to 20 percent of people. A high level is 50 mg/dL and above.

STEP #3: Personalized heart attack–prevention strategy. Work with your doctor or cardiologist to implement Step #1 and address the findings from Step #2.

Important: Soft plaque deposits can be eradicated with lifestyle changes and medication. Plaques that have calcified can't be eradicated, but there are treatments to shrink them and reduce dangerous inflammation.

Your prevention strategy should have the following components…

•**Lower cholesterol.**

Goal: In people with existing atherosclerotic plaques, getting LDL cholesterol under 50 mg/dL can stabilize or shrink them. For others, maintain LDL cholesterol between 50 mg/dL and 70 mg/dL.

Recent finding: HDL, the so-called good cholesterol, does not necessarily correlate with heart disease risk, so the focus has shifted from raising HDL to lowering LDL. Statins have not solved the heart attack epidemic because they lower LDL cholesterol by only about 30 percent…50 percent when taken at a high dose. To achieve optimal LDL levels, you might need to reduce your LDL by 70 to 80 percent. New medications dramatically lower LDL and risk for cardiovascular events. *Cholesterol-lowering medications available now and on the horizon…*

•**Statins** are the first-line medication to lower cholesterol production.

•**Ezetimibe** is a cholesterol absorption inhibitor that has shown to be as effective as monotherapy and when used in conjunction with statin medications.

•**Bempedoic acid,** a prescription medication, also reduces cholesterol production.

•**PCSK9 inhibitor.** PCSK9 is a protein produced in the liver that gets in the way of clearing LDL. When added to statins, a PCSK9 inhibitor helps achieve a further 50 to 60 percent LDL reduction. PCSK9 inhibitors include *evolocumab* (Repatha) and *alirocumab* (Praluent), self-administered by injection every two to four weeks, and *inclisiran* (Leqvio), given twice a year by a health-care provider.

•**Pelacarsen** significantly lowers Lp(a) and is in a late-stage clinical trial.

•Lower triglycerides.

Goal: A normal triglyceride level is under 150 mg/dL…an optimal level is under 100 mg/dL. High triglycerides increase heart attack risk. A clinical trial by researchers at Brigham and Women's Hospital Heart and Vascular Center of Harvard Medical School demonstrated that a highly purified omega-3 EPA ethyl ester (Vascepa) can lower triglycerides by 80 percent. In a study of people with optimal LDL but whose triglyceride levels were high, by Boston University School of Medicine and other institutions, it lowered cardiovascular risk by more than 25 percent.

•**Lower inflammation.** Inflammatory cells produce enzymes called proteinases, which can break down the fibrous cap of an atherosclerotic plaque and cause the plaque to rupture. You can lower inflammation with good lifestyle habits and medications, including the gout medication colchicine, if needed.

Certain Heart Attacks Affect Women More Than Men

C. Noel Bairey Merz, MD, director of the Barbra Streisand Women's Heart Center in the Smidt Heart Institute at Cedars-Sinai in Los Angeles.

Myocardial infarction with non-obstructive coronary arteries (MINOCA) events comprise 10 percent to 12 percent of heart attacks…but up to 30 percent of attacks affecting women. Symptoms are the same as heart attacks caused by blockage—chest pain, shortness of breath, fatigue—but these attacks are often underdiagnosed because the main arteries are not blocked. Patients who are diagnosed with MINOCA are put on a standard post-heart-attack drug regimen.

When Your Heart Skips a Beat

Chris Iliades, MD, a retired surgeon who now dedicates his time to educating people about how to best care for their health. He is a frequent contributor to *Bottom Line Health*.

"My heart just skipped a beat." You have probably heard it or said it. It's called a *premature ventricular contraction* (PVC) or heart palpitation. According to the National Library of Medicine, PVCs are very common. They turn up in 1 to 4 percent of routine electrocardiograms (EKGs), and 75 percent of people will have a PVC over a 24- to 48-hour period. In fact, PVCs are not considered to be frequent unless you have more than 30 in one hour.

> **Stress and Insomnia Could Increase A-fib Risk After Menopause**
>
> According to a recent study 83,000 women, more than one-quarter of postmenopausal women were diagnosed with atrial fibrillation (A-fib), a form of irregular heartbeat. Two major contributing factors are prolonged stress and poor sleep. Women should seek treatment for those conditions, since A-fib increases risk for blood clots and stroke.
>
> Study of 83,000 women led by researchers at Santa Clara Valley Medical Center, San Jose, California, published in *Journal of the American Heart Association*.

What's Going On?

A PVC is an early beat that is out of sync with your heart's regular rhythm. The early beat is followed by a longer pause between beats, like your heart is standing still. When your heart does beat, it beats a little stronger than usual to catch up, which causes the sensation that you feel.

The heart has four chambers: two atria on the top and two ventricles on the bottom. Normally, control of your heart's rhythm starts in the right atrium. An electrical charge starts in the sinoatrial node (SA node) and travels down specialized heart-cell fibers to the lower chambers of your heart (ventricles). This triggers a beat that sends blood from your heart to your lungs and your body. A PVC occurs when the heartbeat is started by fibers in one of the ventricles (called the Purkinje fibers) instead.

Simple PVCs

Most PVCs occur spontaneously and aren't even felt. They can be caused by a variety of things…
- **anxiety.**
- **caffeine.**

- alcohol.
- nicotine.
- not enough sleep.
- heart mineral (electrolyte) imbalance.
- cocaine or amphetamines.

Warning PVCs

Less commonly, PVCs can be a warning sign of a medical problem. Examples include heart disease, high blood pressure, hyperthyroidism, and anemia. You need to have a lot of PVCs to cause heart damage. People who have over 1,000 PVCs per day may develop a condition called cardiomyopathy, in which the heart muscles become soft and weak. This can lead to heart failure.

Frequent PVCs usually cause other symptoms, like dizziness, shortness of breath, a pounding pulse in your chest or neck, or a sensation of almost passing out, called syncope.

Diagnosis

Let your doctor know if you have frequent palpitations or any of the other symptoms of frequent PVCs. A health-care provider may be able to feel or hear a PVC by checking your pulse or listening to your heart, but, in most cases, an EKG is ordered to look for the delayed beat and stronger recovery beat. If an EKG shows that PVCs are very frequent or come in pairs or triplets, it is a possible sign of heart disease. A single EKG may not show any PVCs, but if you have symptoms, you may need to wear a Holter monitor to record your EKG over 24 to 48 hours. If PVCs are worrisome, further testing to find the cause may include blood tests, heart imaging studies, and cardiac stress testing.

Treatment Options

Treatment depends on the cause of the PVCs and could include correcting triggers like stress, anxiety, or lack of sleep, avoiding caffeine or nicotine, treating high blood pressure or hyperthyroidism, correcting electrolyte abnormalities, or treating heart disease.

PVCs that are very frequent may also be treated with medications that control heart rhythm, called *antiarrhythmics*. People who have several thousand PVCs per day may benefit from a procedure called radiofrequency catheter ablation. During this procedure a catheter is threaded into the heart to eliminate the source of the PVCs.

Can PVCs Be Prevented?

There is no way to prevent PVCs, but you may be able to reduce your risk and improve your heart health by maintaining a healthy weight, getting regular exercise, eating a heart-healthy diet, getting enough sleep, and avoiding nicotine, too much caffeine or alcohol, and illicit drugs like cocaine or amphetamines. You can also work with your health-care provider to control anxiety, stress, high blood pressure, or high cholesterol.

When to Get Help

Let your health-care provider know about frequent palpitations or other symptoms, like feeling lightheaded, dizzy, short of

---

Atrial Fibrillation and PVCs

Recent research suggests another reason to let your health-care provider know about any PVC symptoms. Studies show that people with frequent PVCs—more than 1,000 per day—have triple the risk of developing atrial fibrillation (A-fib). A-fib is the most common abnormal heart rhythm in adults. Although it's not dangerous itself, it can cause blood clots to form in the heart that can travel to the brain, causing a stroke. In fact, one in seven strokes are caused by A-fib. A-fib shares many symptoms with frequent PVCs, including palpitations, dizziness, and shortness of breath.

breath, pounding pulse, or syncope. Call 911 if you have trouble breathing or chest pain.

Early Cardiac Arrest Warning Signs

Cedars Sinai Smidt Heart Institute.

Half of people who experienced a sudden cardiac arrest noticed telling symptoms 24 hours before their loss of heart function, investigators learned from a recent study. The symptoms differed by sex. For women, the most prominent symptom of an impending sudden cardiac arrest was shortness of breath, whereas men experienced chest pain. Smaller subgroups of both genders experienced palpitations, seizure-like activity, and flu-like symptoms the day before cardiac arrest.

A Keto Diet Could Hurt Your Heart

Iulia Iatan, MD, PhD, attending physician-scientist at St. Paul's Hospital, Vancouver, Canada, and leader of a 12-year study presented at the American College of Cardiology Annual Scientific Session.

Low-carb, high-fat diets force the body to burn fat by depriving it of carbs.

Recent finding: People who ate a keto-like diet had significantly higher "bad" cholesterol and twice the risk for major cardiovascular events, including heart attack, stroke, peripheral artery disease, and arterial blockages requiring stents.

Note: Not everyone's cholesterol rises on a keto diet. If you want to try it, consult your doctor and monitor your cholesterol.

Should You Treat High Triglycerides?

Sadiya Khan, MD, MSc, the Magerstadt Professor of Cardiovascular Epidemiology at Northwestern University Feinberg School of Medicine.

Cholesterol numbers and their significance often take center stage in discussions about cardiovascular health. However, there's another number that tends to fly under the radar but can be just as important: triglyceride level. These two measures together provide valuable insights into an individual's risk for heart disease.

Cholesterol and triglycerides are both types of lipids, or fats, circulating in the bloodstream. They play pivotal roles in various bodily functions, but when their levels become imbalanced, particularly in the context of heart health, problems can arise. Higher cholesterol and triglyceride numbers are associated with a higher risk of heart disease. However, the interpretation can be more nuanced.

Triglycerides: A Warning Light

Triglyceride numbers over 150 milligrams per deciliter (mg/dL) are associated with a higher risk for heart disease but lowering them doesn't necessarily reduce that risk. They could simply be a marker, and not a cause, of cardiovascular risk.

Elevated triglycerides could represent obesity, uncontrolled diabetes, or lifestyle factors such as excessive alcohol consumption and a high-calorie diet. Triglycerides, often overshadowed by cholesterol, can serve as early warning signs.

In 2022, the published results of the PROMINENT (Pemafibrate to Reduce Cardiovascular Outcomes by Reducing Triglycerides in Patients with Diabetes) trial showed that a medication called *pemafibrate* lowered high triglyceride levels but was not associated with a lower risk for cardiovascular events. These findings prompted some professionals to question whether treating high triglycerides is beneficial.

There are two possible explanations for the study's findings: First, the lower triglyceride level didn't equate to lower risk because triglycerides are a marker, not a cause, of heart disease. The second possibility is that the way that pemafibrate lowers triglycerides was not effective at lowering the risk of heart disease.

Look at Lifestyle

One of the best ways to lower heart disease risk—which may also lower triglycerides—is to focus on diet and physical activity.

The American Heart Association emphasizes the importance of adopting healthy dietary patterns rather than simply focusing on eliminating fats or carbohydrates. The Mediterranean diet, for example, has gained recognition for its heart-protective benefits. (Visit BottomLineInc.com for more on this dietary plan.)

Physical activity, too, is a potent tool. Incorporating a little more movement into daily routines, like parking farther away or using step counters, can make a significant difference. Even if you're not currently meeting the recommended 150 minutes per week, every bit of additional movement counts. The key is to gradually increase activity levels from where you currently are. Any exercise is better than none.

Medications and Controversies

For some individuals, lifestyle changes might not be sufficient, and a physician may recommend trying medications to bring triglyceride levels down. Statins, a class of cholesterol-lowering drugs, are widely prescribed for high cholesterol and have demonstrated effectiveness in reducing heart disease risk, so they should always be first line to lower risk for heart disease.

A newer drug, *icosapent ethyl* (Vascepa), specifically targets high triglyceride levels. Its use is generally reserved for individuals with established heart disease or diabetes who are already on statin therapy. Vascepa can have side effects, such as muscle pain or swelling in the extremities.

Know Your Risk

Regular health check-ups often include cholesterol and triglyceride measurements. Keeping track of these numbers over time provides valuable information about your heart health trajectory. If you're concerned about your levels, discussing them with a health-care provider can lead to a comprehensive plan that considers your heart-disease risk and specifically targets lipid levels and diabetes risk.

Cholesterol and triglycerides are more than just numbers on a report: They are key indicators of heart health. While cholesterol tends to hog the spotlight, triglycerides offer essential insights into metabolic health. Understanding these numbers, making lifestyle adjustments, and, if necessary, seeking medical intervention can contribute to a heart-healthy life.

By the Numbers

Triglyderides are measured with a blood test. You should not eat for eight to 12 hours before the test and avoid alcohol. Some over-the-counter drugs, supplements, and medications can interfere with blood test results. Your doctor will tell you what you'll need to stop taking before the test.

Your results will fall into one of three categories...

- **Healthy:** Below 150 milligrams per deciliter (mg/dL)
- **Borderline high:** Between 150 and 199 mg/dL
- **High:** Between 200 and 499 mg/dL.

Nearly One-Quarter of Coronary Stents Are Unnecessary

Vikas Saini, MD, president and CEO of Lown Institute, a nonpartisan health-care think tank in Needham, Massachusetts. LownInstitute.org

Analysis of more than one million stent procedures at over 1,700 U.S. hospitals shows that 22 percent did not need to be done, exposing patients to unnecessary costs and risks. At some hospitals, more than 50 percent of procedures were unnecessary. Stents are appropriate during or immediately after heart attack...not when coronary disease and angina are stable, predictable and responding to medication.

500 Steps Lowers Heart Disease Risk

University of Alabama at Birmingham School of Public Health.

A new study found that walking an additional 500 steps, or about one-quarter of a mile, per day was associated with a 14 percent lower risk of heart disease, stroke, or heart failure. Researchers analyzed health data for 452 participants with an average age of 78, who used an accelerometer device that measured their daily steps. Compared with adults who took less than 2,000 steps per day, adults who took approximately 4,500 steps had a 77 percent lower risk of experiencing a cardiovascular event.

"It's important to maintain physical activity as we age; however, daily step goals should also be attainable," said Erin E. Dooley, PhD. "While we do not want to diminish the importance of higher-intensity physical activity, encouraging small increases in the number of daily steps also has significant cardiovascular benefits. If you are an older adult over the age of 70, start with trying to get 500 more steps per day."

Climb Stairs for Your Heart

Atherosclerosis.

Climbing more than five flights of stairs each day could reduce the risk of cardiovascular disease by 20 percent. "Short bursts of high-intensity stair climbing are a time-efficient way to improve cardiorespiratory fitness and lipid profile, especially among those unable to achieve the current physical activity recommendations," said Dr. Lu Qi, MD.

Couples' Guide to Keeping Your Heart Healthy

Helen Lavretsky, MD, professor in-residence, department of psychiatry at UCLA...geriatric integrative psychiatrist with a federally funded research program in integrative mental health and well-being...and contributor to the American Heart Association's guideline *Life's Essential 8*. UCLA.edu

Heart disease is a concern for both women and men, and how you work as a couple to ward it off often predicts how successful you will be.

Differences between men and women: Men have heart disease risk factors earlier in life than women. But women catch up after menopause, when estrogen and its heart-protective effects wane. Men tend to die younger from acute events such as heart attack...when women die of heart disease, it tends to be after a lengthy period of living with the condition.

As with men, women's most common heart attack symptom is chest pain or discomfort, but women may experience other symptoms that are less associated with heart attack, including...

- **Uncomfortable pressure,** squeezing, fullness, or pain in the center of your chest that lasts more than a few minutes or goes away and comes back
- **Pain or discomfort in one or both arms,** the back, neck, jaw, or stomach
- **Shortness of breath** with or without chest discomfort
- **Breaking out in a cold sweat,** nausea, or lightheadedness.

When a couple works as a team to fight heart disease, the outcome for both partners improves exponentially. And if one partner has heart disease, having his/her spouse's help encourages a heart-healthy lifestyle.

Good-for-Your-Heart Strategies

First step: Know your risks. Both partners should know if there's any history of heart disease in the family...get screened annually for diabetes, high cholesterol and high blood pressure...and quit if they smoke. Work-related stress also is a risk, and women often face stressors at home because they're tasked with caregiving responsibilities. Other steps...

- **Follow a healthy diet.** Eating more vegetables and fruits is a great start for better nutrition.
- **Lose weight.** It is easier to achieve a weight goal when both partners are on the same page.
- **Be more active.** Make a list of what activities you can do together to reach the weekly goal of 150 minutes. Exercise also is a great way to reconnect with a partner after retirement.
- **Enhance the emotional health of your relationship.** Having strong relationships is as important as quitting smoking. Partners in a happy marriage are more open to including each other in their decisions to practice better habits. They also tend to have lower blood pressure than people who aren't married.

If your marriage is strained: Get help from a counselor or marriage and family therapist.

- **Learn tools for stress reduction and healthy sleep.** Meditate or do breathing exercises or yoga...cultivate joy by engaging in enjoyable activities...listen to or play music...spend time in nature.
- **Change your personal outlook on life.** Having a positive outlook is protective, whereas being a pessimist is linked to a bad outcome for heart disease. Often one person in a couple is more positive than the other. Try to get your partner to see the world in a better light with small but effective practices.

Important: If either partner is depressed, intervention may be needed.

Plant-Based Diet for a Healthy Heart

Stanford Medicine.

A vegan diet improved cardiovascular health in just eight weeks, according to a study of 22 pairs of identical twins. Study authors selected healthy participants without cardiovascular disease from the Stanford Twin Registry and matched one twin from each pair with either a vegan or omnivore diet. Both diets were healthy, replete with vegetables, legumes, fruits, and whole grains and void of sugars and refined starches. The vegan diet was entirely plant-based and included no meat or animal products such as eggs or milk. The omnivore diet included chicken, fish, eggs, cheese, dairy, and other animal-sourced foods.

During the first four weeks, a meal service delivered 21 meals per week. For the remaining four weeks, the participants prepared their own meals. Forty-three participants completed the study. The authors found the most improvement over the first four weeks of the diet change. The participants with a vegan diet had significantly lower low-density lipoprotein cholesterol (LDL-C) levels, insulin and body weight, all of which are associated with improved cardiovascular health, than the omnivore participants. At three time points, at the beginning of the trial, at four weeks and at eight weeks, researchers weighed the participants and drew their blood. The average baseline LDL-C level for the vegans was 110.7 mg/dL and 118.5 mg/dL for the omnivore participants; it dropped to 95.5 for vegans and 116.1 for omnivores at the end of the study. The vegan participants showed about a 20 percent drop in fasting insulin. Higher insulin level is a risk factor for developing diabetes. The vegans also lost an average of 4.2 more pounds than the omnivores.

Heart Shape Predicts Risk

Smidt Heart Institute at Cedars-Sinai.

Investigators from the Smidt Heart Institute at Cedars-Sinai have discovered that people who have round (as opposed to long) hearts are 31 percent more likely to develop atrial fibrillation and 24 percent more likely to develop cardiomyopathy. The shape of one's heart can change, typically becoming rounder over time or after a major cardiac event like a heart attack. The findings point to the potential use of cardiac imaging to diagnose and prevent many conditions.

Beyond Pacemakers

John P. Higgins MD, MBA, professor of cardiovascular medicine and director of sports cardiology at McGovern Medical School, UTHealth Houston. He is also a certified personal trainer and exercise specialist.

The concept of a pacemaker began 200 years ago when Luigi Galvani, the Italian physician and biologist, used an electrical current to make a frog's heart beat. The first pacemaker for humans was introduced in the 1950s. Today, it is estimated that up to 3 million Americans are living with a pacemaker, but pacemakers are not the only implantable electronic heart devices.

Cardiac implantable electronic devices (CIED) restore the natural electrical signals that control the beating of your heart. Conditions that disrupt these signals are called conduction disorders.

A heartbeat starts in the right upper chamber of your heat—the right atrium—in an area called the sinoatrial node (SA node). The signal then travels down a conduction pathway to a node called the atrioventricular node (AV node), which helps control the rate of your heartbeat. Finally, the signal passes to the main pumping chambers of your heart, called your ventricles.

The Pacemaker

A pacemaker helps keep your heart rate at a normal level during rest and exercise. A pulse generator implanted under the skin of your chest or abdomen sends electrical pulses through wires, called leads, which are implanted inside one or more of your heart chambers. An electrode at the end of the lead senses your heart's rhythm and can send an electrical pulse into your heart muscle to control it.

Seventy percent of people living with a pacemaker are over age 65. The main reason for implanting a pacemaker is to control symptoms of a heartbeat that is too slow, called bradycardia. Bradycardia may cause dizziness, weakness, a feeling of passing out called *syncope*, or actual passing out. When your heart beats too slowly, you may start to feel weak and lightheaded if you try to exercise, called exercise intolerance. A pacemaker may also be used to control a heartbeat that is irregular or too fast.

Conditions that cause slow or abnormal heart rhythms can be caused by disease of the SA or AV node, called heart blocks. Abnormal heart rhythms *(arrhythmias)* can be caused by age, heart failure, heart attack, congenital heart defects, or enlarged and thickened heart muscle called *cardiomyopathy*.

The procedure for implanting a pacemaker can be done with local anesthesia and sedation. In some cases, you can go home the same day or the next day. The pulse generator requires a small incision. The leads are passed through blood vessels leading to the heart. Depending on your condition, there may be one or more leads placed.

Since the first pacemaker in 1950, there have been more than 3,000 models. The most recent model is the size of a large pill. This wireless or leadless pacemaker is a small battery-powered self-contained device that is implanted directly into the heart. It does not have the traditional leads. However, the traditional pacemaker generally lasts longer and has more research on its safety and effectiveness.

The Implantable Cardioverter Defibrillator

The main purpose of a pacemaker is to keep your heart's rate and rhythm normal. The main purpose of an implantable cardioverter defibrillator (ICD) is to prevent sudden cardiac death from a dangerous arrhythmia. The first ICD was approved in 1980.

The procedure for implanting an ICD is very similar to implanting a pacemaker. Like the pacemaker, the ICD has an electric pulse generator, about the size of a pocket watch, that is implanted in the chest wall with a lead connected to the heart that constantly monitors the heart rhythm. If it sees a dangerous or fast arrhythmia, like ventricular tachycardia or ventricular fibrillation, it will attempt to restore the normal rhythm by means of a shock.

Abnormal heart rhythms that start in the ventricles are more dangerous because the ventricles are the main pumping chambers of the heart, and they may stop pumping. When the brain does not get oxygenated blood, a person will suddenly pass out. Unless normal rhythm is quickly restored, death will soon follow.

ICDs are for people who are at risk for a sudden cardiac death, including people with serious heart failure and reduced pumping function (less than 35 percent). Other causes are damage from a previous heart attack, cardiomyopathy, or poor blood supply to the heart (myocardial ischemia).

Like the pacemaker, the technology for ICDs has improved. Today, most ICDs also have a pacemaker function. A subcutaneous ICD is the newest type. The pulse generator is implanted under the skin at the side of the chest below the armpit, but the lead is attached to an electrode that runs along the breastbone. Called an S-ICD, it is larger than a traditional ICD and doesn't attach to the heart.

Left Ventricular Assist Device

The left ventricular assist device (LVAD) is a pump that is implanted for patients whose hearts have become very weak (end-stage heart failure). The first LVAD was approved in 1994 as a way to keep someone with heart failure alive long enough to get a heart transplant. Because of the shortage of heart donors for transplant, LVADs are being used more and more as a bridge to a transplant.

We are now in the third generation of these pumps, and the technology has improved enough that an LVAD may be used to keep people alive who don't want or can't get a heart transplant. Recent statistics show that 80 to 85 percent of people living with an LVAD are still alive after one year, and 50 percent are still alive from five to 10 years without a heart transplant.

Unlike implanting a pacemaker or ICD, implanting an LVAD requires open-heart surgery and a stay in intensive care. During this surgery, a pump is placed inside or attached to the outside of the left ventricle. The pump takes over the ventricular pumping function. A tube from the pump comes out through the abdomen to attach to the pump's control device. A person must wear the pump strapped outside along with a battery and a backup battery to keep the pump going.

The newer LVADs are getting better and better, and some patients have survived up to 13 years. People who do receive a LVAD report improved breathing, the ability to resume the activities of daily living, better sleep, and the ability to enjoy leisure time with loved ones.

People with severe renal, pulmonary, liver, or neurological disease or evidence of advanced metastatic cancer cannot receive an LVAD.

CIED technology is keeping millions of people alive who would not have survived a generation ago. If past is prologue, we can expect to see more improvements and innovations in the coming years.

You Can Save a Life

Timothy M. Satty, MD, assistant professor of emergency medicine at Rutgers New Jersey Medical School and medical director of emergency medical services at University Hospital in Newark, New Jersey.

When 25-year-old Buffalo Bills football player Damar Hamlin went into cardiac arrest after a play on the field, his life was saved by the quick reaction of Denny Kellington, one of the team's assistant athletic trainers. Kellington stepped up and performed cardiopulmonary resuscitation (CPR) and used a defibrillator—on national television.

Everyone can and should learn CPR. While people of any age are susceptible to cardiac arrest, as people age and develop certain chronic conditions, their risk increases. So, knowing CPR can be a lifesaver for those close to you. Fully virtual first aid classes are available. However, taking an in-person class can give you a greater sense of confidence. You'll be able to feel the correct hand placement and the timing and depth of chest compressions. You'll also get familiar with how an automated external defibrillator (AED) works.

A portable defibrillator is extremely easy to use because it was designed for people without medical training. As soon as you open its case and press the start button, voice prompts walk you through every step. Inside you'll find self-sticking pads with pictures of exactly where to place them on the person's body. As soon as information is transmitted via electrodes in the pads and analyzed by the computer within the AED, you'll hear voice prompts to press a button to deliver an electrical shock, if needed, and when to pause and restart CPR.

CPR training doesn't take a lot of time. The American Heart Association and American Red Cross have courses that can be completed in a few hours, and there are many options available, making it easy to find a class that fits your schedule.

How to Know When Someone Needs CPR

A sudden collapse is the first sign of cardiac arrest. You're likely to also see that the person...

•**isn't breathing with normal, easy, and obvious breaths.** Be aware that people in cardiac arrest may sometimes gasp, have irregular snoring-like sounds, or have slow breaths at irregular intervals.

•**doesn't respond to their name.**

•**doesn't wake up or move** if you tap their shoulder.

Cardiac arrest might look like fainting. But when most people faint, they continue to breathe and will come around relatively quickly, often within seconds. That's not the case with cardiac arrest. Also, it's no longer suggested that bystanders try taking the person's pulse—you're in a high-adrenaline situation and this measurement can be unreliable.

Err on the side of caution: If someone collapses, it's better to start CPR and find out later if it wasn't needed rather than delay CPR and risk the person dying.

Important: Don't be reluctant to perform CPR on a woman. Studies have found that women in cardiac arrest are less likely to be given CPR by a bystander because the bystander feels awkward about placing their hands on a woman's chest or could be looked at suspiciously. But when someone, man or woman, is in cardiac arrest, there are no higher life-and-death stakes. Trying to save a life will never be viewed as inappropriate.

How Cardiac Arrest Is Treated

The American Heart Association highlights the importance of these crucial steps, done first by bystanders and then medical professionals, for saving the life of someone in cardiac arrest...

1. Recognize cardiac arrest and call 911.

 2. Initiate CPR, with an emphasis on chest compressions.

3. Quickly perform defibrillation with an AED when available.

4. Have emergency responders take over with advanced resuscitation.

5. Administer the right post-cardiac arrest care. Diagnostic tests will be done at the hospital to determine and treat the cause.

6. Deliver a comprehensive recovery plan, which may include additional treatment, needed rehab and emotional support.

Hypertension in Women Linked to Insomnia

Study titled "Sleeping Difficulties, Sleep Duration, and Risk of Hypertension in Women," by researchers at Brigham and Women's Hospital, Boston, published in *Hypertension*.

When we don't sleep well at night, we usually know it the next day. The American Academy of Sleep Medicine and the Sleep Research Society recommend seven or more hours of sleep per night on a regular basis for optimal health. But more people are getting less sleep, according to a new study from researchers at the Channing Division of Network Medicine at Brigham and Women's Hospital in Boston. And their long-term study found a significant increased risk of hypertension in women who sleep less than seven hours on most nights and in women who report symptoms of insomnia.

Insomnia Defined

According to the National Heart, Lung, and Blood Institute, symptoms of insomnia may include difficulty falling asleep, difficulty staying asleep, waking up too early, not being able to go back to sleep, or getting poor-quality sleep. It may also cause sleepiness during the day. The researchers were interested in the effects of long-term insomnia on blood pressure, which is insomnia lasting more than three months that occurs on three or more nights each week.

This specific research uses data from a long-running Harvard study called the Nurses' Health Study II. This ongoing study has been tracking health data in women nurses for decades. Included in the data are age, diet, lifestyles, physical activity, and blood pressure. In 2001, the study started collecting data on hours of sleep and symptoms of insomnia.

The research team notes that both hypertension and sleep problems are common in the United States. Thirty-five percent of adults do not get adequate sleep, 30 percent have symptoms of insomnia, and 45 percent are living with high blood pressure.

The study included over 66,000 women ages 25 to 42 and covered 16 years of data collection. None of the participants had high blood pressure at the start of the study. During the time of the study, just under 26,000 of the women were diagnosed with high blood pressure. *Key findings included...*

•**Women who regularly slept less than seven to eight hours** or had symptoms of insomnia were at higher risk for hypertension risk factors, including higher BMI, lower physical activity, poor diet, more likely to smoke or drink alcohol, and more likely to have gone through menopause during the study.

- **After adjusting for these other hypertension risk factors,** women who slept less than seven to eight hours still had a 10 percent higher risk of being diagnosed with hypertension.
- **Women who reported symptoms of insomnia** had a 14 percent higher risk of being diagnosed with hypertension.

Theories on Insomnia Link to Hypertension

Although the exact relationship between hypertension and sleep is not known, the researchers suspect that lack of sleep may cause increased sodium (salt) retention, stiffening of arterial blood vessel walls, and an increased workload for the heart. Disrupted sleep may also influence the control of constriction and relaxation of arteries, called vascular tone. Arteries are the blood vessels that carry blood away from the heart.

The researchers conclude that insomnia or too few hours of sleep is a significant risk factor and could be used as a reason for primary care doctors to screen patients for hypertension. This may help spot the condition before complications of long-term high blood pressure (such as heart failure and stroke) can develop. Although the current study included only women, they hope to continue their research with studies that include men.

Keep Your Blood Pressure Under Control

Gary Schwartz, MD, head of the hypertension section of the Division of Nephrology & Hypertension at Mayo Clinic in Rochester, Minnesota. He is author of *Mayo Clinic on High Blood Pressure: Your Personal Guide to Managing Hypertension.* MayoClinic.org

High blood pressure—we hear about it every day. Most of us know someone who has high blood pressure, or perhaps you have it yourself. That's not surprising since about half of all U.S. adults have high blood pressure, also known as hypertension.

What you may not know is how dangerous it is. High blood pressure is the single leading risk factor for mortality. In fact, it is the primary or a contributing cause of death for nearly 700,000 people in the U.S. every year, according to CDC estimates. It is a leading contributor to stroke and a range of cardiovascular problems and kidney disease…and it's a major risk factor for developing cognitive impairment. Scary stats, right?

But there is good news, says Mayo Clinic hypertension specialist Gary Schwartz, MD. High blood pressure is extremely preventable and treatable. Just making a few lifestyle changes could dramatically reduce your risk or help control an existing blood pressure problem. In fact, some hypertension self-care strategies are just as effective as medication. But even when drugs are needed, the ones that reduce blood pressure are effective, affordable, and generally very well-tolerated.

The Silent Killer

When people type "hypertension" into a search engine, they often encounter lists of symptoms that include severe headaches, chest pain, dizziness, difficulty breathing, nausea/vomiting, blurred vision, and more. You might conclude that if you don't have these symptoms—and you don't feel physical tension or pressure—you must not have high blood pressure. Don't believe it!

High blood pressure typically is completely asymptomatic—the symptoms listed for the condition generally appear only after hypertension is extremely advanced to very high levels or has caused serious damage to the heart, brain, or kidneys. Much of the harm from high blood pressure occurs before any symptoms appear.

Reality: There is only one reliable way for you to know if you have hypertension—

What Makes Your Blood Pressure Rise

Alcohol Increases Blood Pressure

An analysis of data involving more than 19,000 adults found a clear association between the number of alcoholic beverages consumed daily and increases in blood pressure. Systolic (top number) blood pressure rose 1.25 millimeters of mercury (mmHg) in people who consumed an average of 14 grams of alcohol per day (12 ounces of beer, 5 ounces of wine, or 1.5 ounces of spirits). People who drank an average of 48 grams of alcohol per day (approximately 3.5 servings) saw an average increase of 4.9 mmHg.

American Heart Association.

Road Noise Link to Hypertension

People who live near road traffic noise are more likely to develop hypertension. People who have high exposure to both traffic noise and air pollution had the highest hypertension risk, but noise alone increased risk independently.

American College of Cardiology.

---

have a health-care provider check. Smart watches and phone apps that monitor blood pressure may be useful—if one of these devices reports high blood pressure, it certainly is worth mentioning to your health-care provider. But these devices have not yet been extensively evaluated, so don't depend on their readings alone.

New Blood Pressure Targets

Recent research has led to a reevaluation of what constitutes healthy blood pressure. Historically health-care providers were likely to recommend treatment when systolic blood pressure (the top number) was above 140 and/or diastolic blood pressure was above 90. But the Systolic Blood Pressure Intervention Trial (SPRINT), a large-scale study funded by the National Institutes of Health, persuasively showed that mortality levels are significantly reduced when the lower targets of 130/80 are used instead.

Result: Hypertension treatment now is recommended for many patients who would not have been treated in the past... and the treatments they receive often are more aggressive.

Hypertension Self-Care

The best news is that we all have a substantial amount of control over our blood pressure. An Italian study concluded that genetics contribute only a relatively modest 30 percent of hypertension risk...the remaining 70 percent can be dramatically affected by lifestyle and diet decisions. *Among the self-care options to consider if you are diagnosed with hypertension or wish to avoid that diagnosis...*

• **Lose weight.** Being overweight roughly doubles risk for hypertension...and if you have hypertension, losing weight will lower your blood pressure.

• **Reduce salt consumption.** Multiple studies have identified a link between high salt consumption and high blood pressure. High-salt diets also can reduce the effectiveness of medications prescribed to lower blood pressure. Try to consume no more than 1,500 mg to 2,300 mg of sodium per day.

• **Increase potassium intake.** A recent study by University of Modena and Reggio Emilia, Modena, Italy, in *Journal of the American Heart Association* found that consumption of 3,500 mg to 5,000 mg per day of potassium helps lower the blood pressure of people who have hypertension. For reference, one average-sized banana has around 450 mg of potassium...one avocado, around 500 mg.

Studies also support the notion that a low-sodium, high-potassium diet reduces risk of developing hypertension. In societies that naturally consume such diets, which are rich in fresh fruits and vegetables, hypertension affects a much smaller percentage of the population, whereas in societies like ours that consume a diet high in sodium and low in potassium, almost 50 percent of the population develops hypertension.

Helpful: The Dietary Approaches to Stop Hypertension diet (DASH diet, for short) was created by the American Heart Association to help people who have high blood pressure determine what to eat. It works—studies have found that following this low-sodium, fruit-and-vegetable-rich diet reduces blood pressure as much as any single medication, even without weight loss. Type "DASH diet" into a search engine for details.

• **Engage in aerobic activity.** Many studies have found that aerobic exercise reduces blood pressure—try to get at least 150 minutes per week.

• **Limit alcohol intake.** The evidence is strong that excessive alcohol consumption increases risk for hypertension—and that includes the consumption of red wine, which has sometimes been portrayed as good for heart health. Men who have high blood pressure shouldn't consume more than two alcoholic drinks per day...women, no more than one per day.

• **Limit caffeine intake.** Consuming large quantities of coffee or other highly caffeinated beverages appears to increase blood pressure...at least temporarily. The evidence here is less certain than it is with alcohol, but if you have hypertension, limit yourself to no more than one to two cups of coffee or other caffeinated beverages per day.

• **Try respiratory strength training.** A study by researchers at University of Colorado found that using a "resistance breathing training device" for just 30 breaths a day for six weeks significantly lowers blood pressure. The inhaler-shaped device, which makes it harder to inhale, strengthens breathing muscles when used regularly. These devices are widely available for less than $100.

• **Keep stress under control.** While there is no evidence that stress is a direct cause of hypertension, it can trigger many things that have been found to increase blood pressure, including sleeplessness, overeating, and alcohol use. So using stress-control techniques such as mindfulness training or meditation could make it easier to keep your blood pressure under control.

When Medication Is Needed

Hypertension treatments are not difficult for patients—it is typically one pill once a day. The drug prescribed likely falls into one of three classes—diuretics... calcium channel blockers...or renin-angiotensin-aldosterone system (RAAS) inhibitors. Drugs in this class include *angiotensin-converting enzyme inhibitors* (ACEs) or *angiotensin receptor blockers* (ARBs). Their effectiveness varies from patient to patient for reasons that are still being researched. Affordable generic versions are available...and significant side effects are uncommon.

Patients should not be surprised if their health-care providers later prescribe additional medications—approximately 75 percent of high blood pressure patients respond better to a combination of drugs than to a single drug. But even then, it often is possible to take a single pill because drug companies make tablets that include common combinations of hypertension drugs. The combination pill usually consists of two of the drugs mentioned for single-drug treatment—for example, a diuretic plus a calcium channel blocker or ACE/ARB.

Some patients worry that taking high blood pressure medications could lead to orthostatic hypotension—where blood pressure drops suddenly when the patient stands up, causing dizziness and potentially falls. While orthostatic hypotension is a legitimate concern, health-care providers should test for this risk by taking the patient's blood pressure while he/she is seated and immediately after

Don't Put a Saltshaker on Your Table

According to a recent finding, people who regularly added salt to their food at the table had a 28 percent higher risk of dying before age 75 compared to those who never added salt. In fact, women who salted at the table had a 1.5-year lower life expectancy at age 50 than non-salters...life expectancy for men who salted at the table was 2.28 years lower. Excess sodium boosts risk for cancer, high blood pressure, and stroke.

Study of 501,379 adults led by researchers at Tulane University, New Orleans, published in *European Heart Journal*.

Cut Salt, Cut Blood Pressure

Northwestern Medicine.

Almost everyone can lower their blood pressure by lowering their sodium intake, even people currently on blood pressure-reducing drugs. A new study found that 70 to 75 percent of people who reduced their salt intake by about one teaspoon a day saw a decline in systolic blood pressure by about 6 millimeters of mercury (mmHg). That's as effective as taking medication.

standing. But this is not a reason to not treat hypertension.

New finding: A recent study by a team of researchers at institutions including Harvard Medical School found that intensive blood pressure–lowering treatment actually seems to decrease risk for orthostatic hypotension.

High Blood Pressure When Lying Down

Study of 11,369 adults by researchers at Harvard Medical School, Boston, presented at the Hypertension Scientific Sessions of the American Heart Association in Boston.

High blood pressure when lying down is linked to cardiac risk. Blood pressure usually is measured when you are seated.

Recent finding: People who had pressure above 130/80 mm Hg when seated and when lying down had 1.6 times the risk for coronary heart disease...1.83 times the risk for heart failure...1.86 times the risk for stroke...1.43 times the risk for premature death...and 2.18 times the risk of dying from coronary disease—compared with people who did not have high blood pressure in either position.

Also: People who had high blood pressure when lying down but not while seated had similar elevated risks to those with high blood pressure in both positions. Ask your doctor about taking your blood pressure in two different positions.

Is It Safe to Take Glucosamine If You Also Take a Diuretic?

Jack E. Fincham, PhD, RPh, interim department chair of clinical and administrative pharmacy, University of Georgia College of Pharmacy, Athens, Georgia.

Research indicates that diuretics, such as *chlorothiazide* (Diuril), that are used to treat high blood pressure do not work as well when you take glucosamine, a nutritional supplement used to treat osteoarthritis. It is important to tell your physician if you are taking glucosamine or are considering taking it. If glucosamine and a diuretic are taken together, an increased dose of the diuretic may be needed.

Heart and Stroke Health

Fluctuations in Cholesterol Increase Dementia Risk

Christopher Weber, PhD, director of global science initiatives at the Alzheimer's Association in Chicago, commenting on a study published in *Neurology*.

According to a recent finding, adults whose cholesterol levels moved up or down the most over five years were 19 percent more likely to develop Alzheimer's or a related dementia within 12 years. Fluctuating triglyceride levels in particular boosted risk by 23 percent.

Self-defense: Know your heart-health numbers...get treatment when you need it...live a heart- and brain-healthy lifestyle (for more on that, see page 37).

Another Statin Alternative Proves Effective

Jamal S. Rana, MD, chief of cardiology at Kaiser Permanente Oakland Medical Center in Oakland, California, commenting on a study published in *The New England Journal of Medicine*.

The drug *bempedoic acid* was approved several years ago for lowering LDL ("bad") cholesterol but lacked long-term efficacy data.

Recent finding: Bempedoic acid lowers cholesterol and significantly reduces cardiovascular events compared with a placebo without any increase in muscle aches.

Downside: It increases gout risk. The drug is best for people who have tried multiple statins and dosages and discontinued them due to body aches.

Weight-Loss Drug Improves Cardio Outcomes

Michael Lincoff, MD, professor of medicine at Cleveland Clinic and lead author of a study of 17,604 adults published in *The New England Journal of Medicine*. The study was sponsored by Novo Nordisk, manufacturer of Ozempic and Wegovy.

Overweight or obese non-diabetic patients with cardiovascular disease who took *semaglutide* (Ozempic, Wegovy) had a 20 percent combined reduced risk for heart attack, stroke and cardiovascular death. This adds semaglutide to statins and blood pressure medications as another mechanism that can reduce cardio risk.

Shingles and Your Heart

Paul Goepfert, MD, director of the Alabama Vaccine Research Clinic and professor of infectious diseases at the University of Alabama at Birmingham Marnix E. Heersink School of Medicine.

Shingles causes excruciating, disabling, burning pain that may last for weeks, months, or years. A new study from Harvard researchers shows that it also increases the risk for a heart attack or stroke. The study, published in the *Journal of the American Heart Association*, found a 30 percent increased risk. Called cardiovascular events, these heart attacks and strokes were most likely to occur five to 12 years after shingles.

One in three people over age 50 can expect to get shingles. In view of these findings, the researchers strongly encourage people to get the new vaccine to prevent the misery of shingles and the increased risk of a heart attack or stroke. According to the Centers for Disease Control and Prevention, the vaccine is 97 percent effective in adults ages 50 to 70.

What Is Shingles?

If you've ever had chickenpox, the varicella zoster virus is already in your body. (If you were born before 1979, there is more than a 99 percent chance that you did.) After the chickenpox infection subsides, the virus hibernates in the roots of the nerve cells that supply feeling to your skin. For a variety of reasons, that virus can be reactivated later in life. Possible causes are stress, a long illness, cancer, diabetes, or taking any medication that weakens the immune system. It then travels down the nerve to the skin and causes the painful rash that is shingles.

The rash will appear in the area supplied by the nerve root, usually on one side of the body in the area of your face, neck, chest, or torso. It is extremely painful and lasts for up to four weeks.

How Was the Study Done?

The research team used three long-term, ongoing studies to track how often a stroke, heart attack, or procedure to clear a blocked heart artery (revascularization) occurred after a shingles infection. In these studies, adults between the ages of 25 and 75 have been filling out questionnaires every two years, reporting all their health information.

The studies started between 1976 and 1989 and included about 174,000 women (and 30,000 men). The research team compared cardiovascular events between people who had shingles before the cardiovascular event and those who never had shingles. These were the key findings...

- **There was a 38 percent increased risk of a stroke** five to eight years after shingles, and a 28 percent risk at nine to 12 years.

- **There was a 16 percent increased risk of a heart attack or revascularization** procedures five to eight years after shingles, and a 25 percent risk at nine to 12 years.

The cause of these cardiovascular events is likely inflammation of the large and small blood vessels supplying the heart and the brain. This inflammation, called vasculopathy, slows down blood supply through these blood vessels and may cause a blocked vessel, resulting in stroke or heart attack. Viral inflammation of blood vessels is not only seen in herpes virus, but it also occurs in COVID and other viral infections.

Troubled Vaccine History

Despite the pain and other risks of shingles, less than 50 percent of people over age 60 are getting vaccinated, according to the CDC.

Part of the problem is the old shingles vaccine, Zostavax, which was made from a live virus. It was not very effective and, because it was a live virus, it could cause shingles in people with weak immune systems or chickenpox in unvaccinated babies. It was only about 50 percent effective for people over age 50 and got less effective with age. Zostavax is no longer available in the United States.

An Improved Vaccine

Shingrix, the new vaccine, is an *attenuated* virus, meaning it is made from pieces of the shingles virus. It is approved for adults ages 50 and older. It is also approved for people with a weak immune system, starting at age 19. For adults ages 50 to 69, Shingrix is 97 percent effective. It continues to be over 90 percent effective in people ages 70 and older. Protection lasts for about seven years. Shingrix is given in two injections two to six months apart.

If you already had shingles, you should still get the vaccine because shingles can

> **Other Risks from Shingles**
>
> The most common complication after shingles is *postherpetic neuralgia* (PHN), or severe pain that can last for months, years, or longer.
>
> If you have shingles in the nerve that supplies the face (the facial nerve), you may have facial paralysis, loss of hearing, and dizziness.
>
> If the branch of the facial nerve that goes to the eye is affected, you may have inflammation and damage to the eye resulting in blurred vision. Another common complication is skin bacteria infecting the rash.

come back. The risks and pain of shingles far outweigh any concerns about the new vaccine. Getting the new vaccine should be an obvious choice.

Biologic Therapy for Psoriasis May Reduce Heart Disease

Duke Medicine.

Patients who have psoriasis that is treated with biologic therapy had a significant reduction in high-risk plaque in their heart arteries over a one-year period, according to research from the National Heart, Lung, and Blood Institute. The analysis involved 209 patients ages 37 to 62 with psoriasis. Of these participants, 124 received biologic therapy, and 85 were treated with topical creams and light therapy. The researchers performed cardiac computed tomography (CT) scans on all participants before they started therapy and one year later. After one year of treatment, biologic therapy was associated with an 8 percent reduction in coronary plaque. In contrast, people who did not receive biologic therapy experienced slightly increased coronary plaque progression.

The Cardiovascular Risks of Psoriasis

Nehal N. Mehta, MD, MSCE, the inaugural NIH Lasker Clinical Research Scholar, clinical professor of medicine at George Washington University, and clinical adjunct professor of vascular medicine at the University of Pennsylvania.

The first thing you notice about psoriasis is the telltale skin rash, but the effects of this autoimmune disease are far from being only skin deep. Psoriasis has body-wide effects that can put your overall health at risk in many ways. Chief among them is cardiovascular disease (CVD). Here's what you need to know and how you can protect yourself.

The Psoriasis-CVD Link

Though psoriasis was first identified in the 1800s, its effect on the cardiovascular system is a relatively recent discovery. While scientists suspected a link between psoriasis and CVD, proof came from studies using advanced imaging tests that detected vascular inflammation, the starting point for the kind of plaque that develops along artery walls. Think of it this way: Angry plaques on the outside represent systemic inflammation on the inside.

CVD includes heart disease, heart attack, and stroke. There is emerging evidence that psoriasis can also increase the risk of heart failure, peripheral artery disease (PAD), heart valve problems, and atrial fibrillation. What's more, the more severe your psoriasis, the more severe—and the more accelerated—your CVD risk. Research by Nehal Mehta, MD, has found that these health problems start to develop as early as one's 40s, a decade sooner than they do in people without psoriasis.

There is also a convincing body of evidence that chronic inflammation in the skin can increase the risk for metabolic syndrome, a condition characterized by high blood pressure, high blood sugar, and belly fat. All are independent, additional risk factors for heart disease. It's worth noting that psoriasis has also been linked to depression, inflammatory bowel disease, and even certain cancers. In view of this, other inflammatory diseases, such as atopic dermatitis, are now also being recognized as whole-body diseases.

By the Numbers

Compared with people without psoriasis, those with severe psoriasis and its complication psoriatic arthritis have a 1.5 to two times higher risk of heart attack and 1.5 times higher risk of stroke, PAD, and other forms of CVD.

Severe psoriasis is when just 10 percent of your skin surface has plaques. The palm of your hand is a good visual representation of 1 percent. Up to 3 percent is considered mild and between 3 and 10 percent is moderate. That being said, recent research suggests that even one skin plaque might be enough to drive inflammation.

The good news? Treating psoriasis helps: Clear the plaques on your skin and you can limit the plaque in your arteries.

Get Treated for Psoriasis

If you have (or suspect you have) psoriasis but haven't seen a doctor, your first step is to be evaluated and treated, if needed. Many people still don't appreciate that psoriasis is more than cosmetic. Nearly three-fourths of patients with severe psoriasis are untreated or undertreated and, in turn, underdiagnosed for cardiovascular risk factors.

Psoriasis treatment is based on severity and usually starts with a topical medication, if mild, or methotrexate, if moderate. Stronger psoriasis drugs, such as a TNF inhibitor and doctor-directed UVB phototherapy, improve psoriasis and also have profound impacts on inflammation in the blood, which should improve cardiovascular risk over time. TNF inhibitors may also improve insulin sensitivity and lower your diabetes risk. Phototherapy has also been shown to improve good cholesterol levels.

Get Screened for CVD Risks

If you've been diagnosed with psoriasis but haven't been evaluated for CVD risk factors, get screened and get appropriate treatment. You may need to advocate for yourself: Encourage your health-care provider to consider psoriasis as the equivalent of diabetes when calculating your 10-year CVD risk.

After more than a decade of work by Dr. Mehta's team and others, a 2018 American College of Cardiology (ACC)/American Heart Association (AHA) guideline recognized psoriasis as a driver of inflammation and an independent risk factor for CVD for people with an intermediate 10-year risk.

In particular, you want to be checked for the "3 Bs"…

- **Blood pressure.** High blood pressure must be taken seriously. Research shows that despite having higher risks for cardiovascular diseases overall, people with psoriasis are less likely to have their blood pressure adequately controlled.

- **Blood tests.** Both high cholesterol and high blood glucose need to be managed. The ACC/AHA guideline states that having psoriasis warrants the early initiation of a statin for adults ages 40 to 75 without diabetes and 10-year intermediate risk of CVD.

- **Body mass index.** Obesity drives CVD and diabetes. Separately, psoriasis is often worse in people who are overweight.

Your goals for the three Bs may be stricter than for someone without psoriasis to help mitigate their effects.

The underlying message is that you can clear your psoriasis and protect your heart health in the process.

Cardiac Stents Work for Stable Angina

Study titled "A Placebo-Controlled Trial of Percutaneous Coronary Intervention for Stable Angina," led by researchers at Imperial College London, published in *The New England Journal of Medicine* and presented at the American Heart Association Annual Meeting 2023.

Although heart disease is still the most common cause of death for Americans, deaths from heart attacks have been going down. According to the Centers for Disease Control and Prevention, heart attack deaths have decreased by more than four percent per year over the last 20 years. One major reason for the drop is angioplasty, or *percutaneous coronary intervention* (PCI). In almost all cases of PCI, a cardiac stent is placed into a narrowed coronary artery to help prevent or survive a heart attack.

A new study presented at the 2023 meeting of the American Heart Association, and published in *The New England Journal of Medicine,* finds that PCI can also benefit people with chest pain from coronary artery disease but no immediate danger of heart attack, called stable angina. The main symptom of stable angina is chest pain when you exert yourself, which is relieved by rest or medication. Based on previous research, guidelines have suggested that cardiac stent placement does not offer more benefits than medications for stable angina.

One of the main studies used for the current guidelines is the 2017 Objective Randomized Blinded Investigation with Optimal Medical Therapy of Angioplasty in Stable Angina (ORBITA) trial. Many cardiologists have suspected that the first ORBITA trial did not have enough patients and did not last long enough, and that there are, in fact, benefits from stenting for stable angina. That was the hypothesis of the research team participating in the new trial, called ORBITA-2.

New Trial Could Revamp Previous Guidelines

ORBITA 2 included 301 patients with stable angina. Most of the patients were average age 64. As with the first ORBITA study, the patients were randomly assigned to receive a cardiac stent or a simulated procedure that did not include a stent (the control group). The study was double blind, which means neither the patients nor their doctors knew which patients received the stents.

All the patients were taken off their chest pain medications before the study started. After the procedures, their doctors put them back on medication as needed, and the patients recorded daily chest pain scores using smartphone technology. These were the key results for patients who had stents as compared to the placebo/control patients...

- **They were three times more likely to be free of angina.**
- **They were less likely to require chest pain medication.**
- **They had improved exercise tolerance.**

All these benefits started immediately after the procedure and were sustained through the 12-week follow-up part of the study.

Stents for Unstable and Stable Angina

Until now, there has been controversy about the benefits of PCI and stent placement for patients with stable angina. Stent placement for these patients has been considered unnecessary in many cases. Stent placement is not controversial for people with unstable angina or for those having a heart attack. Unstable angina causes pain that is sudden, severe, and not relieved by rest or controlled by medication.

The researchers conclude that PCI and stent placement to control stable angina symptoms should be an option based on the risk benefit profile of an individual patient. Current European and American guidelines may require updating.

Close to one million stents are placed in the U.S. every year to open a blocked heart artery and restore blood flow to the heart. Unstable angina or heart attack symptoms require a 911 call—individuals should not try to drive to the hospital. In these cases, PCI may save your life or save your heart from serious damage.

Cognitive Decline Is Common After Bypass

David Sherer, MD, a patient advocate and author of *Hospital Survival Guide* and *What Your Doctor Won't Tell You*. DrDavidSherer.com

Up to 42 percent of heart-bypass patients experience deficits to attention span, memory, speech, and thinking, which usually resolve in a few months. The cause is not known—a possible culprit is mini-blockages in the bloodstream that damage the brain. Before surgery, ask what techniques your surgical team will use to filter the blood… and whether patients have experienced cognitive problems after their bypass.

Ablation Protects the Brain

Bahadar Singh Srichawla, DO, MS, of the University of Massachusetts Chan Medical School in Worcester.

Radiofrequency catheter ablation is more brain protective than drugs for atrial fibrillation. In the SAGE-AF study, the odds of developing cognitive impairment over two years were 36 percent lower among patients who had undergone ablation. Different oral medications did not yield significantly different results. The mean age of study participants was 75.

Essential Activities for Post-Stroke Recovery

Joel Stein, MD, professor and chair of the department of rehabilitation medicine at Weill Cornell Medicine and physiatrist in chief at NewYork-Presbyterian Hospital.

Stroke affects each person in different ways, so recovery must be individualized. But one constant is that recovery steps should be started as soon as possible so the brain can begin to adapt and, to some degree, repair itself. The adult brain can't regrow damaged areas, but thanks to brain plasticity, it can repurpose other parts to take on tasks that were previously handled by damaged sections.

Post-Stroke Rehabilitation

Numerous studies have shown that stroke rehabilitation programs lead to the best outcomes. In general, stroke rehab has three main areas of focus: occupational therapy, physical therapy, and speech therapy. How much time a person spends on each depends on how the stroke affected him or her.

Even people who experience a mild stroke should be carefully evaluated by members of their hospital's stroke rehab team, not just the attending doctor or hospitalist, to map out the best course of action. That team might include a physiatrist, a doctor who specializes in rehabilitation; a neurologist who specializes in stroke care; a physical therapist who will work on movement; an occupational therapist who will work on everyday activities, such as getting dressed and eating; a speech therapist who will work on speech and comprehension problems as well as any swallowing difficulty; and possibly a psychologist.

Some people are able to go home directly from the hospital after a few days and start rehab. Some stay in acute care in the hospital for a week or longer, depending on the severity of the stroke, and then

Your Gut and Sleep Patterns Affect Stroke Risk

Inflammatory Bowel Disease (IBD) Increases Stroke Risk

Study participants with IBD had 13 percent greater risk for stroke than the general population. Risk was highest among those with Crohn's disease and with IBD not classified as a particular subtype. Risk was stronger for ischemic stroke (caused by a blockage) than for hemorrhagic (caused by bleeding). IBD's inflammation may damage blood vessel linings, making plaque more likely to cause a blockage.

Jeffrey Berinstein, MD, a gastroenterologist at University of Michigan in Ann Arbor commenting on a study published in *Neurology*.

Insomnia Increases Stroke Risk

A recent study showed that persistent insomnia is associated with a higher risk for stroke—51 percent higher for severe insomnia and 16 percent for those whose insomnia was less severe. The link is strongest for people under age 50. Hypertension, depression, and cardiovascular disease exacerbate the association, but insomnia appears to be an independent risk factor.

Wendemi Sawadogo, MD, MPH, PhD, an epidemiologist at Virginia Commonwealth University, Richmond, and coauthor of a study of 31,000 adults published in *Neurology*.

---

transition to an inpatient rehabilitation unit in the same hospital, a separate rehabilitation hospital, or a skilled nursing facility (also called a subacute rehabilitation program). Once a person is strong enough to go home, they might have home care and then go to outpatient therapy two or three times a week.

The duration of formal stroke rehab varies from weeks to months. Improvement is based on the patient's involvement: You have to do your homework to get all the benefits. You're getting only an hour or less with a physical therapist three times a week. That leaves a large chunk of time where you need to work on your own.

Essential Post-Stroke Activities

Weakness is the most widely known effect of stroke, and exercise is our number-one treatment. A recent study published in *JAMA Network Open* showed just how pivotal physical activity is to successful recovery. The researchers found that people who spent four hours a week exercising after their stroke doubled their chances of a good functional outcome when evaluated after six months.

• **Walking.** Stroke-recovery exercise is different from exercise you'd do at a gym. Walking helps you regain balance and endurance and gets you back in the community. Your physical therapist will also work with you on other aspects of physical rehab, such as range-of-motion and specific motor-skills exercises.

• **Upper body.** For the upper body, focus on doing occupational activities. That might involve opening and closing a drawer and feeding yourself or simply moving the affected arm if that's all you can do at first. Stimulating the recovery of the affected limb is critically important.

• **Cognition and communication.** Other activities address cognitive and communication issues, such as speech disorders and aphasia (difficulty reading, writing, and expressing and understanding language). You may have a hard time focusing your attention or seeing on the left side if you had a stroke affecting the right side of the brain. Outside of formal therapy with a speech therapist, it will help to practice with family members and loved ones.

• **Socializing.** An activity that's often neglected, but that can have a huge impact on recovery, is socializing—spending time in a socially engaged and stimulating environment. More than doing crossword puzzles, Wordle, and Sudoku, you want to engage your mind by chatting with friends and family. Keeping up your end of a conversation uses your brain cognitively. Social engagement also helps with the depression and anxiety that many people feel after a stroke.

If you have barriers to socialization—maybe loved ones live far away or you're homebound, seek out a stroke support group. This is a great way to start connecting with others, sharing best practices, and regaining your self-confidence.

The Plateau Myth

There's a misconception (fueled by some studies) that people reach a plateau after three to six months of rehab. We now know that intense therapy done even a year after a stroke brings results. Most people still have untapped capacity for improvement. Though insurance may cover only a certain number of months of therapy, you can keep challenging yourself. There's no clock ticker that goes off at the three- or six-month mark.

Keep at your post-stroke activities and you'll achieve more than you think. Remember that the brain needs consistent stimulation over time to rewire itself.

Radon Exposure May Increase Stroke Risk in Women

Study titled "Radon Exposure and Incident Stroke Risk in the Women's Health Initiative," by researchers at Brown University, Providence, Rhode Island, published in *Neurology*.

Radon is an odorless and invisible gas. If you breathe in high levels of radon over several years, you may be at higher risk for lung cancer, especially if you smoke. Radon exposure is thought to be the second leading cause of lung cancer after smoking. It may be responsible for about 20,000 deaths from lung cancer in the United States every year.

Get the Care You Need

A 2023 UCLA study found that many patients are missing out on stroke rehab or simply not getting enough, possibly because of logistical barriers, such as not being able to get to a therapy center. If you don't have a caregiver to drive you to outpatient therapy, you may be eligible for free transportation, short-term home care, or telemedicine. It's never too late to contact your physiatrist or to tell your primary doctor that you're not where you want to be and ask for a referral to a rehab physician who can quarterback a program for you.

Radon's Link to Stroke

Stroke, which is a decreased blood supply to the brain, occurs in about 800,000 people every year in the U.S. and is the cause of death in about 140,000. A new study from Brown University has found that radon exposure may be a significant stroke risk. The study is published in the American Academy of Neurology journal *Neurology*.

Researchers took data from a long running study on women's health called the Women's Health Initiative (WHI). The WHI was started in 1991 by the National Institutes of Health (NIH), and is expected to continue through 2026. The purpose of WHI is to collect heath data that may help improve the health of postmenopausal women.

The research team gathered information on stroke occurrence and matched that data with Environmental Protection Agency (EPA) and U.S. Geological Survey data on areas of the country reporting the highest and lowest level of indoor radon. Radon can get into a home through basements, wells, and ground water. Radon gas is measured in picocuries (pCi). The EPA recommends radon home treatment (called radon mitigation) to lower radon gas if the level of radon measures more than 4 pCi per liter of air.

The team divided the radon measurements into high (greater than 4 pCi), intermediate (2 to 4 pCi), and low (less than 2 pCi). The study included close to 160,000 postmenopausal women. They were followed from 1993 through 2020. The average age was 63 at the start, and the average amount of time followed was 13 years. None of the women had any history of stroke at the start. *These were the key results...*

• During the study period there were about 7,000 strokes.

• After adjusting for other stroke risk factors, women living in areas with the highest reported radon levels were 14 percent more likely to be diagnosed with stroke than those in the lowest radon areas.

• Women living in areas of the country with intermediate levels were 6 percent more likely to be diagnosed with stroke than in the lowest radon areas.

Radon Levels Need to Be Lowered to Stop Strokes

This study shows an association between radon exposure and stroke, but it does not prove that radon causes strokes. However, if other studies support these findings, researchers suggest lowering the current EPA remediation recommendation to 2 pCi. The current recommendation of 4 pCi was based on lung cancer studies. This new study suggests that levels above 2 pCi may be too high.

Radon gas dissipates quickly with ventilation. It tends to gather in poorly ventilated areas, such as basements. The EPA estimates that one in 15 U.S. homes test positive for radon gas. Homes and other living areas should be tested with a radon gas kit or by professional mitigation expert. Mitigation procedures are very successful and may include fixing cracks or leaks, blowing air through the area (ventilation), and covering exposed concrete or ground in basements or crawl spaces with plastic.

A-fib Affects Your Cognitive Health Even Without a Stroke

Ijeoma Ekeruo, MD, associate professor of cardiology at McGovern Medical School, UTHealth Houston. Med.UTH.edu

A-fib can contribute to cognitive impairment even without stroke. The link between atrial fibrillation (rapid, erratic heartbeat) and stroke risk is well established.

Recent finding: A-fib patients may be at greater risk of developing reasoning and memory problems even if they did not have a stroke. This could be due to micro-clotting or blood deprivation in the brain.

If you have A-fib: Fix your diet and exercise habits, address sleep problems, and talk to your doctors about the best ways to preserve cognition.

What You Can Do to Reduce Risk of Heart Disease

Study titled "Global Effect of Modifiable Risk Factors on Cardiovascular Disease and Mortality," by researchers with The Global Cardiovascular Risk Consortium, published in *The New England Journal of Medicine.*

An international panel of medical experts and researchers have combined efforts to determine what humans worldwide can do to stop the plight of heart disease. The Global Cardiovascular Risk Consortium has produced a study on how five major modifiable risk factors increase the risk of cardiovascular disease (CVD) and death from CVD or other causes.

In what may be one of the largest studies on CVD risk, the consortium pooled data from 112 studies in 34 countries. These studies included 1.5 million people from eight global geographic regions. None of the participants had been diagnosed with CVD at the start of the study. All the participants had available data on five major CVD risk factors: body mass index (BMI), blood pressure, cholesterol, diabetes, and smoking status.

Most Deaths from Heart Disease Are Preventable

According to the World Health Organization (WHO), CVD is the leading cause of death globally, but most of these deaths could be prevented by managing modifiable risk factors. CVD diseases include heart disease, peripheral arterial disease, blood clots, and stroke. Major risk factors may be the result of unhealthy diet and physical inactivity, which shows up as high blood pressure, high cholesterol, high blood sugar, and obesity.

The results of the study are published in *The New England Journal of Medicine*. The 1.5 million participants were about equally divided between male and female with a mean age between 54 and 55. During the study, about 80,600 people were diagnosed with CVD, and 177,400 died of any cause. According to the WHO, other than communicable diseases, CVD causes about 40 percent of premature deaths, which is death under age 70.

For participants who had all five risk factors, the 10-year incidence of CVD was just over 57 percent for women and almost 53 percent for men. The incidence of premature death from any cause was just over 22 percent for women and 19 percent for men.

High Blood Pressure Kills

The researchers also broke down the CVD risk by each risk factor alone. The highest risk was an elevated systolic blood pressure (the top number). For high systolic blood pressure, the 10-year incidence of CVD was about 29 percent for women and just under 22 percent for men. *For the other individual risk factors, the results were...*

• **High bad cholesterol.** About 15 percent for women and 17 percent for men.

• **Diabetes.** About 15 percent for women and 10 percent for men.

• **Current smoker.** About 15 percent for women and 10 percent for men.

• **High body mass index (obesity).** About 8 percent for men and women.

Among the important associations found in this study was that elevated blood pressure was the largest contributor to CVD risk, confirming the current guidelines to keep the systolic blood pressure (the top number in a blood pressure reading, which measures the pressure in your arteries when your heart beats) at less than 120. Good blood pressure control may offer the greatest potential for risk reduction. The authors note that other modifiable risk factors that could be considered for future studies include physical activity, alcohol consumption, air pollution, climate and noise exposure, education level, depression, mental health, and/or social health issues.

Chapter 9

INFECTIOUS DISEASE

Pneumonia: Prevention Is Your Top Priority

Pneumonia can happen any time—not just during the cold months. And since it can become very serious, even life-threatening, prevention should be your top priority, especially if you're immunocompromised... have long-term health issues...or are over age 65. *We asked infectious disease specialist William Schaffner, MD, what you need to know and how to protect your health...*

•**There is more than one type.** People most often contract pneumonia through exposure to a strain of the pneumococcal bacteria *Streptococcus pneumoniae.*

Secondary pneumonia can develop as a complication of a viral infection.

How this happens: We all carry some bacteria in our throat all the time. Those bacteria come and go, but if you get the flu, for instance, that virus can irritate the throat down to the bronchial tubes—paving the way for the normal bacteria to become more active, move down into the lungs, and cause pneumonia.

Walking pneumonia is community-acquired—you contract it during your normal life. Typically, you walk into your doctor's office feeling awful...he/she diagnoses pneumonia...and you walk out with a prescription for antibiotics. If promptly diagnosed and treated, most people can recuperate at home.

Health-care–associated pneumonia is acquired during or after a stay in a health-care setting, such as the hospital or a long-term-care facility, and often is more antibiotic-resistant.

•**Pneumonia can be prevented.** Some of us are more susceptible to pneumonia—adults age 65 or older...children under age five...anyone with a long-term health issue or a weak immune system...and people who smoke. Prevention, always better than needing treatment, requires a two-pronged approach—a healthy lifestyle and the right vaccines.

•**Vaccines.** The Centers for Disease Control and Prevention (CDC) recommends pneumococcal vaccinations for all adults age

---

William Schaffner, MD, infectious disease specialist, researcher with more than 400 papers to his credit, and professor of preventive medicine in the department of health policy and professor of medicine in the division of infectious diseases at Vanderbilt University Medical Center, Nashville. His work has focused on all aspects of infectious diseases, including epidemiology, infection control, and immunization. VUMC.org

Infectious Disease

65 or older, for children under age five, and for people between those ages with certain underlying medical conditions, including diabetes, heart disease, and lung disease.

There are three different vaccines available, some more appropriate for certain people than others. They are the pneumococcal polysaccharide vaccine *PPSV23*... and the pneumococcal conjugate vaccines *PCV15* (followed a year later by *PPSV23*) and *PCV20*. The numbers indicate how many strains, or serotypes, of Streptococcus pneumoniae are included in the vaccine. The formulas of pneumococcal conjugate vaccines (which use a protein to carry the different serotypes) differ from the polysaccharide vaccine (which uses polysaccharides, or chains of complex sugars, to carry the vaccine).

Which vaccine should you get?

If you have never been vaccinated for pneumonia, the newer PCV20 is the top choice—it covers the 20 most common serotypes now.

If that vaccine is not available in your area, you can get the PCV15 vaccine, followed one year later by PPSV23.

If you had the earlier PCV13 (but not PCV 15), you're likely eligible to get the PCV20 for increased protection.

Best: Because of all the possibilities, talk to your doctor about the most effective approach for you.

Side effects include feeling achy and tired as well as redness, swelling, and soreness at the injection site. If you experience any side effect, ask your provider if it's safe for you to take a pain-relief medication such as acetaminophen.

•**You still need other vaccines.** To avoid getting pneumonia as a consequence of a viral infection, protect yourself with the following vaccines...

•**Flu vaccine.** Each year, the flu vaccine targets the strains projected to be most common. It can reduce risk for illness by 40 percent to 60 percent.

•**Respiratory syncytial virus (RSV) vaccine.** This new vaccine was approved for people age 60 and older (it's now being studied for other age groups including infants). It reduces risk for a lower respiratory tract infection by about 85 percent. If you're not yet 60 but have an underlying chronic heart or lung condition, ask your doctor if you are a candidate for the RSV vaccine.

Note: This off-label use may not be covered by insurance (cost about $300). As of now, only one dose is being recommended.

Possible side effects: There were some "signals" about neuroinflammatory illnesses and atrial fibrillation associated with the RSV vaccine, but the risk is very low.

•**COVID-19 vaccine and boosters.** SARS-CoV-2, the virus that causes COVID-19, can make you vulnerable to secondary pneumonia. The COVID vaccine for the 2023-2024 season had an efficacy rate of up to 95 percent for preventing symptomatic and serious illness. Annual updated vaccines likely will be needed indefinitely to maintain that level of protection.

While vaccines cannot prevent every case of pneumonia (or the other conditions they're given for), people who are vaccinated usually have milder infections, a shorter course of illness, and fewer serious complications than people who don't get vaccinated. The flu, RSV, and COVID booster shots all can be given simultaneously.

•**The same steps to avoid viruses will help you avoid pneumonia.** *Stay away from people who are sick and...*

   •Regularly wash your hands with soap and water.

   •Regularly disinfect common surfaces at home and at work.

   •Keep chronic medical conditions under control, including asthma, high blood pressure, and diabetes.

   •Maintain overall good health and a strong immune system through regular exercise and healthy eating.

   •Don't smoke. Smoking inhibits your lungs from doing their key job—filtering out germs to keep you healthy.

Signs You Have Pneumonia

Despite your best intentions, it still is possible to get pneumonia. Signs of pneumonia that require immediate attention include difficulty breathing or shortness of breath…chest pain when you breathe or cough…coughing with or without mucus (sputum). You may also have classic flu-like symptoms, such as fever and chills, headache, muscle pain, fatigue, nausea and/or vomiting, and diarrhea. If you're an older adult or have a serious illness or a weakened immune system, your symptoms could include a lower-than-normal temperature and feeling weak or confused.

Getting Rid of It

- **Antibiotics.** Most people feel better after one to three days, but take the full course prescribed along with any other medications. Let your doctor know if your symptoms don't improve—you may need a different antibiotic.
- **Pain relievers.** *Acetaminophen* (Tylenol) can help with achiness.
- **Fluids.** Stay hydrated.

Important: Unless your cough prevents you from sleeping, avoid cough suppressants so your body can bring up and eliminate sputum.

For a severe case of pneumonia: You may need treatment in a hospital, where you can get antibiotics and fluids intravenously along with supplemental oxygen.

Painkillers Can Make Infections Last Longer

Daniel Barreda, PhD, professor of immunology, University of Alberta, Canada, and lead author of the study "Fever Integrates Antimicrobial Defences, Inflammation Control, and Tissue Repair in a Cold-Blooded Vertebrate," published in *Immunology and Inflammation.* UAlberta.ca

Opting to run a mild fever rather than control it with painkillers likely reduces the time it takes for your immune system to clear pathogens, decrease inflammation, and heal tissue damage, according to new research.

There has been debate in the medical community for decades about whether running a fever is good or bad for us. It's a surprisingly tricky question to investigate because the inflammation response occurs automatically in warm-blooded animals such as humans.

A team of researchers at University of Alberta and Emory University overcame this challenge by examining fever in cold-blooded teleost fish. Cold-blooded creatures' bodies cannot raise their own temperatures, so when faced with infection, they create "fever" by moving to warmer locations. Researchers discovered that fish that were allowed to swim to warm waters when given bacterial infections—the fish equivalent of running a fever—were able to clear those infections in half the time that fish restricted to static water temperatures cleared the same infections. Fever likely offers a comparable immune system boost to humans.

What to do: When you come down with an infection that is accompanied by a mild-to-moderate fever, think through the trade-off before popping a painkiller.

If your symptoms are mild, the painkiller —either acetaminophen or a non-steroidal anti-inflammatory—might help you feel more comfortable in the short term…but it also might take longer for your health to get back to 100 percent. A painkiller might be worthwhile if you're in significant discomfort or are running a fever above 102°F.

Shingles Vaccine Reduces Dementia Risk

Pascal Geldsetzer, MD, assistant professor of medicine at Stanford University, California, and senior author of a study of 300,000 adults that appeared pre–peer review at MedRxiv.org.

According to a recent study, the shingles vaccination was causally linked to a near-

Infectious Disease

ly 20 percent lower risk for dementia diagnosis within seven years, an effect seen most strongly among women. Since only the Zostavax vaccine was studied, research needs to be done to determine whether the newer Shingrix shot appears equally protective.

COVID-Negative Long Haulers

Igor Koralnik, MD, chief of neuroinfectious diseases and global neurology at Northwestern Medicine.

While the pandemic is largely behind us, millions of people are still experiencing long-lasting chronic pain, brain fog, shortness of breath, chest pain, and intense fatigue. Those who had tested positive for SARS-CoV-2 infection could seek care at post-COVID clinics, but many more people with the same symptoms never received a positive test or treatment for this often-debilitating condition. Many couldn't even get in to a COVID clinic.

Hidden COVID

Researchers at Northwestern Medicine now know than many of the people who initially tested negative for COVID-19 were exposed to the virus after all. By using very sensitive immunologic assays, researchers found that 41 percent of people with long COVID who initially tested negative for COVID-19 have antibody or T-cell responses to the virus, which show that they were infected.

The other 59 percent of people who have long-haul symptoms, but who still test negative, are indistinguishable clinically from those with detectable response, Igor Koralnik, MD, chief of neuroinfectious diseases and global neurology at Northwestern Medicine, told us.

"We call them post-viral syndrome patients, and we care for them similarly to those with a positive test." (There are some similarities between long COVID and chronic fatigue syndrome, but long COVID has distinct characteristics.)

In the study, 93 percent of the people who had initially tested negative were women. "All post-COVID clinics in the United States that I know of have seen a higher frequency of women than men," Dr. Koralnik said. "We think long COVID is a new autoimmune syndrome, and women are more likely than men to develop autoimmune diseases, such as multiple sclerosis, rheumatoid arthritis, and lupus."

Accessing Care

In addition to the challenges of managing a difficult condition like long COVID, patients often face barriers to care. There are only 64 COVID centers in the United States, and of those, only 30 percent will see patients who have not tested positive for COVID-19. That's part of the reason why more than 2,100 people have traveled from 44 states to visit the Northwestern Medicine Comprehensive COVID center, which accepts patients without physician referral and doesn't require a positive COVID test to be seen.

If you have symptoms of long-COVID, whether you've had a positive test result or not, you may need to travel to a specialty clinic for care. In some cases, you can use

> It's estimated that nearly 10 million Americans experienced neurologic manifestations of long COVID without an official COVID-19 diagnosis, due to limited access to COVID testing in the first year of the pandemic or testing outside the window of detection. Millions of people in the United States have been rejected by the medical establishment and stigmatized because they didn't carry a definite diagnosis of COVID-19 when they presented with their long COVID symptoms. We hope those people feel vindicated by our study.
>
> –Igor Koralnik, MD

Healthy Lifestyle May Protect Against Long COVID

Harvard T.H. Chan School of Public Health.

Adhering to six lifestyle factors (maintaining a healthy body weight, not smoking, exercising, sleeping well, eating a healthy diet, and drinking only in moderation) appears to reduce the risk of developing long COVID in women. Researchers found that women who adhered to five or six factors had a 49 percent lower risk of long COVID, compared with those who did not adhere to any. Maintaining a healthy body weight and getting adequate sleep were the most beneficial. The results also showed that, even among women who developed long COVID, those with a healthier pre-infection lifestyle had a 30 percent lower risk of having symptoms that interfered with their daily life. Long COVID is defined as having COVID-19 symptoms four weeks or more after initial SARS-CoV-2 infection. Symptoms can include fatigue, fever, and respiratory, heart, neurological, and digestive issues.

Sleep Well to Stop Long COVID

Study titled "Habitual Short Sleepers with Pre-Existing Medical Conditions Are at Higher Risk of Long COVID," led by researchers at the University of Toronto, published in the *Journal of Clinical Sleep Medicine*.

The daily fear of COVID is history for most of us, but for some the agony lingers. A regular bout of COVID-19 may cause mild symptoms lasting up to two weeks. However, for as many as 40 percent of individuals affected by COVID, at least one symptom will continue for weeks, months, or years. This is long COVID. Risk factors for long COVID include having a severe COVID infection, having multiple COVID infections, and not being vaccinated. People at highest risk are those who also have pre-existing conditions. A new study suggests that these people can lower their risk of long COVID by getting six to nine hours of sleep per night.

The study, from researchers at the University of Toronto, is published in the American Academy of Sleep Medicine's *Journal of Clinical Sleep Medicine*. The study was produced from data available in the 2021 International COVID Sleep Study II. This study surveyed over 13,000 people from 16 counties and included reported data on COVID infections, pre-existing conditions, long COVID symptoms, and sleep habits.

What Is Long COVID?

According to the World Health Organization, long COVID can be defined as the continuation or development of new symptoms three months after the initial SARS-CoV-2 infection, with these symptoms lasting for at least two months with no other explanation. Common long COVID symptoms may include fatigue, fever, brain fog, shortness of breath, cough, headache, palpitations, depression, and anxiety. Long COVID also causes sleep disturbances that may include poor sleep quality, daytime sleepiness, sleep apnea, and insomnia.

Pre-existing conditions that increase the risk of long COVID include being overweight, being female, COPD, fibromyalgia, anxiety, depression, migraine, multiple sclerosis, heart disease, high blood pressure, and diabetes. It is probable that poor sleep is an added risk factor because of the effect that poor sleep has on the body's immune system. For example, a prior study found that people who had poor sleep (less than six hours per night)

Infectious Disease

in the days before getting a flu shot had about a 50 percent reduction in immune response to the vaccine.

What Causes Long COVID...

Based on prior studies, adequate sleep is needed for proper response of the body's immune system. Since long COVID may be a failure of the immune system to respond properly to COVID infection, the objective of the study was to find out if sleep times along with pre-existing conditions play a role in the risk of developing long COVID.

About 2,500 people in the study were diagnosed with COVID-19. Sixty-one percent of these people reported at least one symptom of long COVID. These were the key findings...

•**The risk of developing long COVID was almost twice as high (1.8-fold higher) for average-length sleepers** (six to nine hours per night) with pre-existing conditions compared with people without pre-existing conditions.

•**The risk of developing long COVID was three times higher for short sleepers** (less than six hours) with pre-existing conditions compared with people without pre-existing conditions and average sleep.

The conclusion of the study is that short sleep time increases the risk of long COVID in people already at risk for long COVID due to a pre-existing condition. Along with controlling other risk factors, getting six to nine hours of sleep may help reduce the risk of long COVID for people already at risk. Risk factors that can be changed or managed for any disease or condition are called modifiable risk factors. The researchers suggest that poor sleep is a modifiable risk factor for people at risk for long COVID.

Patient Beware: Hospital Acquired Infections

Charles B. Inlander, a consumer advocate and health-care consultant based in Fogelsville, Pennsylvania. He was the founding president of the nonprofit People's Medical Society.

There's an old axiom that the most dangerous place to be when you are sick is in a hospital. Hospitals and other health-care settings, such as freestanding surgical centers or urgent care facilities, can be quite dangerous, especially for the risk of deadly infections.

In medical lingo, hospital-acquired infections are called nosocomial infections. Prior to the COVID-19 pandemic, up to 80,000 Americans died each year from them. Some studies suggested that up to one in five patients admitted to a hospital acquired an infection they did not have when they entered. Those numbers soared during the first year of COVID. Many of the victims of COVID got the disease when hospitalized for something else.

While hospitals and other health-care facilities worked diligently to enhance their infection control programs, studies have reported that in their effort to redeploy resources, the historic problem infections (such as sepsis, urinary tract infections, and ventilator-related infection, like pneumonia) increased significantly.

There are several steps you can take if you or a family member are hospitalized or receiving treatment at a freestanding surgical or testing center to avoid being a victim of these unwanted souvenirs of the medical system.

•**Tell health-care professionals to wash their hands.** Insist that doctors, nurses, and other facility staff wash their hands before touching you. This simple step cuts the risk almost in half. Simply say, "Please wash your hands." In most cases, they will respond positively, and they will alert other personnel that you are watching them carefully. A similar strategy applies to gloves. If someone walks into your room wearing medical gloves, ask them to wash their hands and put on new gloves. Some healthcare workers wear the same gloves from patient to patient.

- **Beware of catheters and other invasive equipment.** Catheters, ventilators, and other similar equipment should be cleaned and monitored for sanitation regularly. Make sure you, or a family member or friend, frequently ask staff dealing with those pieces of equipment to make sure they are clean.
- **Pay attention to a roommate.** When hospitalized, most of us share a room with another patient. Pay attention to what is going on with that person. If they seem to be getting sicker or you know they have developed an infection, immediately ask if you are at risk. If you get brushed off, ask to see a nurse epidemiologist or the head of the facility's infection-control program. If you feel in danger, ask to be moved to another room.
- **Ask questions.** Don't be afraid to ask questions about infections and infection control. Medical personnel are busy and often overwhelmed, but the risk of infection is high, and you should expect the best care with the lowest risk of infection possible. Establishing that you or your advocate are actively monitoring your care and their actions only increases your chances of having a positive outcome.

Fungal Infections on the Rise

William Schaffner, MD, infectious disease expert, professor of preventive medicine in the department of health policy, and professor of medicine in the division of infectious diseases at the Vanderbilt University Medical Center in Nashville.

Mycosis or fungal infections are caused by a fungus, such as a yeast or mold, rather than a bacterium or virus. There are millions of fungi around the world, in the air and in the soil, and we carry some ourselves in places like the gastrointestinal tract (starting in the mouth) and on the skin. They usually don't bother us unless something triggers their overgrowth.

Fungal infections are often opportunistic: They multiply to problematic levels when the opportunity presents itself, such as when taking antibiotics for another infection changes the body's microbiome.

Anyone can get a fungal infection, but you're at higher risk if you have certain medical conditions, such as diabetes or a weakened immune system from illnesses such as cancer or HIV/AIDS. Fungal infections are more common in areas of the body that trap moisture or are subject to a lot of friction, like the groin. Many affect the skin or nails. For instance, dermatophytes, fungi that live off skin, hair, and nail cells, can cause ringworm. Ringworm takes many forms depending on the location of the infection—athlete's foot and jock itch are two well-known manifestations. Many types of fungi can cause onychomycosis, a fungal infection of fingernails or toenails that often discolors, hardens, and/or cracks them. While unpleasant, these are superficial infections that can be treated with antifungal medications that come as pills, lotions, powders, mouthwash, shampoo, or eye drops, as appropriate.

Candida auris

There are more than a hundred yeasts under the candida fungus umbrella, and many infections that fall under the general term of candidiasis. Most of us know about—and many have had—the more common ones that stem from an overgrowth of the yeast *Candida albicans*, like thrush, which affects the throat, and vaginal yeast infections. Even some cases of diaper rash are from yeasts. While they can be troublesome, treatments can get them under control.

A growing concern currently surrounds the yeast *Candida auris* (C. auris), which was recognized for causing infections in

Infectious Disease

people only a handful of years ago. These infections occur at a very low rate, but that rate has been increasing over the last three years. According to data from the Centers for Disease Control and Prevention (CDC) published in the *Annals of Internal Medicine*, from 2016, when *C. auris* was first reported in the United States, through December 2021, there was a total of 3,270 clinical cases (meaning infection is present) and 7,413 screening cases (meaning the fungus is detected but not causing infection). But 2022 alone saw 2,377 confirmed cases, up from 1,471 in 2021.

An Urgent Antimicrobial Resistance

The CDC calls *C. auris* an urgent antimicrobial resistance threat because it can cause severe infections with high death rates and is often resistant to multiple antifungal drugs, notably echinocandins, the medication most recommended to treat these infections. While *C. auris* is not generally a worry for healthy people, like other fungi, it preys on those who are very sick, frail, and weak from complicated illnesses. Common symptoms of *C. auris* infection include sepsis, fever, and low blood pressure. Diagnosis is through a blood test—the sample is cultured in a lab to make the yeast easier to detect.

It's of particular risk in health-care settings, such as hospital intensive care units, where very ill people are already battling serious medical problems and are getting prolonged antibiotics (or multiple ones) for their underlying problems. These medications give *C. auris* the leg up it looks for. *C. auris* can contaminate surfaces in a hospital and can spread easily unless quickly recognized and addressed. Every hospital in this country has an infection control team that knows about *C. auris*, even if the institution hasn't experienced it. At nursing homes, there's less awareness, though it's less of a threat unless it's brought in by a patient who came directly from a hospital.

Awareness Is Key

Be aware but not alarmed. If you or a loved one is in any type of medical facility, speak up if you don't see staff following effective infection control practices like

---

Lower Your Risk

Practicing good personal hygiene and protecting yourself from various fungi in your environment is key…

- **Always wear shoes in public bathrooms and in gym locker rooms and showers,** places where fungi thrive.
- **Don't share towels or other personal items with other people.** At the gym, wipe down exercise equipment before using it.
- **Choose cotton rather than synthetic fabrics that trap sweat,** at least as a base layer, so your skin can breathe. Consider wearing protective clothing—gloves, boots, long pants, and long-sleeved shirts—when gardening.
- **Promptly change your clothes and shower after gardening,** swimming, and other workouts, and carefully towel off so skin isn't damp.
- **Keep up with self-care.** Keep nails short and clean; if you wear contact lenses, always care for and replace them as directed.
- **Do your best to manage any chronic conditions** and keep all regular appointments with your doctors so they can monitor you and help you be in the best health possible.

If you live in an area with known harmful fungi in the environment, like the fungus Coccidioides that causes the Valley Fever infection and is a problem in California and the Southwest, wear an N95 mask when outdoors when doing dusty work to avoid breathing them in; stay indoors with the windows closed during wind or dust storms, which can blow spores around.

washing their hands before and after each patient contact. Ask if they have measures in place to detect *C. auris* infections early and isolate patients to prevent the spread.

Natural Medicine and Respiratory Syncytial Virus

Jamison Starbuck, ND, a naturopathic physician in family practice in Missoula, Montana, and producer of *Dr. Starbuck's Health Tips for Kids*, a weekly program on Montana Public Radio, MTPR.org. She is a past president of the American Association of Naturopathic Physicians and a contributing editor to *The Alternative Advisor: The Complete Guide to Natural Therapies and Alternative Treatments*.

There has been a lot of talk recently about respiratory syncytial virus (RSV), recognized since 1956 as a mild respiratory virus. It's the culprit for bronchitis, coughs, and what people call a "very bad cold." Almost all of us have had RSV several times in our lives. In fact, 90 percent of children have had at least one bout of RSV by the time they are 2.

Until COVID, doctors, myself included, did not routinely test patients for RSV. Clinical judgment was usually accurate, patients don't like nasal swabs and sputum collection, and RSV symptoms generally resolved before results returned from the lab. But RSV looks a lot like COVID—cough, fever, congestion, sore throat, and fatigue. In 2020, we suddenly needed to know whether our patients were suffering with the potentially deadly, unfamiliar virus, COVID, or with RSV, the mild virus patients' immune systems had likely encountered many times.

In developing rapid tests for COVID, labs also developed rapid tests for RSV. That resulted in lots of RSV diagnoses and a misperception by some that RSV was on the rise. In May 2023, an RSV vaccine became available.

RSV Vaccine Is Available

The FDA has approved two *respiratory syncytial virus* (RSV) vaccines for adults age 60 and older: GSK Arexvy and Pfizer Abrysvo. Both vaccines are recombinant protein vaccines that cause the immune system to produce RSV antibodies. In clinical studies, Arexvy (which contains an adjuvant... Abrysvo does not) proved 83 percent effective against lower respiratory infections and 94 percent effective against severe cases. Most side effects from the vaccine were minor. The Centers for Disease Control and Prevention advises health-care providers to administer the RSV vaccine late summer or early fall. The vaccine is currently (at press) not an annual vaccine. Studies are ongoing to determine whether older adults would benefit from receiving additional RSV vaccine doses in the future.

William Schaffner, MD, professor of preventive medicine and infectious diseases at Vanderbilt University, Nashville. Vanderbilt.edu. Centers for Disease Control and Prevention, Atlanta. CDC.gov

Unchanged about RSV is conventional medical treatment. It remains limited to rest, fluids, and time. If you get RSV, your symptoms will be less severe and you will feel better faster if you add several of these natural remedies to your regimen...

• **Take vitamin C, 500 milligrams (mg) every three hours.** Vitamin C is a powerful antioxidant that boosts immune function. It will help your white blood cells fight the virus and will help reduce fatigue. Vitamin C can irritate your stomach lining, so take it with a small amount of food.

Too much vitamin C can cause diarrhea: Reduce the dose if your stool becomes loose.

• **Take a B complex that contains at least 50 mg of B5—pantothenic acid.** B vitamins support immune health, and B5, in particular, helps adrenal function, necessary to fight an acute health problem. Always take vitamins with food for best absorption and tolerance.

• **Take a respiratory support herbal tincture.** My favorite herbs for RSV are elecampane (*Inula helenium*), cherry bark (*Prunus*), anise (*Pimpinella anisum*), osha (*Ligusticum porter*), and yerba santa (*Eriodictyon californicum*). These are antimicrobial, immune supportive, and decongesting. Follow the manufacturer's directions for dosing, which is typically 60 drops of tincture in water five to six times a day.

Essential oil facial packs are immensely soothing. They decongest the respiratory tract and relax bronchospasms, reducing cough and aiding sleep. Put two drops each of lavender, thyme, and eucalyptus oil (or four to six drops of only one oil) in one cup of very hot water. Pour the water over a facecloth, wring it out, and place it over your nose, cheeks, mouth, and chin, keeping your eyes closed and leaving a gap for breathing. Cover with a dry towel. Leave in place for 10 minutes. Repeat as needed.

• **As with any viral illness, drink plenty of fluids, and rest a lot.** RSV is most risky for infants and the elderly. However, if you have difficulty breathing or a severe, painful cough, see your doctor immediately.

More Severe Strep Throat

Centers for Disease Control and Prevention (CDC), Atlanta. CDC.gov

*I*nvasive Strep A, a severe form of strep throat, has sickened an unusually high number of people, mostly children and people over age 65. Symptoms include fever, difficulty swallowing, swollen tonsils, and telltale white spots in the back of the throat. Confirmation of strep is done by a throat-swab test. The illness must be treated with antibiotics before it enters the bloodstream, a situation that can be life-threatening. Each year, up to 2,300 people die from the streptococcus bacteria that causes strep.

Problem: *Amoxycillin* in liquid form, the antibiotic most frequently prescribed for strep, is experiencing shortages.

What to do: Amoxycillin pills may be available…and Augmentin or penicillin also can treat strep.

When Are You No Longer Contagious?

Kelli McCourt, editor, *Bottom Line Personal*, BottomLineInc.com. Centers for Disease Control and Prevention, CDC.gov

When you've been sick, when is it safe for you to see people again? Here are some guidelines…

Common cold: You are most contagious during the first four days after symptoms onset.

Flu: You likely are no longer contagious after day five.

COVID: You can go out after your fifth day of symptoms if you're fever-free but wear a mask for five more days.

Note: The Centers for Disease Control and Prevention no longer adheres to the five-day isolation protocol for COVID, advising that individuals without fever and other symptoms can return to public after 24 hours. But if you still "feel" sick, it's best to stay home.

Norovirus (stomach bug): You can get out a few days after you are done vomiting and having diarrhea—but continue to wash your hands often.

Respiratory Syncytial Virus (RSV): You are contagious for up to eight days after symptoms start.

Strep throat: You are "safe" 24 hours after starting an antibiotic as long as you are fever-free. Check with your doctor about when you can return to work.

But remember—these are just guidelines. People with weakened immune

Infectious Disease

symptoms may be contagious longer. If you have a fever or symptoms, stay home for as long as you need to so you don't spread your germs.

Travel Health: How to Keep It in Check

Dr. Mark Fischer, regional medical director for International SOS, a leading risk mitigation company that provides health and safety services to clients across the world.

No one wants to get sick while on a long-awaited vacation. Fortunately, pre-planning can help you stay well and enjoy every minute of your trip. Here's a look at how to prepare for some popular destinations.

Cruising Along

Some of the most common health risks on a cruise include gastrointestinal illnesses caused by norovirus, salmonella, E. coli, and shigella, as well as respiratory illnesses, such as influenza.

Before you go, make sure all of your immunizations are up to date and any medical conditions are well controlled. Research what risk mitigation practices the cruise line implements to create a safe environment.

Whenever traveling, make sure you have enough of any prescription medications and, if possible, extra in the event of an unforeseen delay. Talk to your doctor about any medications you should pack, such as anti-diarrheal and anti-nausea drugs. (See the sidebar on sea and motion sickness on page 211.)

While you're there, always practice good hygiene by washing your hands thoroughly and frequently, including before eating, after going to the bathroom, and after coming into contact with high-touch surfaces, like doorknobs and stair railings.

Soap and water are best: Hand sanitizers don't work well against norovirus.

Some Like It Hot

Whether you're going to the beach, the Caribbean, or the desert, you need to prepare for sun exposure and heat.

- **Sun exposure.** Pack sunscreen that has an SPF of 30 or higher, is water resistant, provides broad-spectrum coverage, and is not expired. Apply sunscreen before going outdoors. It takes approximately 15 minutes for your skin to absorb the sunscreen and protect you. The American Academy of Dermatology notes that most adults don't use enough sunscreen. You need about one ounce (think a shot glass) to fully cover your body. Make sure you get all bare skin, including your ears, the tops of your feet, and your scalp if your hair is thinning. Reapply every two hours, or immediately after swimming or sweating. Wearing a hat can provide added protection.

- **Heat.** Prolonged exposure to high temperatures can lead to heat stroke. To help prevent it, stay hydrated; wear lightweight, loose-fitting clothing, and a hat; schedule outdoor activities for early morning or evening, when temperatures are cooler; and if you begin to feel unwell, use fans, cooling towels, or air conditioning to lower your body temperature. Don't try to push through it.

Leaving the U.S.

When traveling outside of the United States, research your destination to understand the required and recommended vaccinations and potential non-vaccine-preventable diseases. The Centers for Disease Control and Prevention website is an excellent resource. It's important to be up to date on all your vaccinations at least a month prior to your departure. You may need to see a travel medicine physician for some of the required vaccinations.

Infectious Disease

Drinking Water

When traveling out of the country, drinking water is one of the most common causes of illness. Drinking water that is contaminated with bacteria (like E. coli, salmonella, and cholera), protozoa, or viruses (like hepatitis, rotavirus, and polio) can lead to everything from inconvenience to a hospital visit and even significant medical complications. You can visit the CDC website for specific information for your destination.

When traveling anywhere with questionable tap water, use only commercially bottled water from an unopened, factory-sealed container for drinking, preparing food and beverages, making ice, cooking, and brushing your teeth. Avoid fountain drinks and ice, which might be made from contaminated water.

Avoid raw food when traveling. Instead, choose foods that are fully cooked and served hot. If you're in an area where you're unsure about the sanitation of the food supply, avoid uncooked vegetables, salads, raw fruit, and unpasteurized fruit juice. Be careful about buying food from street vendors.

Swimming Safety

To reduce the risk of drowning, practice safety around water. If you're on the beach, be aware of water conditions, such as riptides, waves, and other hazards.

> ### First-Aid Basics for Travel
> When traveling, it can be helpful to pack a travel kit with first-aid supplies. Include any medications you take on a daily basis, pain relievers, antihistamines in the case of allergic reactions, antacid medicine, antibacterial hand wipes, bandages, gauze, hydrogen peroxide to clean and disinfect wounds, a thermometer, sunscreen, and aloe in the case of sunburn.

Never swim alone: Always swim with a buddy or in designated swimming areas with lifeguards.

When boating, kayaking, or participating in any water sports or activities, wear a properly fitting life jacket. Don't drink alcohol before or during swimming or water activities.

Don't swim in lakes or rivers after a heavy rainfall. Runoff can contaminate water with sewage, insecticides, and other chemicals.

If you have any open wounds, don't swim in freshwater or seawater without a waterproof bandage.

Insects

A little bug repellent can go a long way. "Mosquitoes and the diseases they spread have been responsible for killing more people than all the wars in history," according to the Illinois Department of Health. Mosquitos can sicken people with viruses like Zika, malaria, West Nile, and many more in almost every country in the world. The only places without them are Iceland and Antarctica.

Ticks can also spread a range of illness, like Babesiosis, Ehrlichiosis, and Rocky Mountain Spotted Fever, to name a few. Some simple steps can reduce your risk at home and abroad.

- **Use an insect repellent with one of the following ingredients:** DEET, picaridin, IR3535, oil of lemon eucalyptus (OLE), para-menthane-diol, or 2-undecanone. Put insect repellent on after sunscreen.
- **Wear long-sleeved shirts and long pants,** and treat outdoor clothing, boots, pants, and tents supplies with 0.5 percent permethrin.
- **To keep mosquitoes at bay,** stay in hotels or rooms with either window and door screens or a mosquito net.
- **To reduce the risk of tick bites,** avoid wooded areas, high grass, and leaf litter. Walk in the center of trails. When you get home, check your clothing and body for ticks. Shower as soon as possible. If you find a tick, remove it as soon as possible.

Infections May Worsen Cognition

Johns Hopkins Bloomberg School of Public Health.

A new study suggests that common infections can contribute to cognitive decline. Researchers found that people who had antibodies to herpes simplex virus type 1, cytomegalovirus, varicella zoster virus (chickenpox and shingles viruses), and Epstein-Barr virus, or the parasite Toxoplasma gondii performed worse on a cognitive test than people without those antibodies did.

"The idea that common infections could contribute to cognitive decline and perhaps Alzheimer's disease risk was once on the fringe and remains controversial, but due to findings like the ones from this study, it's starting to get more mainstream attention," says senior author Adam Spira, PhD.

The pathogens assessed in the study are often encountered in childhood and are either cleared or turned into suppressed, latent infections. As such, the researchers considered significant levels of antibodies against them in the middle-aged and older study participants as likely indicators of their reactivation due to immune system weakening with age.

Managing Motion Sickness

Planes, trains, automobiles (and boats and amusement park rides) can cause motion sickness in some people. *Here are some strategies to try...*

•**Medication.** Over-the-counter remedies like *diphenhydramine* (Benadryl), *dimenhydrinate* (Dramamine), and *meclizine* (Bonine) can help reduce the nausea of motion sickness—but they can also cause sedation. Some medications that are intended to prevent seasickness can interfere with other medications, so talk to your doctor or pharmacist about their use. Furthermore, people with certain medical conditions will need further guidance from a health-care provider before using the above medications.

Non-medication strategies...

•**Look at the horizon.**
•**Avoid reading.**
•**If you're in a car, sit in the front.**
•**If you're on a boat, skip the upper levels.**
•**Choose a window seat on a train.**
•**Try hard ginger candy.**
•**Products like Sea-Bands use acupressure to reduce motion sickness and nausea.**
•**Drink plenty of water,** but limit caffeine and alcohol.

Best Foods to Eat After a Stomach Virus

Jessica Cording, MS, RD, CDN, health coach and author of *The Little Book of Game Changers*. Jessica CordingNutrition.com

Bland foods, such as those in the BRAT diet—bananas, rice, applesauce, and toast. Coconut water, a natural source of electrolytes without added sugar. Pedialyte, an electrolyte-replenishing drink that treats dehydration and is available as a liquid or as a solution or powder to add to water. Yogurt and kefir (plain, unsweetened) to introduce protein and help stabilize blood sugar. Smoothies, which can be made with soy milk, fruit and nut butter—helpful if you have lactose intolerance. Chicken noodle soup, which provides fluids from broth, protein from chicken and carbohydrates from pasta.

Foods to avoid when fighting a stomach bug: Caffeine, alcohol, spicy foods, and highly acidic foods such as tomatoes.

Infectious Disease

Lesser-Known Tickborne Illnesses Are Spreading Fast

Richard Horowitz, MD, medical director of Hudson Valley Healing Arts Center, Hyde Park, New York. CanGetBetter.com

Lyme gets the limelight, but *babesiosis*—potentially fatal and resistant to treatment—is rising rapidly, according to a new CDC report.

Symptoms: Flu-like sweats, chills, headache, nausea, dark urine, and fatigue following a tick bite, blood transfusion, organ transplant, or pregnancy (perinatal transmission). Request antibody (*Babesia microti* and *B. duncani*), PCR, and the *Fluorescence In Situ Hybridization* (FISH) babesiosis tests—standard testing can miss infections.

Why You're a Mosquito Magnet

Men's Health Advisor. Health.Harvard.edu

If you seem more likely to attract these bloodsuckers more than people standing near you, there may be an explanation. Your sweat may have more carboxylic acids, found in the oily substance on skin that keeps it moist—these acids appeal to mosquitoes.

Other factors: A higher normal body temperature...greater amounts of lactic acid and ammonia in your sweat...even what you consume—for instance, bananas and beer seem to be more attractive to mosquitoes...and having type O blood all have been found to make people targeted by mosquitoes.

Mosquitos Like Red!

Mosquitoes locate humans to bite partly by zeroing in on the carbon dioxide we exhale—but they also are drawn to the colors we wear.

Recent finding: A common mosquito species was found to be attracted to red, orange, black, and cyan...but ignored green, purple, blue, and white. While changing your wardrobe may help deflect bites somewhat, all human skin, regardless of pigmentation, gives off a red-orange "signal."

Study by researchers at University of Washington, Seattle, published in *Nature Communications*.

Beware Malaria

William Schaffner, MD, professor of preventive medicine and infectious diseases at Vanderbilt University, Nashville. Vanderbilt.edu

At least eight people (as of summer 2023) have caught malaria on U.S. soil. The Texas and Florida residents had not traveled abroad or acquired the parasite from blood transfusions. About 2,000 malaria cases are imported into the U.S. annually, mostly among U.S. residents with recent travel to areas with endemic malaria, according to the Centers for Disease Control and Prevention. The illness is transmitted when a mosquito bites an infected person and then someone else.

To protect yourself: Wear long sleeves and repellent, use window screens and air conditioning, and remove standing water (where mosquitoes breed) from around your home.

Also: Consult your doctor before traveling to countries with malaria.

Chapter 10

KIDNEY, BLADDER, AND LIVER HEALTH

Your Kidneys Are Fragile

As with many health conditions—high blood pressure and high cholesterol, to name just two—chronic kidney disease (CKD) often flies under the radar until it becomes advanced. In fact, CKD affects an estimated 37 million adults in the U.S., and most don't even know they have it. If left untreated, kidney function can drop to the point where dialysis is needed to do the work of the kidneys...or a kidney transplant becomes necessary. It also can have cardiovascular complications like hospitalization for heart failure.

But there is good news: When detected early, even if your kidney function has started to decline, you can take steps to slow or even stop further loss.

A Condition of Stages

Your kidneys are constantly removing waste and extra fluid from your blood as urine as well as filtering natural wastes from protein metabolism. If your kidneys aren't working at optimal capacity, that waste and extra fluid can flow back into your bloodstream, causing swelling of your hands and feet, fatigue, itching, muscle cramps, and more. Natural wastes in the blood stream also can contribute to these symptoms.

CKD has different degrees, or stages, depending on how much kidney function has been lost or how much albumin, a type of protein, is in the urine. There are two simple tests to determine your kidney function or filtration...

•**Urine test that measures the ratio of albumin to the waste product creatinine.** A normal reading is 30 mg/g or under. Any protein in your urine signals the first stage of CKD, even if your eGFR test (see below) is within normal range.

•**Blood test that measures estimated glomerular filtration rate (eGFR)**—how many milliliters of blood your kidneys are able to filter per minute. The higher your eGFR, the better your kidney function. In adults age 18 and over, a normal eGFR usually is between 90 and 120, but eGFR declines with age, even in people who do not have kidney disease. *The stages of CKD are identified by your eGFR...*

Joseph A. Vassalotti, MD, clinical professor of medicine in the Division of Nephrology at Icahn School of Medicine at Mount Sinai, New York City, chief medical officer of the National Kidney Foundation and co-editor of *Nutrition, Fitness, and Mindfulness: An Evidence-Based Guide for Clinicians.* Kidney.org

Stage 1: *eGFR 90 or higher* with an increase of albumin in the urine test means possible kidney damage with normal function.

Stage 2: *eGFR 60 to 89* with an increase of albumin in the urine test means mild loss of kidney function.

Stage 3a: *eGFR 45 to 59,* mild-to-moderate loss of kidney function.

Stage 3b: *eGFR 30 to 44,* moderate-to-severe loss of kidney function.

Stage 4: *eGFR 15 to 29,* severe loss of kidney function.

Stage 5: *eGFR under 15,* kidney failure.

Managing CKD

A diagnosis of CKD doesn't mean that dialysis is inevitable. In fact, that's not the case for most people. Your first step is to make lifestyle changes that can preserve your kidney function and protect your heart. CKD is a risk factor for heart disease and heart attacks. *Healthy lifestyle steps to take to reduce or prevent CKD...*

• **Control blood pressure and blood glucose levels.** Elevated levels harm the kidneys. You may need a comprehensive medical team to help you address all three chronic conditions. A nephrologist—a kidney specialist—can give you strategies to prevent further kidney function loss...a cardiologist will help manage high blood pressure...and an endocrinologist will guide your diabetes treatment.

• **Revise your diet.** A registered dietitian can recommend a diet that reduces salt intake—to help manage high blood pressure—and manage levels of electrolytes, minerals including potassium and phosphorus. Having CKD can make you prone to imbalances in electrolytes, which can cause problems from muscle weakness to heart trouble. Also limit alcohol intake...avoid ultra-processed foods...and lose unwanted pounds. If you have diabetes, a certified diabetes educator (CDE) can help you with meal planning to keep your blood sugar under control.

• **Be more physically active.** Aim for at least the recommended 150 minutes of moderate activity a week.

• **Get enough sleep.** Your kidneys are influenced by the wake–sleep cycle.

• **Stop smoking if you smoke.** Among its other ills, smoking is associated with worsening kidney function, heart disease and many cancers. (For more on the dangers of smoking, see page 279.)

• **Take your medications as prescribed—** but avoid those that can hurt kidneys, such as naproxen, ibuprofen and other nonsteroidal anti-inflammatory drugs (NSAIDs). Review any drugs you take with your kidney-care team.

• **Create a support network.** If you have advanced CKD, you may experience anxiety or depression. Advice from a therapist and/or a support group can provide the encouragement you need to care for yourself. Check out the National Kidney Foundation's Online Communities page at Kidney.org/online-communities to find resources near you.

Treating Late-Stage CKD

When kidney function is very low, you should start preparing for kidney failure treatment with dialysis or a kidney transplant.

• **Dialysis.** There are three types of dialysis that most patients should be able to participate in. *Each treatment has benefits and risks that should be discussed with your care team...*

• *In-center hemodialysis.* This is the traditional approach in which your blood is filtered through a dialysis machine. Minor surgery is needed first to create an access point in your arm where the tubing will be connected so that blood can flow into the dialysis machine and, after being filtered, be returned to your body. It is common to go to a dialysis center, usually three times a week for four hours at a time, but there also is home hemodialysis that usually requires a caregiver to assist you. People who do hemodialysis at home can do it more frequently, which can bring better results. New, more convenient approaches include doing daily but shorter home sessions and doing dialysis while you sleep.

• *Peritoneal dialysis* involves filling the abdomen with a solution that filters your blood internally. Minor surgery is needed to create an access point near the belly button. *There are two methods for peritoneal dialysis, both of which are done at home...*

Continuous ambulatory peritoneal dialysis (CAPD). You place the solution into your abdomen through the access point, wait a certain period, then drain it. This is done three to five times a day.

Automated peritoneal dialysis (APD). You connect the tubing of a cycler machine to the access point, and it delivers and drains the solution for you. You usually can do this while you sleep.

For any type of home dialysis, you'll receive training and be monitored regularly. Home treatments allow you to set your own schedule, and you won't have to look for a dialysis clinic when you travel. But you must be willing to participate in your care rather than simply going to a dialysis clinic.

• **Kidney transplant.** Age is not a barrier to a kidney transplant. If there is a kidney available from a living donor or a recently deceased kidney donor, it can be an alternative to dialysis. Care is needed afterward, and you will have to take anti-rejection medications for the rest of your life. Kidney transplant offers a better quality of life and longer survival for most patients.

• **Palliative care or symptom management.** For those who are frail, have numerous medical conditions or have dementia, simply managing CKD symptoms might be appropriate. Symptom relief allows people to lead a meaningful life without the strain of dialysis.

On the horizon: The interactive web-based tool *Decision Aid for Renal Therapy* (DART), designed to communicate the choices available to older people with end-stage CKD. Developed by researchers from Tufts University and other institutions and tested at eight kidney centers across the country, DART helped patients better assess treatment options. You can access it at Patient.health-ce.wolterskluwer.com/DART/programs.

Added Salt Linked to CKD

JAMA Network Open.

A study that looked at data from 465,288 individuals showed that people who reported always adding extra salt to their food had an 11 percent higher risk for developing chronic kidney disease (CKD) compared with those who never or only rarely added salt. The association did not take into account salt used in cooking, only salt added at the table. People who reported usually adding salt had a 7 percent higher risk, and those who only sometimes adding salt had a 4 percent higher risk.

Is Your Chicken Dinner Causing Your UTI?

Janet Bond Brill, PhD, RDN, FAND, a registered dietitian nutritionist, a fellow of the Academy of Nutrition and Dietetics, and a nationally recognized nutrition, health, and fitness expert who specializes in cardiovascular disease prevention. Based in Hellertown, Pennsylvania., Dr. Brill is author of *Intermittent Fasting for Dummies, Blood Pressure DOWN, Cholesterol DOWN,* and *Prevent a Second Heart Attack.* DrJanet.com

You may have heard of *Escherichia coli (E. coli),* the bacteria that can result in food-borne illness. Some *E. coli* strains also have the capacity to colonize in the urinary tract. A new study (June 2023) has linked the consumption of these strains of *E. coli* in chicken and pork to hundreds of thousands of painful UTIs annually. *Here is what you need to know about UTIs and how to prevent them...*

• *Urinary tract infections.* A UTI is an infection in any part of the urinary system. The urinary system includes the kidneys, ureters, bladder, and urethra (the tube that releases urine from the bladder out of the body). Most infections involve the lower urinary tract—the bladder and the urethra. A UTI occurs when a bacterium enters the urethra. It is easy to contract a UTI, especially in women. Women are at greater risk for a UTI because they have a shorter urethra than men do, so it's easier for bacteria to travel to the bladder. Most women experience more than one UTI during their lifetimes.

• **Risk factors.** *Risk factors for UTIs in women include...*

• *Sexual activity.* Frequent sexual intercourse tends to lead to more UTIs. Having a new sexual partner also increases risk.

• *Certain types of birth control.* Using a diaphragm for birth control and spermicides may increase the risk of UTIs.

• *Urination frequency.* Holding it in for lengthy periods of time and incomplete bladder emptying increases the risk.

• *Menopause.* After menopause, a decline in circulating estrogen causes changes in the urinary tract. These changes can increase the risk of UTIs.

• **Symptoms of UTIs.** UTIs can be painful. Common symptoms include discomfort when urinating, urgency and frequency of urination, tenderness above the bladder area, cramps, fatigue, or a stinging sensation during sex. Most UTIs are mild and easily treated with antibiotics. In rare cases, a UTI can be severe and even fatal.

• **Preventing UTIs.** Prevention of UTIs includes drinking lots of water, emptying the bladder often, wiping from front to back, urinating as soon as possible after sex, drinking cranberry juice, and washing your hands often.

• **Preventing food-borne UTIs.** *E. coli* acquired from the consumption of undercooked meat is one way a UTI can be contracted from food. A food-borne UTI occurs when *E. coli* bacteria is consumed, excreted, and then migrates from the anus to the urethra. Poultry is a major source of the bacteria that cause urinary tract infections in people. Pork, but not beef, is also associated with increased risk. The best way to prevent UTIs from *E. coli* acquired from the consumption of undercooked meat is to cook the meat extremely well. Safe food handling is also important. Be sure you wash your hands with soap and hot water after handling raw poultry as well as the surfaces it has touched. Another way to acquire a UTI from food aside from ingesting it is touching the raw food and then transmitting the bacteria to yourself or others. (*E. coli* can contaminate food, but humans and animals can also carry and transmit the bacteria to one another.) Good hygiene is your best bet for warding off foodborne UTIs.

First New Antibiotic for Urinary Tract Infections

Study titled "Oral Gepotidacin Versus Nitrofurantoin in Patients with Uncomplicated Urinary Tract Infection (EAGLE-2 and EAGLE-3): Two Randomized, Controlled, Double-Blind, Double-Dummy, Phase 3, Non-Inferiority Trials," by researchers at Justus Liebig University, Germany, published in *The Lancet*.

Over half of all women and about 10 percent of men will experience an uncomplicated urinary tract infection (UTI). Uncomplicated means the infection does not involve the kidneys. Due to antibiotic resistance, many will suffer recurrent infections. Even when taking a first-choice antibiotic, up to 80 percent of recurrent UTIs consist of breakthrough infections. A recent report on two studies finds that a new antibiotic for stubborn UTIs may soon be available.

New Antibiotic for UTIs on the Horizon

The two studies are reported in the February 2024 medical journal *The Lancet*. The new first-line, oral antibiotic that may soon be approved avoided antibiotic resistance and was more effective than the current first-line options. If approved, this new antibiotic will be the first new option for UTIs in over 20 years.

The name of the new antibiotic is *gepotidacin*. It works by preventing bacteria DNA from replicating. The two phase III studies reported in *The Lancet* are the EAGLE 2 and 3 studies. A phase III study is the final phase before possible approval by the FDA. Researchers from Justus Liebig University led the study that was a collaboration of researchers at 219 sites worldwide.

These were randomized, double-blind studies comparing gepotidacin (1500 mg, twice per day for 5 days) to the antibiotic nitrofurantoin (100 mg, twice per day for 5 days). Randomized means that people in the study were randomly assigned to one drug or the other. Double-blind means neither the patients or the researchers knew which patients received which drugs.

Women Get Relief from Gepotidacin

All the patients in the study were women, with an average age between 50 and 52. All the patients had two or more symptoms of UTI that could include painful urination (dysuria), frequent urination, a strong urge to pass urine, or lower belly pain. They also had urine positive for nitrites or white blood cells (both are signs of UTI). Successful treatment (therapeutic response) was complete relief of symptoms and negative microbiological test for bacterial infection. These were the key findings...

In EAGLE-2, 320 patients were assigned to gepotidacin and 287 to nitrofurantoin. Therapeutic response was 4.3 percent better for the gepotidacin group.

In EAGLE-3, 277 patients were assigned to gepotidacin and 264 to nitrofurantoin. Therapeutic response was 14.6 percent better for the gepotidacin group.

Gepotidacin was effective against the most common cause of UTI *(E. Coli)*, even when the bacteria were resistant to nitrofurantoin.

Gepotidacin was also effective against less common bacteria, including those commonly resistant to common antibiotics.

Side effects of treatment were about the same for each drug and included mild nausea and diarrhea in about 25 to 35 percent of patients.

For FDA approval, a new drug must show that it is equally as effective as other drugs available for treatment. Because gepotidacin was more effective, the drug developer (GlaxoSmithKline) plans to apply for U.S. and European approval later in 2024.

The research team concludes that gepotidacin is effective and safe against bacteria that cause uncomplicated UTIs, including drug resistant bacteria, and has the potential to offer substantial benefits to patients. According to one recent review, more than 90 percent of bacteria that cause UTIs are resistant to at least one commonly used antibiotic, so the addition of a new option is very good news.

Keep Your Gallbladder Healthy

Stephen Pereira, MD, chief of the division of general surgery and director of robotic general surgery at Hackensack University Medical Center and founder of One Surgical Specialists in Hackensack, New Jersey. OneSurgicalSpecialists.com

The gallbladder—it's fair to say that most of us know very little about this small organ...until something goes wrong, and then it can cause big pain.

Good news: There are ways to keep your gallbladder healthy, says Stephen Pereira,

MD, chief of the division of general surgery at Hackensack University Medical Center, and just as important, there are ways to recognize signs of a problem before it turns serious.

• **What is the gallbladder?** The gallbladder is about the size and shape of a pear, nestled under your liver and connected to the pancreas, liver, and small intestine via a complex ductwork. It concentrates and stores between 10 percent and 25 percent of the one liter of bile your liver makes every day. When you eat fatty food, the gallbladder contracts to release bile into the intestines to break down that fat as part of the digestive process.

How to keep it happy: The same steps you take for overall health will keep your gallbladder healthy. Eat a nutritious diet that includes high-fiber whole grains, legumes, fruits and vegetables, and healthy fats from olive oil and fatty fish. Avoid refined carbs (white flour-based and sugar-laden foods), saturated fats, and high-cholesterol foods. Maintain a healthy weight, and get 150 minutes of moderate-intensity exercise every week. Don't smoke—smoking increases risk for many types of cancer, and though rare, gallbladder cancer often is not discovered until later stages.

The Big Problem—Gallstones

For reasons we don't yet understand, sometimes the gallbladder just doesn't work as it should.

• **The most common problem.** Small stones that form within the gallbladder. About 80 percent are cholesterol gallstones, which form when your bile has too much cholesterol, typically from a high-fat diet, although family history and genetics also play a role. The rest are called *pigment gallstones,* and they form when the balance of certain natural body chemicals—bile acids and *lecithin*—is off. The cause of this imbalance is primarily hereditary, but it is a poorly understood phenomenon. (Diet plays no role in this type of gallstone formation.) It's possible to have anywhere from a few to hundreds of gallstones, and each can be as tiny as a grain of sand or as big as a golf ball.

About 20 percent of adults develop gallstones at some point in their lives, but they become troublesome for only about 20 percent of those people. Many people with so-called silent gallstones learn that they have them only when they get an ultrasound (the most likely test to detect them) for another reason. When gallstones are found incidentally on an imaging study, such as an ultrasound, and the patient has no symptoms, intervention generally is not required.

Many factors increase risk for gallstones…some are modifiable, others are not. They include increasing age…being a woman and having been pregnant…being genetically disposed to gallstones…eating too many simple sugars and saturated fats and too little fiber…being obese…having high levels of cholesterol in your blood…and carrying a lot of belly fat.

While slowly losing excess weight can reduce your risk, be wary of losing weight too quickly. That can *increase* risk for gallstones, so keep an eye out for subtle symptoms (see below). Up to 40 percent of people who have bariatric surgery develop gallstones within the following year or two, and gallstones will be problematic for up to 15 percent of them.

One explanation for the link: Changes to your digestive system from the surgery in turn change the composition of your bile and affect gallbladder function. If you already had gallstones, they may act up. (Work with your bariatric doctor on steps to help you avoid problems.)

When gallstones attack: It is possible to experience a mild attack that feels like indigestion or reflux. You might take Tums or Pepcid and think the medicine made the pain go away—but what actually happened was the stone moved on its own, stopping the spasms. If you experience this kind of upset stomach regularly, it's worth mentioning to your primary care doctor. Gallstones are easy to see on a simple ultrasound.

If you have diabetes: Your symptoms may be less intense if you have diabetic neuropathy, which affects how much pain you experience, but still report such an episode to your doctor.

A gallstone can quickly become a health threat if it lodges in the duct or tube that drains the gallbladder, halting the outflow of bile. When this happens, the gallbladder will go into spasm, causing sharp, stabbing pain. You'll feel the classic "gallbladder attack" in your upper abdomen, sometimes radiating to your back. It typically happens shortly after eating a fatty meal since fat triggers the gallbladder to contract or squeeze the bile out to the intestines. You may feel bloated and nauseated, and possibly have some vomiting. An attack can last for a number of hours until the stone moves and relieves the blockage. Pain that persists beyond a few hours may mean that the stone is stuck. This life-threatening situation can lead to infection, fever and chills...as well as inflammation and/or damage to the gallbladder.

An even more serious complication of gallstones is if a gallstone passes out of the gallbladder and into the bile ducts or tubes that drain the bile from the liver. This can cause bile to back up into the liver causing jaundice, which can lead to severe pain and the life-threating infection of the biliary system called *cholangitis.* Signs include the skin turning yellow because the flow of bile is blocked, dark urine, and light-colored stools. If you experience hours of pain, don't wait for it to pass—call 911 or go to the ER.

Another severe condition that can be caused by gallstones blocking the bile duct is pancreatitis (inflammation of the pancreas), when the duct to the pancreas is blocked. When this happens, severe upper abdominal pain comes on very suddenly and quickly. Call 911 or go immediately to the ER for treatment.

What not to do if you develop gallstones or have a gallstone attack: Any type of gallbladder "cleanse" or home remedies that claim to dissolve gallstones—studies have shown that these unapproved remedies don't dissolve or "cleanse" gallstones.

•**One attack usually is just the beginning.** Doctors often advise gallbladder removal after just the first attack. That's because gallbladder attacks are very likely to recur, and there's no way of knowing whether a stone will move along the next time...or get stuck. Even when stones do become dislodged or unstuck, repeated attacks can cause inflammation and scarring of the gallbladder, affecting its functioning and making surgery more complex with a higher risk for complications.

Another reason not to wait: The younger and healthier you are, the better you'll sail through the surgery.

When It Is an Emergency

Of course, it's a medical emergency any time a stone is stuck. If a gallstone passes out of the gallbladder into the bile duct that drains the liver, a specially trained surgeon may insert a scope through your throat to your digestive tract to retrieve the stone...or he/she may remove your

GLP1 Agonists May Be Good for the Liver

GLP1 agonists such as *semaglutide* (Ozempic, Wegovy) are associated with a reduced risk of developing cirrhosis and liver cancer in people with type 2 diabetes and chronic liver disease.

These drugs reduce blood sugar levels and are mainly used to treat type 2 diabetes and, increasingly, obesity.

Results from early clinical trials also suggest that people who take the drugs long term have a lower risk of later developing severe forms of liver disease such as cirrhosis and liver cancer. The results need to be confirmed in clinical trials.

Karolinska Institutet.

gallbladder and extract the stone that has lodged in the bile duct.

Doctors often advise *cholecystectomy* (gallbladder removal) after a first episode. Thanks to advances made in robotic 3D surgery, the gallbladder can be removed through a single incision in the navel. What's more, the surgery can be guided by a dye called *indocyanine green fluorescence,* which makes it possible to visualize the gallbladder and surrounding structures before any incisions are made. This makes the operation safer, especially when there's inflammation, infection, or serious scarring, and reduces risk for serious complications. These innovations have drastically reduced the need to convert midway through the procedure to open (large-incision) surgery, which can happen during any type of minimally invasive surgery.

Most people have no post-op issues after their gallbladder has been removed. About one in five patients will experience bloating, gassiness, or loose stool after meals as their bodies adjust—often within a few weeks or, on rare occasion, a few months—to no longer having a gallbladder.

Life Without a Gallbladder

You can do just fine without that jolt of bile from the gallbladder for digestion. Remember that the liver supplies a continuous flow of bile into your intestine. Usually there's nothing you need to do other than enjoy life without any more gallbladder attacks.

Chapter 11

NATURAL REMEDIES AND SUPPLEMENTS

The Power of Prebiotics

You probably know about probiotics, the friendly bacteria in your gut that promote good health. But you may not know much about prebiotics, the nutritional compounds in your diet that are the food supply for probiotics. Getting more prebiotics into your daily diet is one of the most important actions you can take for better health and healing.

The Gut Microbiome

Your colon is the primary home of a complex ecosystem of 100 trillion bacteria collectively called the *gut microbiome.* Many of those hundreds of species of bacteria are probiotics—friendly, health-giving bacteria that aid digestion, strengthen the immune system, improve metabolism, and energize the brain. Other gut bacteria are unfriendly and health-threatening, like *C. difficile,* which can multiply after the use of antibiotics, causing diarrhea, stomach cramps, kidney damage, and, in the most severe cases, death.

When unfriendly gut bacteria dominate the gut microbiome, you have a condition called *dysbiosis*—an intestinal imbalance that sparks chronic inflammation throughout the body.

Scientific research shows that dysbiosis plays a key role in causing or contributing to many inflammation-linked conditions and diseases, including high blood pressure, cardiovascular disease, type 2 diabetes, autoimmune disease, asthma, allergies, glaucoma, depression and anxiety, and cognitive decline.

Prebiotics are the food for the microbiome. Having more prebiotic-rich foods in your diet can prevent or clear up dysbiosis—making them one of your best nutritional tools for preventing, treating or reversing inflammation-based health problems.

Short-Chain Fatty Acids

The probiotics in your gut are picky eaters, with a diet that consists mainly of fiber (like the inulin found in asparagus, chia seeds, and bananas), unrefined carbohydrate (like the oligosaccharides found in kale and pears), and polyphenols (like the colorful

---

Elizabeth Lipski, PhD, author of *Digestive Wellness (4th Edition),* academic director of nutrition and integrative health programs at the Maryland University of Integrative Health, a faculty member of the Institute for Functional Medicine, and founder of Innovative Healing Inc. LizLipski.com

chemicals found in blueberries and tomatoes). When these compounds reach the colon, they are gobbled up by the gut microbes. Simultaneously, the plant polyphenols and other colorful substances in food decrease inflammation and signal our genes that all is well. As the well-nourished probiotics grow and thrive, they generate *short-chain fatty acids* (SCFAs)—a biochemical superstar that nourishes the health of the gut, cooling chronic inflammation throughout the body. *There are three main SCFAs: butyrate, propionate, and acetate...*

- **Butyrate** energizes and repairs the colon, balancing the gut microbiome, activates genes that strengthen the colon wall, promotes growth factors that strengthen the bones and brain, and inhibits the toxic chemical histone deacetylase (HDAC), the same mechanism of a new class of anti-cancer drugs.

- **Propionate** helps with mineral absorption, regulates appetite, normalizes cholesterol levels, decreases excess fat in the liver, and improves sensitivity to insulin (the hormone that regulates blood sugar levels).

- **Acetate** helps gut bacteria create butyrate, improves oxygen uptake in the colon, helps synthesize cholesterol, which is used to make key hormones like cortisol, estrogen, progesterone, and testosterone, and travels to the muscles and brain, providing energy and decreasing inflammation.

A scientific paper published in *Advances in Immunology* summarizes the importance of SCFAs: "Given the vast effects of SCFAs, and that their levels are regulated by diet, they provide a new basis to explain the increased prevalence of inflammatory disease in Westernized countries."

In other words: Eat more prebiotic-rich foods if you want to reduce inflammation and be healthier.

Prebiotic-Rich Foods

The most effective way to balance the gut microbiota and generate plenty of SCFAs is with prebiotic-rich whole foods. On the other hand, ultra processed foods, with added sugar, salt, fat, starches, and artificial colors, flavors, and preservatives, cause dysbiosis.

Fortunately, a wide variety of foods supply prebiotics: artichokes, asparagus, avocados, bananas (underripe), barley, beet root, bran, burdock root, chia seeds, chicory, Chinese chives, cocoa, cottage cheese, dandelion greens, eggplant, flax seeds, fruit, garlic, green tea, honey, Jerusalem artichokes, jicama, kefir, leeks, legumes, lentils, maple syrup, nuts and seeds, onions, peas, plantains, potatoes, radishes, root vegetables, rye, sea vegetables, soybeans, herbs and spices, sweet potatoes, tomatoes, vegetables, Yacon root, yams, and yogurt.

Choose the foods from the list that you like, and eat seven to eight servings a day. But don't start eating all those servings tomorrow. Most of these foods are fiber-rich, and the gut does best slowly adjusting to a higher intake of fiber.

To avoid gas and bloating, start with two to three servings daily. Add one to two servings per week, taking two to three weeks to reach eight daily servings. Each day, try to get one to three tablespoons of fresh (or one to two teaspoons of dried) herbs and spices. For example, you could grow mint on the windowsill and drink mint tea daily. Or add rosemary, thyme, sage, or parsley to stews, casseroles, and soups. Put a sprinkle of cinnamon on your oatmeal. Make a smoothie with ginger and fresh turmeric.

A Look at the Evidence

There's plenty of evidence that these prebiotic-rich foods are doing their job. One scientific study showed that dandelion greens stimulated the growth of 14 strains of probiotics. Scientists at Louisiana State University Health Sciences Center found that walnuts increased the diversity of probiotics like *Lactobacillus*. Researchers at the University of Massachusetts Amherst found that xyloglucan—a prebiotic in cranberries—is a favored food of *bifidobacteria,* a probiotic.

"We already know we have beneficial microbes in our guts, so let's feed them," said

David Sela, PhD, the lead researcher in the cranberry study. "Let's give them the things that they like."

Prebiotic Supplements

Prebiotics are available in supplement form, often packaged with probiotics in a supplement called a synbiotic. But supplements aren't the best way to get your prebiotics. That's because the prebiotics found in supplements are extracts from food—compounds like fructans, galacto-oligosaccharides, and glucose-derived oligosaccharides. While helpful, they don't supply the diversity of prebiotics you get when you eat a variety of food. For example, ginger delivers more than 300 bioactive compounds. Which of these are the best to help feed probiotics and balance the gut microbiome? No one really knows. It's far better to rely on food itself to supply your body with the prebiotics it needs.

Healing with Prebiotics

However, some health conditions may benefit from targeted supplementation with a synbiotic supplement. Nearly 1,000 clinical studies have been conducted on the power of prebiotics to heal disease. *Studies conducted in just the last year show that prebiotics (often in a synbiotic supplement) can improve three common conditions...*

• **Parkinson's disease.** Researchers from Rush University Medical Center in Chicago treated 20 Parkinson's patients—10 newly diagnosed and not on medication and 10 who were receiving medication—with prebiotics. After 10 days, the study participants had less dysbiosis (a characteristic of Parkinson's disease, according to the researchers), more SCFAs, less inflammation, and lower levels of a protein biomarker for neurological damage. They also had less severe symptoms of the disease.

• **Irritable bowel syndrome (IBS).** This digestive problem affects an estimated one in seven Americans, with symptoms including constipation and/or diarrhea, abdominal pain and cramping, bloating, flatulence, depression, and lower quality of life. In a study published in *Gut and Liver*, researchers gave 67 IBS patients either a synbiotic (a combination of probiotics plus prebiotics) or a placebo. After four weeks, those taking the synbiotic had significantly less abdominal pain and more psychological well-being than the placebo group.

• **Stress.** Chronic stress can cause a wide range of physical and mental health problems. In a study published in *Molecular Psychiatry* in February 2023, researchers studied 45 people, dividing them into two groups. One group was given a diet rich in prebiotics and probiotics (fermented foods), and the other ate their standard diet. After four weeks, the group eating the prebiotic/probiotic diet had a 32 percent reduction in perceived stress, compared with a 17 percent reduction in the control group.

Disease-Busting Prebiotics

Studies from the past year show many health problems can be improved by increased prebiotic or synbiotic intake...

• **Anemia in late-stage kidney disease.**
• **Schizophrenia.**
• **Infectious complications after liver transplant.**
• **Mild cognitive impairment** (a potential precursor to Alzheimer's disease)
• **Systemic lupus erythematosus.**
• **Metabolic syndrome** (a group of risk factors for cardiovascular disease and type 2 diabetes)
• **Menopausal symptoms,** including hot flashes, anxiety, and depression
• **Cardiovascular disease** (lessening of inflammatory biomarkers, depression, and anxiety)

Natural Remedies and Supplements

Ginger Stimulates the Immune System

Molecular Nutrition & Food Research.

The spicy flavor of ginger comes from a compound called [6]-gingerol. In a recent study, researchers gave participants one liter of ginger tea and then tested their blood. Significant amounts of the compound entered the blood about 30 to 60 minutes after drinking tea. The white blood cells that were exposed to the ginger reacted 30 percent more strongly to a peptide that simulates a bacterial infection. In short, ginger appears to boost immunity.

The Pet Prescription

Carrie Nydick Finch, LCSW, a licensed clinical social worker and Deputy Director of Programs & Strategy at PAWS NY (Pets Are Wonderful Support, New York). Ms. Finch is certified in animal-assisted activities, therapy, and learning. PawsNY.org

What's one of the strongest prescriptions for better health? According to decades of scientific research, it may be owning a pet. There is a wide range of proven health benefits.

- **Better heart health.** In a study published in the *Mayo Clinic Proceedings,* researchers looked at health data from more than 2,000 people collected over five years. On average, those who owned a pet—particularly a dog—had higher cardiovascular health scores. In another study, from researchers at the Stanford Cardiovascular Institute at Stanford University in California, dog owners had a 31 percent lower risk of dying from heart-related problems compared to nonowners—and a 65 percent lower risk of dying after a heart attack.
- **Less obesity.** Pet owners are less likely to be overweight or obese, according to a study from the University of Utah.
- **Slower rate of cognitive decline.** Seniors who own pets have a slower rate of cognitive decline and better memory than seniors who don't, according to a study reported at the American Academy of Neurology's 74th Annual Meeting in 2022. The study looked at 1,369 older adults with an average age of 65. More than half owned pets (with 32 percent owning pets for five years or more) and 47 percent did not. The long-term pet owners had the slowest rate of cognitive decline, significantly outscoring all the other groups on cognitive tests.

The Alabama Brain Study on Risk for Dementia, published in *Frontiers in Aging Neuroscience*, looked at 56 pet owners and 39 nonowners, ages 20 to 74. Pet owners had higher levels of cognition (memory and attention) and larger brain structures. All in all, the researchers estimated that the brains of the pet owners were 15 years younger than the nonowners'.

- **Less wear and tear from stress.** *Allostatic load* is a biological measurement of wear and tear on the body from chronic stress. It takes into account factors like blood pressure, levels of the stress hormone cortisol, and heart rate variability. One study found that dog owners were more likely to have a lower allostatic load than nonowners.
- **Less anxiety.** In a study published in the *International Journal of Geriatric Psychiatry,* dog owners had less anxiety than nonowners.
- **Greater ability to cope with trauma.** In a study of people with post-traumatic stress disorder (PTSD), 84 percent who were paired with a service dog reported a significant reduction in symptoms, and 40 percent were able to decrease their medications, according to a report from Johns Hopkins Medicine.
- **Fewer doctor visits.** Seniors who owned and regularly walked a dog had fewer doctor's visits in a study from researchers at the University of Missouri.

Preparing for a Pet

Sixty-seven percent of American households already have one or more pets. If you're among them, you already know many of the benefits of having an animal companion. *If you're new to pet ownership, there are several factors to consider…*

- **Young animals can be a lot of work.** Sure, puppies are adorable, but they also require a lot of work, including housetraining (they have to go outside several times at night), behavior training, frequent vet visits, and more. A slightly older dog is easier to care for, and there are countless senior pets in shelters looking for homes. If you're interested in a young animal, a kitten is easier to care for than a puppy.

- **Match the pet's energy level and interests to your own.** Before getting a pet, consider what you'd like to do together. Are you looking for a dog to run or hike with or a lap dog? A cuddly cat or one that's more independent? Just like you have to think of your needs (do you have time for a morning walk before work every day?), you need to consider the animal's, too. Some animals are anxious or lonely if they're left too long. Further, dogs can only "hold it" for so long.

- **Consider the cost.** Pets can be expensive, with outlays for food, veterinary care, pet sitting, and more. Before buying a pet, carefully evaluate your budget and make sure you can afford the additional expense, which involves timely preventive and emergency care. You can expect to spend anywhere from $600 to $1,800 per year on a healthy pet, and illnesses can drive that figure up quickly. (Pet insurance can help with unexpected costs.) If finances are an issue, you can experience the joy of pets without the cost by serving as a foster pet parent for a pet rescue.

- **Spay and neuter.** You'll also want to make sure to neuter your pet. Neutering benefits your pet's health, lowering or eliminating the risk of reproductive cancers and improving behavior. It also reduces the number of homeless pets that end up in shelters. Nearly 1 million cats and dogs are euthanized every year.

- **Take your time.** Most importantly, don't make the decision of pet ownership impulsively. Carefully consider if you have the time, money, and energy to engage an animal companion. Pets develop strong emotional bonds with their owners, and it's painful for them to be left at a shelter if the fit isn't right.

- **Longer life.** Dog owners had a 24 percent lower risk of death from any cause in a study published in the journal *Circulation* that looked at nearly 4 million people.

Soothing Companions

Pets provide companionship and decrease loneliness with their presence and, in the case of dogs, when you go out and interact with other dog owners. A report from the Centers for Disease Control and Prevention showed that social isolation increases the risk of premature death from all causes—rivaling smoking, obesity, and physical inactivity as a risk factor. Social isolation, says the report, is also linked to a 50 percent increased risk of dementia, a 29 percent increased risk of heart disease, and a 32 percent increased risk of stroke. Similarly, loneliness is linked to higher rates of depression and anxiety.

As you interact with an animal companion—playing with a dog, stroking a cat, delighting in an aquarium—there are a wide range of positive biological responses…

- **Blood pressure and heart rate fall.**

- **There are lower levels of cortisol, the stress hormone.**

- **There are higher levels of oxytocin,** a feel-good hormone released during touch, warmth, and stroking in trusting relationships (and also during labor, breastfeeding, and sex).

Natural Remedies and Supplements

- **There are higher levels of dopamine,** the neurotransmitter released during pleasurable activities.

The end result is positive feelings of happiness, self-esteem, calm, and purpose.

And let's not forget perhaps the greatest benefit of all: receiving the unconditional acceptance and love that people value so highly in their animal companions.

Maximizing Benefits

Pets—particularly dogs and cats—communicate with their human companions in many ways. Although you don't have to become a behavioral expert to figure out your pet, it's good to have a basic knowledge of dog or cat behavior so you can understand what they're trying to "say" to you.

Seeing your pet as a sentient being with its own wants and needs—and seeing yourself more as a guardian than an owner—will benefit you and your companion, ensuring your pet is happy and healthy.

Finally, a relationship with an animal companion is a relationship: Take the time to develop it. Spend time with your companion every day. Take your dog for a walk; play games with your cat.

Plan for an Emergency

Imagine this unfortunate but not uncommon scenario: Your dog is at home waiting for your return, but you're injured in a car accident and have to go to the hospital. Who is going to take care of your pet? The best way to handle this possibility is to have a friend or relative who has agreed to take care of your pet in case of an emergency. Make sure there's a financial agreement as to how the pet care will be paid for.

Similarly, plan ahead for the possibility of evacuation in the event of a natural disaster. Identify where you can go with your pet, and have a go-bag ready for you both.

This will build a strong bond and provide the best health for you and your friend.

Supplements: An Inflation-Friendly Nutrition Strategy

Sherry Torkos, BScPhm, RPh, a pharmacist, author, and health advisor, who integrates conventional and complementary therapies. She is the author of *The Canadian Encyclopedia of Natural Medicine and Saving Women's Hearts*. Torkos has received national pharmacy awards and serves as an advisor for Probiotics.com and Wakunaga. SherryTorkos.com

Eating healthfully is already a daily struggle for many individuals. Adding the extra stress of inflation and unpredictable food prices at the grocery store can make it even more challenging to shop for nutritious choices. This is where strategic use of dietary supplements can help.

Supplements are designed to complement your diet, so if you are having trouble getting all the nutrients you need through food, supplements are your best budget-friendly asset. By incorporating quality supplements into your routine, you can bridge the nutrient gap and ensure that your body receives the essential vitamins and minerals it requires.

Food and Supplements

While it is widely acknowledged that a nutritious diet forms the foundation of good health, there is a growing body of research that shows the role of dietary supplements is an important adjunct to achieving optimal nutrition.

With the quality of food being less than optimal today, I believe it is necessary to include dietary supplements daily, along with the most wholesome diet you can afford. Strive to include fruits, vegetables, whole grains, lean proteins, and healthy fats in your diet to help reduce the risk of chronic diseases, support a healthy weight, enhance energy levels, and improve overall well-being.

Multipurpose Supplements

One effective budget-friendly strategy is to opt for multipurpose supplements that offer a range of benefits. Combination supplements offer a holistic approach to nutrition by integrating a variety of nutrients, vitamins, and minerals into a single capsule. These supplements are designed to address multiple health issues simultaneously, offering convenience, cost-effectiveness, and targeted support for specific concerns.

Using combination supplements gives you extra bang for your buck, and you also don't have to take as many pills. By investing in quality, science-supported supplements, you not only save money now, but also take preventive steps toward your future health, potentially reducing health-care costs in the long run.

Overall Health

A multivitamin supplement can cover many nutritional bases, but not all supplements are the same. Read labels carefully. A multivitamin should include calcium, iron, magnesium, potassium, thiamine, riboflavin, niacin, B-6, B-12, folate, selenium, zinc, and vitamins A, C, D, E, and K. Choose a multivitamin with 100 percent of the recommended daily intake (RDA) of most of its ingredients. (Not everything will be 100 percent or the pill would be too large.)

Immunity, Bone, Heart Health

Though heart and immune health top the list of biggest health concerns for men and women, bone health is equally important, especially as you age. All three of these health issues can be addressed with the right combination supplement. *Here are some ingredients to look for in combination products…*

- **Aged garlic extract (AGE).** Although AGE is a form of garlic, it's not the same garlic you use when cooking. AGE is made through an aging process that enhances the powerful antioxidant compounds in garlic and eliminates the odorous sulfur compounds. I recommend 1,200 milligrams per day.

- **Omega-3 fish oil.** If you don't eat fish, consider adding a fish oil supplement. Omega-3 fatty acids may help lower blood pressure and prevent and manage heart disease, lower inflammation, and boost immunity. The American Heart Association recommends taking about 3 grams per day.

- **Vitamin E** helps the immune system fight infections, widens blood vessels, and helps prevent clots. (RDA: 15 milligrams [mg].)

- **Vitamin D-3.** A large number of people have vitamin D deficiencies, and that may harm their health. Vitamin D is important for bone health and may reduce the risk of heart failure, but the heart-health benefits require additional research, says the American Heart Association. (RDA: 600 international units [IU] for people under age 70 and 800 IU for those over age 70.)

- **Vitamin K-2** is linked to bone strength, and supplementation has been associated with improved cardiovascular outcomes, according to a study published in *BMJ*. (RDA: 90 micrograms [mcg] women and 120 mcg for men).

- **Vitamin B complex.** The B vitamins have many important roles in the body. In particular, vitamin B-12 plays a crucial role in energy metabolism and neurological health. Since vitamin B-12 is found primarily in meat, eggs, and dairy, if you are cutting back on expensive proteins or trying out a plant-based diet, you may be lacking in this valuable nutrient. Having your vitamin B-12 levels measured is important so you know if you are low or deficient. (RDA: B-1: 1.1 mg; B-2: 1.1 mg; B-3: 14 mg; B-5: 5 mg; B-6: 1.3 mg; biotin: 30 mcg; folic acid: 400 mcg; B-12: 2.4 mcg.)

Gut and Urinary Tract Health

As a holistic pharmacist, I have received many questions from women throughout my career on how to prevent urinary tract infections (UTI). Cranberry has a long history of use for bladder health. However, drinking cranberry juice is not only costly, but it adds a lot of calories, and studies have been inconsistent on whether cranberry juice can actually help.

One form of cranberry that has been found to be beneficial for fighting UTIs is cran-max, a concentrated cranberry extract that is sold by a variety of manufacturers.

A combination product that combines cran-max with probiotics can enhance both gut and urinary tract health. Working synergistically, probiotics and cranberries support urinary tract health by promoting a balanced gut microbiome, aiding in the normalization of the gastrointestinal system, and preventing bacteria from adhering to the bladder wall.

Stress and Fatigue Support

Who doesn't have concerns about stress and fatigue these days with inflation and economic pressures? Most of us do. Finding a combination supplement that targets both stress and fatigue while supporting your immune system is important, since stress is a primary cause of fatigue and compromised immunity. This brings me back to my recommendation on aged garlic extract (AGE). Combining AGE with several B vitamins, including B-1, B-6, B-12, as well as the amino acid GABA, which can calm the nervous system and promote relaxation, can help fight fatigue, tame stress, and support the immune system.

> ### Be Selective About Supplements
>
> When selecting dietary supplements, it is crucial to choose those backed by science, supported by studies, and proven to be effective in the correct doses. You don't want to spend money on cheaper supplements, especially if they haven't been proven effective. Indeed, they could be a waste of money. Quality is key when it comes to dietary supplements, so seek out companies that have gone the extra mile to do clinical research and are using the proven dosages.

The Sunshine Vitamin: Vitamin D Is Even More Important Than You Think

Ouliana Ziouzenkova, PhD, researcher and associate professor of human nutrition in the department of human sciences at The Ohio State University, Columbus, and one of the scientific reviewers for the *Frontiers in Immunology's* special research topic, "The Role of Vitamin D as an Immunomodulator." EHE.OSU.edu

---

Research on the varied roles of vitamin D is continuing at a rapid clip. We already know that vitamin D is essential for bone health...and now we're learning more about the ways it contributes to overall good health as well as the perils we face when we don't get enough of the vitamin.

We asked nutrition researcher Ouliana Ziouzenkova, PhD, to parse through the findings of recent studies from around the world supporting the role of vitamin D for our health. Most of the studies used daily supplements of 2,000 international units (IU). This is higher than the recommended dietary allowance (RDA) of 600 IU for adults up to age 70 and 800 IU for adults over age 70 but still in line with what experts recommend for optimal health.

Caution: Before starting to take supplements, talk with your doctor and a nutritionist about the appropriate dosage for you, especially if you have kidney disease or atherosclerosis. Your endocrine and mineral status, bone density, dietary habits, and age all should be taken into account.

•**Vitamin D lowers risk for autoimmune diseases.** This Harvard study looked at the potential for vitamin D supplements, taken on their own as well as with omega-3 fatty acids, to prevent autoimmune diseases such as rheumatoid arthritis (RA), polymyalgia rheumatica, autoimmune thyroid disease, and psoriasis in middle-aged and older people.

Finding: Participants who took 2,000 IU of vitamin D-3 (cholecalciferol) every day for five years, with or without a daily supplement of 1,000 mg of marine-derived omega-3s, reduced their risk for autoimmune diseases by 22 percent compared with participants who received only placebos. The reduction was the highest for RA at 40 percent. Because the preventive effects of vitamin D increase over time, the researchers are continuing to follow participants for two more years to see whether the benefits will continue to go up.

•**Vitamin D reduces risk for type 2 diabetes complications.** The deadly complications of type 2 diabetes, notably heart disease, often stem from inflammation in blood vessels. Blood cells known as platelets stick to inflamed blood vessels and form clots. This can have a snowball effect that ultimately could lead to heart attack, stroke, amputation and/or loss of kidney function. To investigate the health effects of vitamin D on people with diabetes, researchers from the National Institute of Pharmaceutical Education and Research in Guwahati, India, gave study participants 60,000 IU of vitamin D-3 per week for three months followed by 60,000 IU per month (2,000 IU daily) for three months as maintenance.

Finding: Having a sufficient circulating level of vitamin D reduced platelet activity and oxidative stress. In particular, the serum levels of the well-known inflammatory proteins IL-18 and TNF-alpha were lower—a key factor in reducing or preventing many type 2 diabetes complications.

> **Best Ways to Get Your Vitamin D**
>
> **Morning sun,** especially when combined with fresh air and exercise.
> **Diet**—in particular, shiitake mushrooms, fatty fish, eggs, yogurt with live cultures.
> **Supplements**—the recommended dietary allowance is 600 IU daily up to age 70...800 IU over age 70. Check with your doctor for the appropriate dosage.

•**Vitamin D helps women avoid clots after stroke.** Having a vitamin D deficiency is more common in middle-aged and older women than men because of diet, less sun exposure, estrogen loss, and other factors. Separately, women have a higher risk than men of developing serious blood clots in a deep artery, most often in a leg, a condition called *deep vein thrombosis* (DVT). This study, led by researchers at China's Wenzhou Medical University, looked for a connection.

Finding: Having vitamin D levels higher than 75 nmol/L (which many experts consider an optimal level as opposed to a "sufficient" level of 50 nmol/L) is linked with lower risk for DVT, and supplementing with vitamin D could help make up for the gender difference in DVT risk.

•**Vitamin D deficiency hurts heart and circulatory health.** Researchers from the South Australian Health and Medical Research Institute in Adelaide found that people with vitamin D deficiency are more likely to suffer from heart disease and high blood pressure than people whose levels of vitamin D were above deficiency.

Finding: Participants with the lowest concentrations of vitamin D had double the risk for heart disease than those with sufficient concentrations. Just increasing vitamin D levels in the blood to 50 nmol/L offered effective protection from heart disease. (Higher levels of vitamin D didn't seem to offer further protection for this health threat.) The study also found a positive association between adequate vitamin D levels and systolic and diastolic blood pressure levels.

• **Vitamin D helps protect athletes from the perils of overexertion.** Exercise is essential to maintain health and counteract inflammatory processes, but too much exercise can increase inflammation, decrease immune function, and expose you to a higher risk for diseases. This is especially true in the face of vitamin D deficiency, which accompanies calcium loss during the stress and excitement of athletic training and competitions, according to researchers in the Department of Movement, Human and Health Sciences at University of Rome in Italy. Some athletes who become vitamin D deficient experience higher levels of oxidative stress and inflammation as well as respiratory infections, fractures and muscle injuries.

Finding: Having enough vitamin D counteracts inflammation and balances calcium metabolism. This, in turn, enhances the body's immune defense and improves the health of muscles, bones, and the bone marrow blood cells that work in concert to improve healing, prevent fractures, and maintain endocrine health.

• **There's more evidence that vitamin D helps you fight off infections.** This was a lab-based study conducted by researchers from University of Eastern Finland in Kuopio. It took a close look at vitamin D's role in fighting off threats to the immune system.

Finding: While vitamin D is used as co-therapy for certain conditions, such as psoriasis, for the best immune defense it's important to be proactive and get your vitamin D level optimized before you get sick, particularly in winter or whenever your exposure to sunlight is scant.

• **Vitamin D-3, not vitamin D-2, may be the supplement of choice.** Researchers at University of Surrey, University of Brighton and Newcastle University, all in the UK, compared the effects of the two readily available forms of vitamin D supplements—vitamin D-2 *(ergocalciferol),* found in plant foods such as mushrooms, and D-3 *(cholecalciferol),* found in animal-based foods. Participants took daily supplements of 15 micrograms (600 IU) of either vitamin D-2 or D-3 over a 12-week period in winter. The researchers then used blood samples to examine the difference in the regulation of genes implicated in the immune response.

Finding: Vitamin D-3, but not D-2, helped prepare genes for a more robust immune defense. In other words, supplementing with vitamin D-3 was better at enhancing the body's immune response against bacterial and viral diseases.

The Future of Vitamin D Research

These insights into the health benefits of vitamin D raise new questions about the vitamin's importance in special population groups, such as how much vitamin D do vegetarians and vegans and people who fast need. *Also…*

With advances in genetic testing, we're now finding that there are mutations in the genes responsible for converting vitamin D to its hormonally active form. Research is needed to find out what levels of the vitamin are needed by people with such mutations.

Blood levels of vitamin D are used to diagnose an overall deficiency, but deficiencies can develop autonomously within the bones, immune cells, kidneys, and other organs and lead to diseases. Tissue-specific diagnostics of vitamin deficiencies is key to identifying more preventive strategies in the future.

Valid clinical studies comparing the effects of vitamin D produced with different levels of sun exposure to the dietary and supplemental forms of vitamin D also would be beneficial. This would ensure vitamin D sufficiency based on where you live, the local diet that you follow and the pollutants you might be exposed to.

Benefits from Specific Kinds of Massage

Cleveland Clinic Arthritis Advisor. ArthritisAdvisor.com

Swedish massage calms the nervous system and is gentle and relaxing. *Lymphatic massage* helps lymph fluid flow more freely to get rid of waste through the kidneys and can help people with arthritis and other inflammation-related diseases. *Deep tissue massage* is useful during times of high stress or when muscles are tight. *Trigger point massage* targets specific areas, such as knotted muscles, using direct pressure to boost blood flow and release tension. *Myofascial release* kneads connective tissue under the skin—usually used on the back, shoulders, and neck. *Craniosacral therapy* focuses on membranes and tissue surrounding the organs, glands, nerves, brain, and spinal cord—it is especially effective for neck pain and body trauma.

You Need More Procyanidins

William W. Li, MD, president and CEO of the Angiogenesis Foundation, and author of *Eat to Beat Disease: The New Science of How Your Body Can Heal Itself*. He has served on the faculties of Harvard Medical School, Tufts University, and Dartmouth Medical School, and his scientific publications have appeared in leading journals such as Science, *The New England Journal of Medicine*, and *The Lancet*. DrWilliamLi.com

Tanmeet Sethi, MD, clinical associate professor at the University of Washington in Seattle, senior faculty for the Center for Mind Body Medicine, and author of *Joy Is My Justice*. TanmeetSethiMD.com

Bite into a Red Delicious apple and you've bitten into a juicy universe of health and healing. The apple is rich in pectin, a soluble, gel-like fiber that lowers cholesterol and balances blood sugar; vitamin C, which strengthens immunity, helps preserves the integrity of skin, and improves iron absorption; and potassium, an essential mineral that regulates blood pressure, nourishes muscles, and lowers the risk of colon cancer. But there's another nutritional compound found in Red Delicious apples that you may not know about (or even heard of) that is equally effective in preventing and treating disease: *procyanidins*.

Procyanidins are one of the bioactive compounds in plants called *flavonoids* that endow plants with their bright, deep, vivid colors. Procyanidins are behind the blue in blueberries, the red in strawberries, the purple of plums, the red and green of grapes, and the deep brown of

---

Herbs for Stress

- **Siberian ginseng** may improve memory, thinking ability, and resistance to stress. Take 2 to 3 grams of dried root daily or 2 to 4 milliliters (mL) of a tincture two to three times daily.
- **Rhodiola rosea** can relieve feelings of stress, anxiety, anger, confusion, and depression in people under severe stress. Look for a product standardized to contain 2 to 3 percent of rosavin and 0.8 percent salidroside rhodiola. Take 200 to 400 milligrams (mg) daily, ideally in a formula that combines rhodiola and Siberian ginseng.
- **Ashwagandha.** This gentle, balancing adaptogen can lower levels of the stress hormone cortisol. Take 1 dropperful of a tincture (about 40 drops or one teaspoon) three times a day in a shot of water or take a 500 mg capsule twice daily.
- **Tulsi.** This gentle adaptogen is useful for insomnia and mild anxiety. Take 1 to 2 tablespoons of tulsi tincture in a 12-ounce cup of water.

Herbs can interact with medications or medical conditions, so talk to your physician before trying these or any other supplements.

Jamison Starbuck, ND, a naturopathic physician in family practice in Missoula, Montana.

cocoa (the primary ingredient in chocolate). Along with apples, grapes, berries, plums (and prunes), and cocoa, you can also find procyanidins in legumes (beans and lentils) and nuts.

But procyanidins do a lot more than provide a palette for plants. They are powerful antioxidants, capable of containing the oxidative damage—a kind of cellular rust—that causes and complicates the chronic conditions that afflict millions of Americans, like heart disease, type 2 diabetes, and Alzheimer's disease.

Here are the many ways that procyanidins can protect or restore your health, and how to get just the right amount in your daily diet.

High Blood Pressure

About 45 percent of American adults have high blood pressure—systolic blood pressure (the top number) of 130 mmHg or higher or diastolic blood pressure (the bottom number) of 80 mmHg or higher. It's *the* leading risk factor for heart disease and stroke. Procyanidins can help you bring high blood pressure under control.

In a recent study published in *Pharmacological Research,* scientists analyzed the results from six studies on procyanidins and high blood pressure, and found that high intake reduced diastolic blood pressure by an average of 4.6 points and reduced systolic blood pressure by an average of 2.8 points. Procyanidins, wrote the researchers, could be a "useful treatment of hypertensive patients as well as a preventive measure in prehypertensive and healthy" people.

Procyanidins improve circulation by strengthening the endothelium, the lining of blood vessels that controls whether these flexible tubes are relaxed or tight. They also help prevent the arterial plaque that clogs blood vessels. In addition, procyanidins stimulate the stem cells that renew and repair damaged blood vessels. And they help control an immune compound called NLRP3 that triggers the inflammasome, which generates numerous inflammatory (and cell-damaging) compounds called cytokines.

Cancer

Cancer is the number-two cause of death in America, with nearly 2 million people diagnosed every year, and 610,000 dying. In a laboratory study from the Institute of Food Research, procyanidins in apples were used to starve a cancer by depriving it of blood.

Here's how: Tumors can't grow to any substantial size without their own blood supply, which is dependent on the growth of new blood vessels (angiogenesis). Procyanidins block a compound that powers angiogenesis.

In a laboratory study from Georgetown University Medical Center, researchers combined a procyanidin in chocolate with breast cancer cells, and the breast cancer cells stopped dividing or *proliferating,* the core process in cancer. There was also far less activity in a gene that drives breast cancer.

Dozens of laboratory and animal studies suggest that extracts of black raspberries—rich in procyanidins—can inhibit many cancers in laboratory studies.

A scientific paper in the *Journal of Berry Research,* from researchers at the Ohio State University, presents five studies that show black raspberry extracts are

> ### Should You Drink More Red Wine?
>
> Red wine has lots of procyanidins, but that doesn't mean it's good for you. That's because it also delivers ethanol, which is toxic to the body. For women, even small amounts of alcohol are linked to an increased risk of breast cancer. Just one drink a day (six ounces of wine) increases risk by up to 50 percent. Feel free to enjoy red wine in the context of occasional social gatherings and enjoyment, but don't look to red wine as a steady, daily source of a healthful bioactive like procyanidins.

effective in treating precancerous rectal polyps in patients with a high risk for colon cancer; colon cancer; oral dysplasia, a precancerous condition for oral cancer; and Barrett's esophagus, a disease that increases the risk for esophageal cancer.

Type 2 Diabetes

One out of every four adults ages 65 and older has type 2 diabetes (T2D), a disease of chronically high blood sugar. People with T2D have a higher risk for cardiovascular disease, kidney disease, and Alzheimer's disease, and complications of T2D include nerve damage, problems with vision, and leg and foot ulcers that can lead to amputation. Another 88 million American adults—about one in every three of us—have prediabetes, blood sugar levels that put you at a much higher risk for developing T2D.

Scientists reported in the journal *Antioxidants* that the procyanidins in cocoa can help control diabetes in many ways. They boost the secretion of insulin, the hormone that ushers blood sugar out of the bloodstream and into muscle, fat, and other cells. They improve insulin sensitivity, the ability of cells to make use of insulin. They lower cholesterol and triglycerides, heart-hurting blood fats. And, of course, they decrease oxidation and inflammation. "Cocoa or dark chocolate," write the researchers, "might be a potential preventive tool useful for the nutritional management of TD2."

Procyanidins also directly stimulate the sympathetic nervous system, activating the burning of excess fat and improving metabolism—lowering the risk for TD2 and helping manage the disease if you have it.

Cognitive Decline

More than six million older Americans have Alzheimer's disease. And an estimated one in five older adults have mild cognitive impairment (MCI), the mental decline that is characterized by poor memory, judgment, focus, and trouble finding the right words when speaking or writing.

In a study titled *Procyanidins and Alzheimer's Disease,* scientists write that procyanidins are a "potentially effective" way to prevent and treat Alzheimer's disease. They point out the compounds can prevent or reduce the amyloid-beta plaques and tau tangles in the brain, the cellular pathologies that are a feature of the disease; improve the "plasticity" of neurons in the brain, or their ability to change and adapt; and improve cognitive function itself. Procyanidins also work to improve cognitive function by improving blood flow to and decreasing inflammation in the brain.

In a recent study, researchers from the USDA Human Nutrition Research Center on Aging at Tufts University gave either freeze-dried strawberry powder (the equivalent of two cups a day of strawberries) or a placebo to 37 people aged 60 to 75. After 12 weeks, the strawberry group had significantly improved memory and learning ability compared with the placebo group.

And in a study in the journal *Hypertension,* researchers looked at 90 people with MCI, giving them a daily cocoa drink with either high, intermediate, or low levels of procyanidins and other flavonoids. After eight weeks, those getting the high-procyanidin drink performed better on several tests that measure cognitive impairment, including the Mini Mental State Examination. They also had lower blood pressure, less insulin resistance, and lower levels of oxidized cholesterol. "Regular consumption" of procyanidin-rich cocoa "might be effective in improving cognitive function" in people with mild cognitive improvement, write the researchers.

Getting More Procyanidins

The key to getting a healthful daily dose of procyanidins from the diet is to eat a wide variety of colorful foods every day: one or more servings of berries, grapes, apples, chocolate, legumes, nuts, and tea (black and green). The more diverse the menu, the more likely you'll be to get all the procyanidins you need.

Cooking at home rather than eating out is another good strategy for maximizing your intake of procyanidins—simply because you have more control over the menu. And don't forget spices! Cinnamon, for example, is a particularly rich source of procyanidins, and also excellent for balancing blood sugar.

A social network and friends is also a good way to meet your goals for healthy eating—perhaps having a dinner with friends once or twice a week where everyone brings a procyanidin-rich dish. Even if you can't have dinner together, you can network with people who want to eat healthier and encourage each other in your goals—sending pictures of your favorite procyanidin-rich snacks or meals or sharing a checklist of the procyanidin-rich foods you ate that day.

Getting procyanidins from supplements—like green tea extract, pycnogenol (pine bark), or resveratrol (grape extract)—is *not* the best way to guarantee a steady, healthful level of procyanidins. Supplements are potentially a good *addition* to any diet, but shouldn't be used to meet your nutritional goals.

The Good Medicine of Onions

Jamison Starbuck, ND, a naturopathic physician in family practice in Missoula, Montana.

When I was 6 years old and suffering with a bad cold, my mother told me that my grandfather always swore by raw onion sandwiches. While I opted for chicken noodle soup and hot tea, I never lost my curiosity about the healing power of onions. Decades later, I can say that my grandfather was right. Onions have been a staple of my nutritional medicine protocols for over 30 years.

As with their cousins garlic, chives, and leeks, onions are in the *Allium* family, a plant group known for its medicinal properties. *Alliums* contain strong antioxidants called flavonoids and lots of vitamin C. Both can help prevent cancer and heart disease. Onions also contain folate, B-6, calcium, potassium, and iron, nutritional inflammation fighters.

Onions are mucolytic: The same compounds that make your eyes water also work to break up mucus and congestion in your nose, sinuses, and lungs. Onions also nourish healthy bacteria in the gut, reduce inflammation in the walls of the gastrointestinal tract, and are an excellent source of plant fiber.

•**For acute illnesses,** such as a cold, sinusitis, bronchitis, cough or sore throat, onions are a great go-to medicine. Most folks have one or two in the kitchen and can quickly sauté a batch. To help reduce fever and mucus production, speed recovery time, and suppress a cough, eat ½ cup of sautéed onion at two meals per day until well. For ease of preparation, keep freshly sautéed onions in the refrigerator and add them to broth, soup, or serve as a vegetable with a small portion of protein such as chicken or fish. Cooked onions will retain their medicinal value for up to three days if kept cool in a tightly covered container.

•**To reduce a cough and relieve shortness of breath** from bronchitis and acute asthma, use an onion poultice. Wrap hot sautéed onions in a moist cotton cloth and place over the upper back (lungs) for 15 minutes. Cover the person receiving the poultice with several blankets so they stay warm. Repeat as often as needed for symptom relief.

•**For sore throats and respiratory congestion,** onion syrup is helpful. You can make your own to have on hand. Layer thin slices of raw onion alternating with thick layers of honey in a pint-size glass jar. Cover with a tight lid and store in the refrigerator for up to two months. To use, stir one tablespoon of honey/onion syrup into 8 ounces of hot water and sip as a tea or eat the syrup directly off a spoon several times a day until symptoms resolve.

•**For long-term good health, eat onions regularly.** You don't have to eat platesful; just try to make onions a part of your diet at least three times a week. Put a slice on a burger, dice them for a salad or on a baked potato, grill them on the barbeque, or add some to soup, spaghetti sauce, or an omelet. Maybe even follow my great-grandfather's advice and try a raw onion sandwich the next time you have a cold.

Does Melatonin Really Help You Sleep?

Michael J. Breus, PhD, clinical psychologist and a fellow of The American Academy of Sleep Medicine. He is author of *The Power of When: Discover Your Chronotype—and the Best Time to Eat Lunch, Ask for a Raise, Have Sex, Write a Novel, Take Your Meds, and More.* SleepDoctor.com

People struggling to sleep are increasingly turning to melatonin, the so-called "sleep hormone," as a solution.

In fact, the use of melatonin supplements by American adults more than doubled during the decade ending in 2018, according to a study by researchers at the Mayo Clinic...and melatonin use has no doubt increased even further still since 2018, as the pandemic years caused widespread sleep issues.

Problem: Melatonin supplements might not be as safe as people think and may not be as helpful for their sleep problems as they hope.

Melatonin supplements are available over the counter in the U.S., creating the impression that they're low risk...but in other countries, they're available only with a prescription, and those countries' caution might be merited. Here's why...

•**Melatonin is a hormone,** like testosterone or estrogen, and messing with the body's hormone levels is serious business. Multiple studies have shown that short-term use of melatonin generally is safe for adults—but no large-scale research has been done on the effects of taking melatonin supplements daily for longer than six months.

•**Taking melatonin supplements can alter the effectiveness of other medications,** including certain antidepressants and antihypertension medications.

•**Excessive dosages may be dangerous.** Research suggests that 0.5 to 1.5 milligrams of melatonin is all that's needed to aid in sleep, yet the vast majority of the melatonin supplements on the market are 3 milligrams or more. And because melatonin supplements are not regulated by the FDA, consumers can't even be confident that the supplements they purchase contain the dosages claimed on the packaging.

•**Melatonin supplements may be risky for children.** Children's bodies produce tremendous amounts of melatonin naturally—much more than should be necessary for sleep.

Biggest concern now: Many melatonin users fail to reap any meaningful benefit from taking these supplements, because they take them at the wrong time and/or to overcome sleep problems that melatonin won't solve.

People who take melatonin tend to do so right before they go to bed—but in pill or gummy form, it's best taken 90 minutes before bedtime...or in liquid form, 30 minutes before bedtime.

And while melatonin supplements may be effective for people hoping to reset their sleep schedules after traveling to different time zones—and potentially also for people hoping to adjust their circadian rhythms to work a night shift—the evidence suggests that melatonin does not help with chronic insomnia and other sleep problems. Other treatments, such as cognitive behavioral therapy for insomnia (CBT-I), are shown to be more effective.

Inhaling Fragrances During Sleep Boosts Memory

Study of 43 adults by researchers at University of California, Irvine, published in *Frontiers in Neuroscience.*

Every night for six months, healthy study participants ages 60 to 85 used diffusers and cartridges filled with scented natural oils to emit pleasant fragrances, one per night, for two hours. The fragrances were combinations of resinous, flowery, fruity, and aromatic odors. Compared with a control group, those using full-strength cartridges performed 226 percent better on a word-list test used to evaluate memory. Researchers say this is further evidence of a link between olfactory sense and cognition.

Look to Bees to Boost Your Health

Jamison Starbuck, ND, naturopathic physician in family practice in Missoula, Montana.

Most of earth's inhabitants need bees to survive and live healthy lives. Nuts, seeds, fruit, grains, flowers, trees—75 percent of agricultural crops and 90 percent of wild plants—rely on bees for pollination and successful growth. But the health benefits of bees go far beyond pollination.

•**Honey** is a naturally occurring sweet food. Like white sugar, it contains calories and can contribute to weight gain and blood sugar imbalances. But honey contains antioxidants and nutrients that improve blood vessel and cellular health. Because honey tastes sweeter and metabolizes more slowly than sugar, people often need less honey than sugar to feel satisfied. Reduce calories and improve health by substituting ⅔ cup honey for one cup sugar in your recipes.

Honey is also a great medicine. Simply spoon honey directly on a clean wound or burn, cover with sterile, non-stick gauze. Monitor the wound for infection and re-apply fresh honey. *Note:* If your wound is deep or your burn severe, seek medical help immediately and before using honey.

I also prescribe honey to patients with ulcers, gastritis, and bowel inflammation. Take honey as medicine for these conditions in a medicinal herbal tea. Use one tablespoon of dried herb (peppermint, spearmint, catnip, or chamomile) per 16 ounces of boiled water. Let it steep five minutes, and then add one tablespoon of honey. Drink up to 32 ounces of hot, honeyed tea daily, taken at least an hour away from meals and at bedtime.

As a cough suppressant: Eat it slowly, directly off a spoon, or add a liberal amount to a cup of hot tea.

•**Bee pollen** boosts immune health, can reduce allergic reactivity, and may help in heart, liver, and bone health due to its easily absorbable nutrients.

Take bee pollen as a food: Buy loose bee pollen (it should be yellow/brown granules) and add a spoonful to a serving of yogurt, cereal, fruit salad, or a smoothie.

Caution: If you are allergic to weeds, flowers, or fungi, avoid bee pollen and honey as they may contain these allergens. Also, children under one year of age should not consume honey due to a risk of botulism.

Chapter 12

PAIN RELIEF AND AUTOIMMUNE DISEASE

The Pain Gap: Women Experience More Pain Than Men

More than one in five U.S. adults live with chronic pain, defined as unrelenting pain that lasts longer than three months. *The majority of these patients are women who are living with pain from one or more conditions such as...*

- Cancer.
- Migraine.
- Hip, back, knee, and pelvic floor pain.
- Osteoarthritis and rheumatoid arthritis.
- Irritable bowel syndrome.
- Endometriosis (a condition in which the uterine lining grows outside the uterus and in other areas throughout the body.)
- Interstitial cystitis (a chronic bladder condition).
- Fibromyalgia (a chronic condition including widespread pain and tenderness, disrupted sleep, and cognitive troubles).

Women and Pain

Women are more likely to experience *high-impact chronic pain,* pain so severe it interferes with the ability to work or enjoy life. Why do women suffer disproportionately? *There are a few reasons...*

- **Women experience pain differently.** Women feel pain more intensely than men, perhaps due to having more nerve receptors throughout the body, an increased tendency toward inflammation, and different ways of processing pain in the central nervous system.

- **Women are often not believed.** Medical gaslighting, a phrase used to describe the phenomenon of having one's symptoms minimized or ignored, overwhelmingly impacts women, who leave their appointments with either Band-Aid solutions or subpar treatments. Women of color—Blacks and Asians in particular—are particularly vulnerable. They may be subject to the false belief that they should be

---

Monica Mallampalli, PhD, MSc, a biomedical scientist, women's thought leader, and expert on women's pain. She is a member of the Healthy Women Women's Health Advisory Council and chair of the Healthy Women Chronic Pain Advisory Council. HealthyWomen.org

more physically stoic or misperceived as drug-seeking.

- **Poor sleep worsens pain.** Women of all ages are disproportionately affected by sleep disorders—perimenopausal and postmenopausal women especially so—due to hormone-induced insomnia and night sweats or anxiety. Without refreshing sleep, you'll wake up fatigued, which makes pain feel more acute. Bouts of insomnia are likely to precede painful flare-ups of fibromyalgia, migraine, and other pain conditions. Fractured sleep also interferes with the body's ability to calm inflammation, further stalling efforts to heal. Poor sleep increases the risk of, or worsens existing mood disorders like anxiety and depression, keeping the pain cycle in motion. Yet pain can make sleep feel impossible.

How to Move Forward

Some types of pain, like migraine and endometriosis pain, tend to diminish with age as estrogen levels decrease. Other types, like arthritis and pelvic pain, increase with the wear-and-tear of age. Treatments exist, but patients first need to be believed for those treatments to be in reach.

- **Find your voice so you can advocate for yourself and your pain.** Women need to let their doctors know they are hurting. Unfortunately, they need to be strategic in their communication so they aren't perceived as complaining or coming across as overly emotional. (Even though they have every right to be emotional. It's incredibly difficult to live with day after day.)

- **Empower yourself with information regarding your condition.** When you go to your medical appointment, carry detailed notes of medications and treatments, along with list of written questions to ask your health-care provider to ensure you get the care you need.

One patient advocate I've worked with who lives with chronic migraine, fibromyalgia, anxiety, and depression carries a letter from her specialists stating she has these conditions whenever seeing a new provider. She shouldn't need to, but she has learned that doing so, especially as a Black woman, ensures she is believed.

- **Assemble an interdisciplinary team of health-care professionals to address your pain.** Possibilities include a rheumatologist, pain specialist, orthopedist, gynecologist, physical therapist, acupuncturist, psychologist, or psychiatrist. Ask friends or colleagues who've dealt with chronic pain for referrals, or ask your primary care physician to connect you with additional experts. Start by describing some strategies that ease your pain (e.g., medications, avoiding certain foods, exercise, meditation) to help point them in the right direction.

- **Take steps to reduce underlying inflammation,** which may be affecting your chronic pain. Pay attention to how diet affects your pain. Some migraineurs find that wine, gluten, or dairy make their headaches flare up. Many pain sufferers experience some relief by following an anti-inflammatory diet protocol.

- **Exercise.** It seems counterintuitive that moving would ease pain in the back, hip, shoulder, or knee, but exercise eases stiffness and sends healing nutrients and lubricating fluids to the affected area. (There's a saying that describes the pain-relieving potential of physical activity: "Rest is rust, motion is lotion.")

Certain types of exercise offer specific benefits: Strength-training builds muscle to increase endurance; stretching loosens stiff joints and muscles; walking outside gets the blood flowing and helps clear the mind.

- **Get a handle on stress.** Stress and pain go hand-in-hand. One-third of adults with arthritis have anxiety or depression, for example, and acute bouts of stress can trigger debilitating fibromyalgia flare-ups. Managing stress, even just a bit, can have a meaningful effect on how you experience life. Different techniques work for different people, so experiment with everything from meditation and guided imagery to nature walks and volunteering. If it helps get your mind off your pain, it counts.

• **Therapy is a tremendous asset.** Two types of therapy that work well with chronic pain are cognitive behavioral therapy (CBT) and acceptance and commitment therapy (ACT). CBT teaches you how to reframe negative thoughts and behaviors that would otherwise intensify and fuel pain. ACT is more about separating yourself from your thoughts, accepting your situation, and focusing on what you would like to be different. Both are usually covered by insurance and should be used alongside other treatments, not instead of. Therapy can also help process trauma you've endured that may contribute to your continued pain.

• **Prioritize sleep.** Tossing and turning all night can lead to a nasty cycle of heightened pain, worsened sleep, and more pain. Try to go to bed at the same time every night, ideally by 10 p.m. A regular sleep routine with a reasonable bedtime helps regulate your circadian rhythm, promoting more and better rest. Avoid or minimize the use of electronics in the hours before bed, as the blue light emitting from the screens will interfere with your ability to fall asleep. If menopause-induced insomnia or night sweats are interrupting your sleep, ask your doctor if you're a candidate for hormone therapy.

• **Ensure you're on the right type of pain medication.** Women respond differently to opioids than men and are also more prone to becoming addicted to them. Ask your doctor about over-the-counter or prescription anti-inflammatory meds. Acetaminophen can be helpful for osteoarthritis and low back pain, while nonsteroidal anti-inflammatory drugs may be better for rheumatoid arthritis. Other options include muscle relaxants, antidepressants (some may help relieve chronic pain, plus they have the added bonus of easing depression and anxiety), acupuncture, and more.

> ### Pain on the Brain
> Past trauma; current anxiety, depression, or post-traumatic stress disorder; and other psychological dynamics can increase pain, as do social factors such as age, ethnicity, and marital status. Depression can worsen pain or interfere with coping mechanisms, and women are nearly twice as likely as men to experience depression. Similarly, people who are divorced or widowed experience more chronic pain than those who are married or live with a partner.
>
> –Monica Mallampalli, PhD, MSc

New Nasal Spray for Migraine Approved by the FDA

Rashmi B. Halker Singh, MD, FAHS, FAAN, an associate professor of neurology at Mayo Clinic, Scottsdale, Arizona, commenting on a study published in *The Lancet Neurology*.

Fast-acting *zavegepant* (Zavzpret) nasal spray is for people whose migraine attacks cause nausea and/or vomiting, making it difficult to take pills. In trials, 24 percent of patients taking zavegepant were pain-free after two hours—slightly less effective than with triptans, but triptans can't be taken by people who've had a heart attack or stroke.

New Ways to Fight Migraine Pain

Brian M. Grosberg, MD, FAHS, director of the Hartford HealthCare Headache Center of Ayer Neuroscience Institute in West Hartford, Connecticut, professor of neurology at University of Connecticut School of Medicine, and an international speaker on migraine. HartfordHealthcare.org/services/headache-center

Researchers still are trying to unravel the mystery of the intense form of head pain known as migraine. If you suffer from this debilitating neurological condition, relief is never as simple as taking aspirin, NSAIDs, or other painkillers. Migraine is a highly individualized disorder that needs a personalized medication regimen...and even that may not work all the time. But there is hope—new classes of drugs are emerging along with new ways of using existing medications. We spoke with migraine specialist Brian M. Grosberg, MD, to learn more about the new treatments and what is coming in the future.

Two Ways to Treat

There are two prongs to migraine treatment—medications that work to reduce frequency...and acute medications to relieve attacks once they occur.

A migraine-prevention regimen is appropriate if...

•**You have frequent or long-lasting migraines.** Frequent means having headaches more than four days per month. Long-lasting means not getting consistent benefit (90 to 100 percent relief) within two hours of migraine onset and complete functionality following treatment.

•**Your migraine causes significant disability** or loss of quality of life.

•**You don't get relief from acute migraine medicine**...the medicine causes unbearable side effects...or you can't take NSAIDs because of gastrointestinal ulcers or triptans because of heart disease. (A triptan may narrow coronary blood vessels.)

•**You're at risk for medication-overuse headaches**—when you take acute medications more than two days a week over an extended period. Medications that may result in this risk are opiates and barbiturate-containing combination analgesics, such as Fioricet and Fiorinal.

•**You have menstrual migraines,** which can be very severe, longer lasting, and less responsive to acute treatment.

•**You have depression and anxiety, obesity, other pain disorders, or allodynia,** sensitivity to things that aren't normally uncomfortable such as brushing your hair or wearing glasses. With any of these conditions, you are at higher risk for increased migraine frequency.

Preventive medications typically are aimed at people with episodic and chronic migraine, and they can help prevent episodic migraine from becoming chronic. Nearly 40 percent of people with migraine could benefit from preventive therapy, but only about 10 percent have tried it.

Game changer: CGRP antagonists are drugs that block calcitonin gene-related peptide (CGRP), a protein that causes blood vessels in the nervous system to dilate, triggering pain. They have been proven effective for chronic and episodic migraine prevention.

The four large-molecule CGRP antagonists—called *monoclonal antibodies*—are *erenumab* (Aimovig), *fremanezumab* (Ajovy), *galcanezumab* (Emgality) and *eptinezumab* (Vyepti). Aimovig, Ajovy and Emgality are self-administered injections. Vyepti is given intravenously in a hospital or outpatient infusion center every three months.

Small-molecule CGRP antagonists, known as *gepants* and available in pill form, were first used for treatment of acute migraine. *Atogepant* (Qulipta) was the first gepant developed exclusively as a preventive treatment for episodic migraine. In three- and 12-month studies on episodic migraine, it was shown to be safe and effective, reducing monthly migraine days by more than four days. Also, participants needed less medication to stop an attack and were able to cut monthly sick days by half or more. Another gepant, *rimegepant* (Nurtec), is approved to prevent episodic migraine and can be taken every other day.

What's new in preventive treatment: In April 2023, *atogepant* (Qulipta) was approved for prevention of chronic migraine. It reduced monthly migraine days by an average of seven when participants took 60 mg daily. Separate research found that Qulipta is a viable treatment for people who weren't helped by other classes of preventive medications.

In the pipeline: Ongoing research includes the first head-to-head comparison of a small-molecule CGRP drug versus a large-molecule one. In contrast to large-molecule CGRP antagonists, which have a half-life (the time it takes for the drug's active substance in your body to reduce by half) lasting about a month, small-molecule CGRP antagonists are oral medications with shorter half-lives that leave the body more rapidly, so you need less medication.

When You Have a Migraine

Preventive medications don't work for everyone or don't work all the time, so sufferers need to have migraine-relief medications in their arsenals. These drugs can take one to two hours to work, so they should be taken at the first sign of a migraine and in the exact dose prescribed. Gepants have replaced triptans for many sufferers, especially those with heart disease who can't take triptans because of potential effects on blood vessels.

What's new in acute treatment: *Ubrogepant* (Ubrelvy) received FDA approval for treatment of acute migraine in adults in December 2019. Approved in March 2023, *zavegepant* (Zavzpret) became the latest gepant and first fast-acting nasal spray. It comes premeasured to deliver 10 mg into one nostril and can be used once a day. Studies have found that zavegepant can start to ease pain in 15 minutes, allow people to function normally in 30 minutes, and feel pain-free in two hours—an effect that lasted 48 hours.

Nasal sprays are good for people who don't respond to oral drugs. Within the last few years, nasal sprays have become a more popular delivery method for older migraine medications as well, including *sumatriptan* (Tosymra) and *dihydroergotamine mesylate* (Trudhesa).

Nondrug Treatment

Give yourself the best possible chance of relief by making lifestyle changes that will have the greatest impact...

• **Keep a comprehensive journal of your migraines, medications, etc.** Include a food diary—many foods have been linked to migraine, but they differ from person to person—and a record of your activities, including not only work absenteeism but also presentism, when you're where you're supposed to be but not functioning at your normal capacity.

• **Stick to a schedule.** Lifestyle factors that impact migraine are exercise or lack of it, missed sleep and sleep disturbances, and stress. Beware of the letdown phenomenon—the level of endorphins, released when you are under stress, is high during the week but come Friday, those endorphins drop, you stay out late, your sleep schedule is off...and you get a migraine.

• **Consider losing weight.** Weight loss from bariatric surgery has been linked to less frequent migraines. Research is underway to study whether medical weight loss, achieved with a drug such as Ozempic, has the same effect.

• **Try mind-body practices.** Cognitive behavioral therapy (CBT) teaches you to change thought patterns and behaviors. Biofeedback, relaxation therapies like deep breathing and mindfulness mediation, and yoga also are helpful.

You Don't Have to Live with Chronic Pain

Pain medicine specialist and anesthesiologist Taralin Hollins, MD, physician in the department of pain management at Cleveland Clinic South Pointe Hospital in Warrensville Heights, Ohio. My.ClevelandClinic.org

America has a pain problem. A National Institutes of Health study revealed that Americans are more likely to devel-

> **To Treat Sunburn Pain...**
>
> Cool down skin that is warm or hot to the touch with a lukewarm shower. Apply moisturizer while skin is still damp—use pure aloe vera or a product that lists aloe among the first ingredients. Ibuprofen or aspirin can help reduce swelling and redness and alleviate discomfort. Sunburn dehydrates the rest of the body as moisture is pulled to the skin surface, so drink extra water. Stay out of the sun until the burn heals...and be more careful about sun protection in the future. Repeated burns age skin and increase risk for skin cancer.
>
> *Avoid:* After-sun sprays may relieve pain but also irritate skin...and petroleum jelly products can hold in heat.
>
> Consumer Reports. CR.org

op chronic pain than they are to develop diabetes, high blood pressure, or depression.

This is no shock to pain experts like Tara-lin Hollins, MD, from Cleveland Clinic South Pointe Hospital. She routinely sees patients battling pain described as unrelenting aching, stabbing, burning, and more. In fact, one in five Americans live with chronic pain, defined as pain experienced on most or all days for three months...and nearly one in 10 have high-impact chronic pain that has lasted three months and is severe enough to limit at least one work or day-to-day activity. *We asked Dr. Hollins why we have chronic pain and what we can do about it...*

When the Pain Alarm Is Stuck

Pain is the body's warning that whatever you're doing will likely cause injury. When you unwittingly grab the handle on a hot pan, nerve cells in your hand detect the heat and release neurotransmitters that shoot a pain signal up the spinal cord to the brain screaming, *Danger! This will burn you!* When your brain hears this message, it makes you feel pain in your hand and prompts you to yank your hand away from the handle. Whether you're left with a bit of lingering redness and sensitivity or an angry blister, the pain has accomplished its goal—to get you out of an unsafe situation. Other examples of acute pain—temporary pain that starts suddenly for a logical reason and stops once the injury has healed—include a stubbed toe, broken bone, herniated disk, or even surgical pain.

The problem occurs when the pain-signaling neurotransmitters continue to fire back and forth for months even after the injury has healed, revving the brain in a way that perpetuates the pain. Your wound, broken bone or surgical site may be healed, but you still feel pain there. That pain actually is being created and sustained by the brain.

Chronic pain isn't always due to injury —it is a symptom of many conditions, including osteoarthritis, back pain, fibromyalgia, migraine, and irritable bowel syndrome. And there even are times when the pain lacks a clear cause.

Who's at risk? Women, Native Americans, and people of multi-racial ethnicity are at greater risk for acute pain that morphs into chronic pain. Also at greater risk are people who have experienced emotional trauma in the past, live with depression and anxiety, and/or whose pain started in a traumatic way.

When does pain become chronic pain? Chronic pain physically and chemically changes the nervous system, heightening a person's sensitivity to pain. With the brain's pain alarm stuck in the "on" position, the individual becomes hyper-vigilant to pain in other areas of his/her body (a migraine patient may report higher-than-usual pain after knee surgery, for instance) or may start perceiving things that would otherwise not cause discomfort, such as a hug, as painful stimuli.

About 25 percent of people with chronic pain develop chronic pain syndrome, when recurrent pain creeps into other areas of life in the form of depression, anxiety, insomnia, alcohol or drug use, and other stress-related symptoms.

Breaking the Cycle

Chronic pain is notoriously difficult to treat. For decades, doctors tried to dull chronic pain with powerful opioid medications, including *oxycodone* (OxyContin), *hydrocodone*, codeine, and morphine. But these drugs are designed for only short-term use to ease acute pain, such as post-operative pain. They usually don't help chronic pain. In fact, long-term opioid use can *worsen* chronic pain—by making the opioid receptor sensitive, opioids cause a paradoxical response. (Opioids also have side effects and are highly addictive.)

Some smarter treatment options for chronic pain...

• **Diclofenac gel** (Voltaren), a topical nonsteroidal anti-inflammatory gel, relieves pain where you apply it. Even though chronic pain originates in the brain, there can be local inflammation and muscle irritation that respond to topical products. Unlike oral nonsteroidal anti-inflammatory drugs (NSAIDs) such as ibuprofen and naproxen, diclofenac is well-tolerated by people with poor kidney function. Applying it topically also prevents the side effects of long-term NSAID use, such as peptic ulcer and gastrointestinal bleeding. Diclofenac also is available in a prescription-only patch called a Flector patch. The gel can be applied up to four times a day...the patch is changed daily. Both can be used for several months, with less needed over time.

• **Antidepressants and anti-seizure medications.** Many chronic pain sufferers find relief with drugs that act on the brain or spinal cord—not by blocking the pain but by calming neurotransmitter activity to ease pain. Certain antidepressants treat pain by ramping up production of serotonin and other pain-relieving neurotransmitters. These drugs work double duty for patients with depression and anxiety, both of which fuel the chronic pain cycle. *Examples of pain-relieving antidepressants and anti-seizure medications (these drugs all take several weeks to deliver relief)...*

• *Venlafaxine* (Effexor) This antidepressant, a serotonin and norepinephrine reuptake inhibitor (SNRI), is used to treat pain associated with osteoarthritis, rheumatoid arthritis, and lower back pain.

• *Duloxetine* (Cymbalta), another SNRI, can help with fibromyalgia, diabetic peripheral neuropathic pain, chronic back pain, and arthritis.

• *Pregabalin* (Lyrica), an anti-seizure medication, is a synthetic form of gamma-aminobutyric acid, an anti-inflammatory neurotransmitter that dampens nerve pain, including pain that occurs after shingles (postherpetic neuralgia).

• *Gabapentin* (Neurontin) is an anti-seizure drug used to treat nerve pain.

Powerful pairing: Sometimes an antidepressant and an anti-seizure medication are needed.

Example: A combination of *pregabalin* and *duloxetine* can ease chemotherapy-induced pain experienced by breast cancer patients.

• **Acupuncture.** According to this traditional Chinese medical practice, inserting needles into points throughout the body unblocks energy, called Qi (pronounced "chee"), helping to resolve pain and other chronic conditions. Stimulating the acupoints triggers production of pain-relieving *endogenous opioids*—the body's version of prescription opioids—which can offer a reprieve from discomfort while reducing the need for pain medication. Western medicine is catching onto acupuncture's power to alleviate chronic neck, back and shoulder pain, osteoarthritis knee pain, chronic headache, and more.

Fascinating: Acupuncture lowers circulating levels of the inflammatory, pain-inciting enzyme cyclooxygenase-2 (COX-2). Oral NSAIDs such as ibuprofen (Advil) and naproxen (Aleve) work, at least in part, by inhibiting COX-2.

- **Pain Reprocessing Therapy (PRT).** With this mind–body approach, patients work with a pain-management therapist to change how they think about their chronic pain. PRT teaches patients to view long-term pain as a real yet harmless sensation created by the brain, not as a sign of a physical abnormality. They learn how the pain–fear cycle intensifies pain and work with the therapist to gather evidence that shows the pain is not due to a physical problem.

Example: A back pain patient may see on an MRI that she has no bulging disks, or the therapist may point out that her pain began during a very stressful time in her life. Reframing thoughts, beliefs, and fears about pain often leads to a reduction in that pain.

PRT is most effective with pain that has no obvious physical cause (in other words, it is not related to a prior injury). You can find a pain psychologist at the website of the American Association of Pain Psychology (AAPainPsychology.org/find-a-provider).

> ### Breakthrough Therapies for Chronic Pain
>
> There are several new, nondrug therapies that show promise in the relief of chronic pain.
>
> - **Scrambler therapy.** This FDA-approved therapy transmits impulses into nerve fibers that "scramble" pain messages, reducing pain. It's most effective in chronic nerve pain (neuropathy). The painless signals are intended to scramble the pain signals and prevent them from reaching the brain. Clinical trials have shown that scrambler therapy can significantly relieve pain in 80 to 90 percent of patients with chronic pain.
> - **Radiofrequency ablation.** This procedure temporarily disrupts pain signals from arthritic joints to the brain, and the benefits can last for six months or more. It's very helpful for neck, midback, and sacroiliac (low back) pain.
> - **Regenerative medicine.** This type of therapy focuses on repairing, replacing, or regenerating damaged or diseased tissues and organs. The most popular and effective regenerative therapy for chronic pain is platelet-rich plasma (PRP) therapy, which uses injections of the platelet-rich portion of a patient's blood to target chronic pain, usually in a joint or tendon.
>
> Jennifer Hankenson, MD, a physiatrist (specialty of physical medicine and rehabilitation), an assistant professor of orthopedics and rehabilitation at Yale School of Medicine, and program director of the physiatry residency.

Halt Lower Back Pain with Exercise

Mitchell Yass, DPT, doctor of physical therapy, president and cofounder of Yass Global Enterprises, Inc., Jacksonville, Florida. He is author of *The Yass Method for Pain-Free Movement: A Guide to Easing Through Your Day Without Aches and Pains.* LiveWithoutPains.com

It sounds counterintuitive, but exercise—strength training, in particular—is one of the best ways to alleviate joint pain. Why? Because in most cases the tissue causing the pain is muscle...even when structural abnormalities such as herniated discs and arthritis are identified by diagnostic tests. For patients with painful hips, knees, and backs, the root cause often is a weakness or imbalance of strength between the muscles in the front and the back of the body...or in the muscles surrounding the painful joint. Strengthening the weaker muscles often can resolve the pain. Mitchell Yass, DPT, creator of The Yass Method for pain-free movement, suggests the following two strengthening moves to help with one of the most common pain scenarios—lower back pain.

MOVE #1: Hamstring curls. If you have access to a gym, use the seated leg curl machine. Position yourself so that your ankles are resting on top of the padded bar. Press the bar down with your legs, imagining your power coming from the contraction of your hamstrings (the muscles at the back of your thighs). Once your knees are bent at a 90-degree angle, slowly raise your legs back up until they're nearly straight but your knees aren't locked. Repeat for 10 reps for one set. Rest...then repeat. Do a total of three sets.

Reminder: The weight should be heavy enough that the first eight reps feel doable but challenging and the final reps feel difficult.

Working out at home? Perform the same exercise with a resistance band in lieu of the machine. Make a loop with the band and anchor the ends of the band (knotting the ends together helps) between the door and frame. Sit in a sturdy chair far enough from the door to provide resistance for the band—the band should hold your leg off the ground when that foot is placed in the loop. Then proceed following the same moves as with the machine. Repeat for 10 reps for each foot for one set. Perform three sets.

MOVE #2: Hip extensions. Despite the name, this move works the gluteus maximus muscle—the outermost muscle of the buttocks—not the hips. Standing near a solidly built door, loop a resistance band behind your right knee and anchor the loose ends between the door and frame at knee height when standing. Facing the door, step back about two feet—far enough that the band has moderate tension. Place your hands on the door, and lean slightly forward. Once stable, shift most of your weight to your left foot and raise your right knee, bending it to a 90-degree angle with the sole of your foot facing away from the door. Extend your bent right leg back about 10 degrees behind the hip—imagine leading with your right heel. When you reach the band's end point, return to the start position. Do 10 reps on each side for one set. Perform three sets. If you are doing this exercise at a gym, use a cable system to perform the exercise.

Spinal Cord Stimulation Does Not Provide Long-Term Relief

Adrian Traeger, PhD, senior research fellow at the Institute for Musculoskeletal Health, a division of the School of Public Health, University of Sydney.

Researchers analyzed the results of 13 clinical trials that compared spinal cord stimulation treatment with placebo or no treatment for low-back pain and found that spinal cord stimulation is no better than a placebo. The researchers also found that adverse side effects to the surgery were poorly documented overall, preventing them from estimating the level of risk involved. Harms from spinal cord stimulation could include nerve damage, infection, and the electrical leads moving, all of which may necessitate repeated surgeries. The majority of clinical trials looked only at the immediate impact of the device, and none investigated the long-term (more than 12 months) impact.

5 Strategies to Protect Your Back

Mara Vucich, MD, a spine specialist at Mercy Medical Center, Baltimore, Maryland.

Back problems are incredibly common, striking people of all ages. There are a multitude of causes of back pain, from sprains and strains to degenerative disks, inflammatory conditions, osteoporosis, and more. While no strategy can guarantee that you'll never develop back pain, there are a few tried and true guidelines that will reduce your risk, says Mara Vucich, DO, from the Maryland Spine Center at Mercy Medical Center.

1. Maintain a healthy weight. Back pain is more common in people who are overweight. Excess weight puts pressure on our bones, joints, cartilage, ligaments, tendons, and muscles. Studies show that people who are overweight have higher rates of degenerative disk disease as well as systemic chronic inflammation that may contribute to or worsen pain.

2. Exercise regularly. When it comes to a healthy back, there are two types of exercises to prioritize: low-impact aerobic exercises and core-strengthening strategies.

•**Aerobic exercise** increases the blood flow and nutrients to the soft tissues in the back, which promotes healing and reduces stiffness. Exercise can also reduce the sensation of pain by increasing the production of pain-fighting endorphins. For the most protection, get your heart pumping with a low-impact activity like walking, biking, swimming, or using an elliptical machine. Jogging and running put extra force on the spine, which could increase pain. Aim for 150 minutes (such as 30 minutes per day for five days) of moderate-intensity activity each week.

•**Core strengthening** protects your back by building support all the way around your midsection.

The core includes several muscle groups: In the front, there's the rectus abdominis (what you think of as "abs") and the deeper transverse abdominis. On the sides, you have internal and external obliques. In your back lie the erector spinae and multifidi. The core also includes the diaphragm, pelvic floor, hip flexors, and gluteal muscles. There are several simple core exercises you can do at home.

•**Planks.** Kneel on all fours. Pull in your abdomen and move your feet back until your legs are straight. Keep your neck straight and your hands directly under your shoulders. Hold your abdomen and legs tight, and keep your back straight so it's not sagging or lifting. (You can use a mirror to check your position.) To make the exercise easier, lower your knees. To make it more challenging, rest your forearms on the ground. Hold for 30 seconds. If that's too long when you start, do what you can and work your way up to that time. Make sure you breathe.

•**Alternating leg extensions.** Kneel on all fours. Tighten your abdominal muscles and reach one arm out in front of you. Then extend the opposite leg behind you. Repeat on the other side for a total of 10 repetitions on each side.

•**Bent knee raises.** Lie on your back, with your knees bent. Tighten your abdominal muscles and lift one leg a few inches from the floor. Return to the starting position and switch sides. Aim for 10 repetitions per side.

It's important to use what's called good form when doing any exercise. If you're new to exercise—or just want a refresher—a physical therapist can help you master using safe and correct positions. If you go to a gym, a personal trainer can help as well, but they don't have the same kind of training that a physical therapist does.

3. Avoid smoking. Smokers have more low back pain and more degenerative disk disease in the lumbar spine than nonsmokers. A 2016 study found that the prevalence of back pain was 23.5 percent in never smokers, 33.1 percent in former smokers, and 36.9 percent in current smokers. Smoking impairs the delivery of oxygen-rich blood to your bones and tissues.

4. Avoid heavy lifting. If you don't have to lift something heavy, don't risk it. But when it's unavoidable, lift with your legs, not your back. That means bending at the hips and knees instead of rounding your back to lean forward. Tighten your core muscles and hold the object you're lifting close to your belly button. Avoid twisting while lifting.

5. Avoiding repetitive bending and twisting. If you're working on a task that requires bending or twisting, look for either tools or techniques to reduce those motions. For example, if you're working in the garden, instead of bending, sit with your legs folded under you or use a little stool. When bending, tighten your core muscles and bend through the hips—like a hinge—instead of rounding your back.

When Is the Right Time for Back Surgery?

Amit Jain, MD, MBA, chief of minimally invasive spine surgery in the department of orthopaedic surgery and associate professor of orthopaedic surgery at Johns Hopkins Medicine in Baltimore. HopkinsMedicine.org

Have you tried medication, exercise, even physical therapy for your back pain but nothing is helping? Perhaps your doctor has recommended spinal surgery, but your fears about the outcome are holding you back.

Problem: Delaying surgery can create its own cascade of negative events—your back pain worsens...your overall heath declines because you aren't able to move and exercise comfortably...and in turn, you're in worse condition to handle surgery when it becomes inevitable.

Fear of surgery and negative consequences, such as nerve damage or even paralysis, keep some people from considering surgery—perhaps they have a loved one whose procedure didn't correct their problem or made it worse...or they are concerned because older procedures were less exacting. But recent advances have led to minimally invasive approaches that reduce healing time and pain, and sophisticated imaging techniques now allow surgeons to visualize the anatomy of the back in ways that weren't available not that long ago. These also have made it possible for people to have successful surgery even into their 70s.

Still, unless your condition is so severe that surgery is the only option—perhaps you have severe myelopathy (spinal cord compression), severe spinal stenosis (nerve compression), spinal tumors, or you've had an accident or other trauma—a skilled orthopedist will try all possible conservative measures to ease your pain before suggesting surgery. These include physical therapy to help you move and exercise more easily as well as medication.

Signs that you need back surgery: Your back pain is constant and getting progressively worse...your symptoms indicate nerve damage—tingling, numbness, or weakness in the arms or legs, including foot drop (difficulty lifting the front

Causes of Back Pain

- **Spinal stenosis.** This occurs when the combination of disk degeneration and arthritis narrow the canal or openings that nerves travel through. Leg pain, numbness, or weakness are often worse than back symptoms. Position changes may provide temporary relief.
- **Muscle or ligament strain.** Sudden movement or repeated heavy lifting can strain back muscles and spinal ligaments.
- **Bulging or herniated disks.** Disks act as cushions between the bones in the spine. If they bulge or herniate, they can press on a nerve and cause pain.
- **Arthritis.** Osteoarthritis can affect the lower back and, in some cases, contribute to spinal stenosis.
- **Osteoporosis.** When bones become porous and brittle, the vertebrae can develop painful breaks.
- **Ankylosing spondylitis.** An inflammatory disease, AS can cause some of the bones in the spine to fuse, causing pain and stiffness.
- **Sciatica.** This nerve pain travels through the buttocks into the leg.
- **Desk work.** If you work at a desk all day, poor posture and sitting for too long can cause back pain. To reduce risk, sit up straight and don't slump your shoulders. Keep your ears over your shoulders, shoulders over your hips, and hips over your ankles. Take frequent breaks to stand and walk.

part of the foot) or difficulty with grip strength...and/or loss of bowel or bladder control due to pressure in the cervical or lumbar spine. Physical changes that require surgery, such as nerve or spinal cord compression or a herniated disk, should be visible on an MRI as well.

Having a necessary surgical procedure will help you avoid more physical damage, and you'll be able to enjoy a future without back pain. Of course, any surgery's risk increases as we move into our 70s (mostly because of other health issues that develop as we age), but many seniors still can benefit from back surgery when it's warranted.

Working with the right doctor should help allay your fears. Both orthopaedic spine surgeons and neurosurgeons with specialized training in spine surgery can perform spinal procedures. Don't be afraid to get a second opinion if you have any concerns or want to see if other surgical techniques are available for your condition. Above all, make sure you have a clear understanding of what outcome you can expect.

Types of Spinal Surgery

There are many different spinal procedures. The right one for you depends on your specific condition. Most fall into one of the following categories...

Decompression surgery relieves chronic pain or loss of function due to a bone spur, injury, herniated disk, narrowing of the spinal canal from spinal stenosis, or a tumor pressing on spinal nerves. Two of the most commonly performed decompression surgeries...

Laminectomy is surgery to remove all or some of the lamina (part of the bone that makes up each vertebra), bone spurs, and/or thickened ligaments. This is done to create more room in the spinal column and, in turn, ease pain.

Discectomy is surgery to remove all or part of a herniated disc. Normally, discs act as shock absorbers to cushion vertebrae, but when a disc slips out of place or is damaged from wear and tear and bulges out, it can put pressure on nerves and cause pain. A common symptom is sciatica, a sharp, shooting pain along the sciatic nerve that runs down the back and the length of a leg, usually on one side of the body.

Spinal fusion. Variations of this procedure are used to fuse or attach specific vertebrae to one another with special cement and/or hardware to stop the pain that occurs when they move.

Spinal fusion can correct conditions such as instability in the spine, scoliosis, and/or severe disc degeneration.

The procedure you have, as well as whether it can be done using minimally invasive, possibly robotic procedures or a more traditional open surgery with a large incision, depends on your condition and how many vertebrae are involved. With minimally invasive surgery, the surgeon makes a few small incisions through which special surgical instruments can reach the spine. This often spares surrounding tissues and leads to a shorter recovery. Advances in robotics for spinal procedures can assist with more precise placement of necessary surgical hardware, such as rods and screws, in the spine.

Recovery from Back Surgery

Some minimally-invasive surgeries are done on an outpatient basis, while traditional procedures could require a few nights in the hospital. Your recovery time will depend on the type of surgery you had.

In general, recovery from decompression surgery—laminectomy and discectomy—is relatively quick. You should be able to get back to work and many activities within a few weeks. Pain, numbness and/or weakness along the path of the nerve that was under pressure should improve within this time, although healing may continue for a year or more.

For spinal fusion, you likely will be out of work for four to six weeks...longer if your job is strenuous. If you're older and had extensive surgery, it could take four to six months before you can return to certain activities.

Follow all the instructions you're given, especially concerning movement. Lifting, bending, going up and down stairs, physical activities, and driving likely will be off limits for a few weeks to a few months. You'll need to be conscious of how you sit and your sleeping position. You will probably be told to take short walks every day for the first few weeks after surgery and then slowly increase how far you walk.

If your surgeon prescribes physical therapy, attend these sessions—you'll learn how to move in ways that prevent pain, keep your back in a safe position, and prepare you for getting back to all the activities you love.

Tummy Troubles

Brijen Shah, MD, a professor of medicine and gastroenterology at the Icahn School of Medicine at Mt. Sinai in New York and a Fellow of the American Gastroenterological Association.

We all get bellyaches, but stomach pain comes in many different forms. It can be occasional or daily, a minor discomfort or a major disrupter. The pain can be dull or sharp and be accompanied, or not, by a long list of other symptoms.

Most causes of stomach pain, defined as discomfort in the upper abdomen, are not serious. But it's important to pay attention to the pain so you can figure out what's going on, how to get relief and, if possible, prevent it in the future.

Here are a few of the most common causes and what you need to know about them...

When Stomach Pain Is an Occasional Problem, It Might Be...

•**Indigestion.** Indigestion, or what your doctor might call dyspepsia, is the familiar discomfort most people have had after a holiday feast or other large meal. Some people get indigestion more often. When it happens, your stomach may feel uncomfortably full and you may feel some heat, burning, or pain. You also might feel gassy, bloated, or nauseated.

While indigestion alone isn't a sign of serious illness, if it lasts for more than two weeks or you also have bleeding, weight loss, or trouble swallowing, you should get checked out by a doctor.

While indigestion has different causes in different people, there are things you can try to prevent future trouble. They include limiting alcohol, caffeine, and carbonated drinks and eating smaller meals at a slower pace. It's also a good idea to avoid eating too close to bedtime. Taking a walk after dinner might also help you digest your food more comfortably.

•**Heartburn.** While some people with indigestion also have heartburn, they aren't the same thing. Heartburn refers specifically to a burning feeling in your chest or throat resulting from stomach acid backing up into your esophagus, the tube that runs from your stomach to your throat. It can be worse when you are lying down or bending over, and it often occurs right after eating.

Some of the habits that prevent indigestion also can help prevent occasional heartburn. They include eating smaller meals and avoiding eating at night. Many people also find it helpful to avoid certain foods, including fried foods, coffee, and chocolate. When heartburn is an occasional problem, most people can get relief with over-the-counter remedies that reduce stomach acid. But when it becomes chronic, you may need to talk to your physician.

•**Stomach viruses or food poisoning.** If you have stomach discomfort along with vomiting or diarrhea, and maybe a fever, a virus may be to blame. While some people call such illnesses "stomach flu," doctors refer to them as viral gastroenteritis. You can pick up stomach bugs from close contact with an infected person or from contaminated food or water. Some stomach viruses, such as norovirus and rotavirus, are especially common among young children and people in close contact with them. Such viruses sometimes cause outbreaks in group settings, such as hospitals, cruise ships, and nursing homes.

Another possible cause of such symptoms is food poisoning from bacteria. Symptoms usually start just a few hours after you eat the tainted food.

Most healthy people recover within a couple of days from either kind of infection. The best treatment is plenty of fluids. Look for beverages containing electrolytes. But if you have trouble staying hydrated, have bloody stools or fevers above 102°F, you should seek medical advice.

When Stomach Pain Is Frequent, It Might Be...

• **Gastroesophageal reflux disease (GERD).** If you have frequent heartburn that interferes with your life, you might have GERD. That means acid and other contents from your stomach back up into your esophagus. In addition to heartburn, you might have symptoms such as persistent sore throat, hoarseness, and cough.

If you haven't gotten relief from over-the-counter remedies and life-style changes, such as avoiding certain foods and eating smaller meals, your doctor can suggest other treatments. If you still don't get relief, you might need a more extensive workup from a gastroenterologist, especially if your doctor suspects complications, such as damage to your esophagus. Your workup might include an upper endoscopy, a test in which a viewing tube is passed through your mouth to your esophagus and stomach. Worrisome signs include trouble swallowing and weight loss.

• **Ulcers.** If you have frequent burning pains in your stomach, it could be a peptic ulcer, a sore in the lining of your stomach or the topmost part of your small intestine.

Could Your Stomach Pain Be a Heart Attack?

Not all heart attacks announce themselves with crushing chest pain. Some people, especially women, experience symptoms that might mimic stomach trouble, including nausea and pain that seems to be coming from the top of the stomach or lower rib cage. Some people vomit, according to the American Heart Association.

Clues that such symptoms might signal heart trouble might include shortness of breath and heart palpitations. Other heart-attack signs can include uncomfortable pressure, squeezing, or fullness in the middle of the chest, or pain in one or both arms, the back, the neck, or the jaw.

If you think you might be having a heart attack, call 911 and get to a hospital right away.

Some ulcers hurt when you eat; others actually feel better after a meal. Some ulcers cause no pain at all. The first sign may be blood in your stool or other signs of blood loss, such as excess fatigue and shortness of breath. Any of those symptoms should prompt a medical workup.

Contrary to long-held beliefs, ulcers aren't caused by spicy foods or stress. In the United States, the most common causes are medications that can damage the stomach lining, especially nonsteroidal anti-inflammatory drugs (NSAIDs), such as aspirin and ibuprofen. Blood-thinning drugs, taken by many older adults, increase the risk that NSAIDs will cause ulcers. The second-leading cause is infection with *Helicobacter pylori (H. pylori)* bacteria.

If your ulcer is caused by bacteria, it can usually be cured with antibiotics and acid-blocking drugs. If your ulcer is medication related, you will need to change your medication habits and use acid-blocking drugs.

- **Gallbladder problems.** What seems like stomach pain might be coming from your gallbladder, a pear-size sac in the upper right side of your abdomen. The gallbladder stores bile, used in digestion. Substances in bile sometimes form stones, which can lead to abdominal pain. The pain can come in attacks that last a few minutes or a few hours. Some people vomit and sweat during gallstone attacks. Some gallstones cause no symptoms at all, so you might find out about them only if they show up on unrelated medical imaging tests. Gallstones can be surgically removed or, in some cases, dissolved with medication.

- **Less common causes.** A few less common causes of pain in the upper abdomen include inflammation of the pancreas, celiac disease (an immune system reaction to gluten in food), and, rarely, cancer. Early stomach cancer often has no symptoms. When it does have symptoms, they can include common problems such as indigestion, mild nausea, and bloating. If you also have blood in the stool, unexplained weight loss, or trouble swallowing, see a doctor.

When Is Constipation Pain Serious?

Niket Sonpal, MD, internist and gastroenterologist, Wyckoff Heights Medical Center, Brooklyn, New York City, and Rudolph Bedford, MD, gastroenterologist, Providence Saint John's Health Center, Santa Monica, California.

Occasional pain from constipation—usually just slight abdominal discomfort—is common, should not interfere with normal quality of life and should resolve within a few days to one or two weeks. Drinking coffee or a lot of water, getting some exercise or using an over-the-counter laxative often brings relief. Frequent constipation may point to a need for lifestyle changes, such as increasing fiber intake by eating more fruits and vegetables...adding a high-fiber bran-based cereal...increasing the amount of water you drink...and increasing how much you exercise.

Constipation with severe pain or that does not resolve after two weeks: See a gastroenterologist.

If pain is overwhelming: Go to an emergency room immediately, especially if you develop a fever while constipated or if you see blood in the toilet or on toilet paper.

Food Dye Can Trigger IBS

Canadian Institutes of Health Research.

Long-term consumption of Allura Red food dye (also called FD&C Red 40 and Food Red 17) can trigger off inflammatory bowel disease, including Crohn's disease and ulcerative colitis. The dye directly disrupts gut barrier function and increases the production of serotonin, a hormone/neurotransmitter found in the gut that subsequently alters gut microbiota composition leading to increased susceptibility to colitis. The dye is commonly used in candies, soft drinks, dairy products, and some cereals. Other studies suggest that the dye also affects certain allergies, immune disorders, and behavioral problems in children, such as attention-deficit/hyperactivity disorder, the researchers noted.

Exercise Eases Arthritis Pain

Stephen P. Messier, PhD, professor and director of the J.B. Snow Biomechanics Laboratory at Wake Forest University, Winston-Salem, North Carolina, and lead author of the study "Effect of Diet and Exercise on Knee Pain in Patients With Osteoarthritis and Overweight or Obesity: A Randomized Clinical Trial," published in *JAMA*. WFU.edu

For people with arthritis, life is governed by pain. You may not even realize how much you've given up if you've been slowly adapting to each progressive "new normal"—each adaptation likely represents a narrower range of what you used to be able to do.

Stephen P. Messier, PhD, director of the J.B. Snow Biomechanics Laboratory at Wake Forest University, led a study to determine what really works for arthritis pain.

His conclusion: Exercise—specifically a plan that includes walking and some resistance training.

But what types of exercise really work? That's what the WE-CAN (Weight-Loss and Exercise for Communities with Arthritis in North Carolina) trial tested. Participants went to community centers for group workouts for 18 months, enough time to make their new routine a permanent habit.

The exercise component: 60-minute sessions three days a week consisting of aerobic walking for 15 minutes…20 minutes of moderate resistance-training for the lower body using weight machines…a second walking phase for 15 minutes…and a cooldown of 10 minutes. Many people think they can't do resistance training if they have arthritis, but developing the muscles that support joints improves mobility with less pain. In a prior study called START, researchers found that low-intensity workouts with less resistance and more repetitions than high-intensity programs were as effective and easier.

The diet component: In the WE-CAN trial, participants followed a low-calorie diet—1,100 calories for women and 1,200 calories for men with 15 to 20 percent protein (at least 1.2 g of protein per kilogram of ideal body weight)…less than 30 percent fat with less than 10 percent saturated fat…and 45 to 60 percent carbohydrates. The control group did not get a diet-and-exercise plan, but both groups received five one-hour nutrition-and-health-education sessions over 15 months and a phone session every other month.

Results: At the end of 18 months, the exercise-and-diet participants had, on average, a 30 percent reduction in pain and lost more weight than the control group.

Applying the Lessons Learned

• **Work with a trainer experienced in resistance training** who can personalize a program based on your abilities and challenge you without causing pain. Exercises can be done with free weights and/or machines, starting with a low number of repetitions and building up to three sets of 10 to 15 reps.

• **Find or create an exercise group,** even if it's just one other person. The group dynamic is important for sticking with an exercise program.

To find a group: The Arthritis Foundation (Arthritis.org)…Silver Sneakers (SilverSneakers.com).

• **Find activities you like.** Being active throughout your lifespan happens only when you do exercises you enjoy.

• **Start slow if needed.** When you start walking for fitness, your pain may increase

Ginger Fights Autoimmune Symptoms

Ginger supplements reduce autoimmune disease symptoms. According to a recent study, people who took a 20-mg supplement of ginger daily for 20 days increased levels of the chemical cAMP in a white blood cell called the neutrophil. This improves these cells' resistance to an inflammation-promoting condition called NETosis that is believed to drive symptoms of autoimmune diseases including rheumatoid arthritis and lupus. Ginger has long been used as an anti-inflammatory in traditional therapies.

Study by researchers at University of Colorado School of Medicine, Aurora, and University of Michigan, Ann Arbor, published in *JCI Insight*.

at first. But once you get into the habit, you'll be able to walk with more ease. Start with five or 10 minutes at a comfortable pace, and build from there.

• **Back off if you're having a bad day.** Don't tax yourself during a flare-up, or perhaps replace weights with elastic bands such as Theraband.

• **Don't forget your diet.** Weight reduction reduces stress on joints, and that translates to less pain.

• **Other types of body work help, too.** Almost any exercise is going to reduce pain by 20 percent to 25 percent. To improve flexibility, consider yoga, tai chi, and stretching classes.

Music Soothes Pain

Study of 63 adults by researchers at McGill University, Montreal, Canada, published in *Frontiers in Pain Research*.

Listening to your favorite music reduces pain. During an experiment to measure response to pain when listening to music, volunteers who listened to their favorite music experienced less pain than those who heard other or no music. The favorite music also lowered anxiety and reduced the perceived intensity and unpleasantness of painful touches.

If you need to have a potentially painful procedure: Bring along your favorite music to listen to during the procedure—even if supposedly relaxing music is provided to patients.

Is It Gout...or Pseudogout?

Arthritis Advisor. Arthritis-Advisor.com

Both conditions are marked by the formation of crystals that cause pain and swelling within the joints—the difference is what forms the crystals.

Gout: Crystals are formed by uric acid from consuming foods high in purines, such as red meat, certain seafoods, alcohol, and high-fructose corn syrup. Avoiding these foods and drinks can limit flare-ups.

Pseudogout is caused by crystallization of calcium pyrophosphate dihydrate, which does not come from food and is present in everyone's body. Diet is not involved in flare-ups.

Give Foot Pain the Boot

Johanna S. Youner, DPM, board-certified foot surgeon and a Fellow of the American College of Foot and Ankle Surgeons. ACFAS.org

Virtually all of us experience foot pain at some point in our lives. Feet are like car tires—but unlike tires, feet are not replaceable. Even simple foot discomfort can have far-reaching consequences—when our feet hurt, we become more sedentary, which can increase our risk for life-altering health problems such as obesity, heart disease, and diabetes.

With 33 joints and 26 bones in each foot, there's a lot that can go wrong.

Good news: Foot pain sometimes has surprisingly simple solutions, says podiatric surgeon Johanna S. Youner, DPM. Here are her suggestions for things you can do to avoid and solve foot pain...when to see a podiatrist...and simple solutions to a few common foot issues.

Vital First Step: Wear the Right Shoes

Wearing supportive, properly sized footwear will reduce the odds of developing foot pain in the first place and solve many foot problems that do occur.

• **Get sized properly.** Unfortunately, most shoe stores don't provide sizing these days.

Best: Look for a shoe store that specializes in running shoes or orthopedic shoes. Salespeople at these specialty stores usually understand that providing a proper fit is essential, and they are trained to help you with that.

Contrary to what you might think, supportive, comfortable shoes can be attractive. *The best brands that combine support and style...*

Cole Haan for men's and women's shoes (ColeHaan.com)

Allen Edmonds for upscale men's shoes (AllenEdmonds.com)

Vionic for women's and some men's shoes (VionicShoes.com)

Dansko, best known for its women's clogs but it offers other shoes for women and men as well (Dansko.com).

Alternative: Wear sneakers rather than more formal footwear. Seniors may fear that giving up on formal or stylish shoes will make them seem even older—but what really makes people seem older is hobbling around in painful footwear. Wearing sneakers that help you move more often, more rapidly and more steadily will help you maintain your youthfulness. Besides, sneakers are increasingly fashionable these days. Sneaker brands that do an excellent job of providing support...

Asics (Asics.com) for people who have narrow feet.

Hoka (Hoka.com) for people who have somewhat wider feet.

Helpful: If you have unusually low or high arches, slip orthotic insoles into your shoes. Insoles made by Superfeet are excellent and affordably priced—often less than $30 per pair. Check the "Insole Finder" tool at Superfeet.com to select appropriate insoles. It is best to have a separate pair in each of your shoes.

Also: You may need to go up a half size in shoes to accommodate your orthotic.

For athletic shoes: PowerSteps (PowerStep.com) are orthotic support options for athletic shoes. Replace the liner in the sneaker with the Powerstep.

If these don't help, a podiatrist can have custom orthotics made, typically for $300 or more. Medicare or health insurance might pay part of the bill.

Foot and Ankle Stretches

Doing a few very easy foot and ankle flexibility exercises dramatically reduces the odds of a wide range of foot problems. You don't have to join a gym or buy expensive workout gear to do these exercises—you don't even have to get off your couch. *Do each of the following every day with both feet...*

• **Ankle circles.** While seated, extend one leg out in front of you with no part of the foot touching any surface. You could do this by extending the foot beyond the edge of an ottoman or by placing a rolled-up towel on a coffee table under your lower calf/upper ankle. Without moving your leg, rotate your foot and ankle in the largest circles you can manage. Do at least a few clockwise and then counterclockwise.

• **Foot alphabet.** While seated, extend one leg out in front of you—as above, no part of that foot should be resting on a surface. Use this foot to spell out the alphabet, letter by letter.

• **Towel stretch.** While seated, extend one leg out in front of you—the heel of this foot can be resting on a surface. Fold or roll a towel so that it's relatively narrow in width...grip one end of the towel in each of your hands...then loop this towel under the toes and ball of your outstretched foot. Gently pull the towel while keeping your leg straight, so that the foot points somewhat back toward your head.

When to See a Podiatrist

If you experience acute foot pain and/or pain that persists for more than a week, it's time to see a podiatrist. Foot pain that lasts longer than a week may cause you to alter your stride in a way that leads to more foot, leg, knee, hip, and/or back problems.

Caution: If a podiatrist recommends surgery, be extremely wary...and get a second, even a third, opinion. There is no such thing as minor foot surgery—virtually any foot operation has the potential to cause lifelong mobility problems.

It's distressingly common for podiatrists and orthopedic foot surgeons to recommend surgery for issues that could have been solved with better footwear choices, physical therapy, exercise, or other treatment options—surgery generates significantly more revenue for surgical practices.

Best: Try all other options before resorting to foot surgery, and never get foot surgery for purely cosmetic reasons. I know a professional dancer who thought she was having minor surgery on her pinky toe and ended up never being able to dance again.

Solutions to Common Foot Problems

Here are some common foot problems and what to do about each...

•**Plantar fasciitis** is essentially inflammation of the band of connective tissue that runs along the sole of the foot, providing support for the arch. This condition can be extremely painful—the pain is typically felt near the heel. It often can be successfully treated without seeing a doctor, but you have to act quickly—the longer plantar fasciitis lingers, the longer it's likely to take to resolve.

What to do: Ice the painful area at night before bed—at least two cycles of 10 minutes with the ice on, five minutes with it off. Also ice it during the day as needed. Gently stretch the foot and the back of the lower leg—the towel stretch mentioned earlier is a good choice here. Wear only supportive, cushioned footwear.

•**Calluses** can form where our feet rub against our shoes. Over time, callouses can start to feel like pebbles inside the shoe, and that can affect our stride in ways that sometimes lead to foot, knee, hip, leg, and/or back pain. This is increasingly likely to occur as we get older—young adults shed old skin cells every 20 or 30 days, but by the time we're in our 70s, it can take 75 days or longer, dramatically increasing the odds that calluses will develop.

What to do: To remove calluses, soak the foot...dry it...gently rub a pumice stone over the callus. Then apply a urea cream or lactic acid callus-removal cream. Over-the-counter creams are available, or a doctor can prescribe a cream with a higher acid content for especially stubborn calluses.

Warning: "Morton's neuroma" could be confused with a callus. Like a callus, it can feel like a pebble in the shoe. But a neuroma is overgrown nerve tissue inside the foot, not excess skin cells. Morton's neuromas typically occur in the forefoot, often between the third and fourth toes. They're usually painful. Sometimes placing a pad on the bottom of the foot between the metatarsal heads can alleviate discomfort. Shoes that are wider across the forefoot may help as well. A podiatrist can offer nonsurgical treatment options, such as "radiofrequency ablation"—high-frequency radio waves delivered via a needle that destroy the problematic nerve tissue.

•**Verrucae** are a type of wart that typically appears on the bottoms of the feet. Like other warts, these are caused by a virus and should be treated promptly—they'll spread if allowed to linger, both around the body and to other members of the household. Verrucae often are contracted by walking barefoot in hotel rooms or gym showers that have not been properly cleaned.

What to do: Over-the-counter salicylic acid–based wart-removal products are less effective than the stronger products a doctor can prescribe. Your primary care physician might recommend applying liquid nitrogen to freeze warts as well as salicylic acid. Avoid walking barefoot until the problem is resolved to reduce the odds of transmitting the virus to other household members.

Pain Relief and Autoimmune Disease

Knee Arthritis: Questioning the Standard of Care

Chris Iliades, MD, is a regular *Bottom Line Health* contributor. He is a retired ear, nose, throat, head, and neck surgeon.

If you have pain and stiffness in your knees that isn't caused by a recent injury, you may have knee osteoarthritis (OA), often called "wear and tear" arthritis. OA pain is caused by thinning and wearing away of the cartilage that protects the bones of your knee joint.

There are several telltale symptoms of knee OA: joint stiffness that affects one or both knees, morning stiffness that lasts about 30 minutes, morning knee pain and stiffness that is more noticeable with activity, especially going up stairs or bending up and down, and knee pain and stiffness that gets better with rest and swelling that responds to ice and nonsteroidal anti-inflammatory drugs (NSAIDs).

Treatment Options

For some people, knee replacement surgery is necessary, but there are several treatments and lifestyle changes that may reduce your risk of needing surgery.

- **Exercise.** After reviewing more than 600 studies, an expert panel of scientists determined that the strongest evidence supports using an exercise program to strengthen knee muscles and reduce stiffness, which can include supervised, home, or aquatic exercises.
- **Over-the-counter pain relief.** There is also strong support for the use of topical or oral NSAIDs or acetaminophen (Tylenol) to improve pain and function. Narcotic medications (including tramadol) should be avoided.
- **Injections.** The team found that the use of injections has only moderate scientific support. For about 10 percent of people, injecting a corticosteroid or a substance called hyaluronic acid (HA) into the knee joint (intra-articular injections) is beneficial. Steroids block inflammation that causes pain and stiffness, although they do not stop or reverse wear and tear.

HA is a substance found in the lubricating fluid inside the knee joint, called the synovial fluid. Synovial fluid decreases with OA, so adding HA may help restore fluid and lubrication, although this has not been strongly supported by clinical studies.

According to the guidelines, HA is not recommended for routine use. Steroids are recommended for only short-term relief of pain and swelling.

Chapter 13

PHYSICAL INJURY AND BONE HEALTH

Getting a Grip on Carpal Tunnel Syndrome

The carpal tunnel is a narrow passageway that runs from the wrist (the carpus) to the hand. Its bottom and sides are formed by small bones, and the top is a band of rigid connective tissue. Running through this tunnel is the median nerve, one of the main nerves in the hand, and nine flexor tendons that allow you to bend and flex your fingers. Carpal tunnel syndrome occurs when the median nerve becomes compressed, reducing its blood supply.

Common Causes

Carpal tunnel syndrome comes from doing activities that involve frequent, repetitive movements or extreme flexion or extension of the hand and wrist for long periods of time. These motions can aggravate any of those nine tendons and lead to swelling that puts pressure on the nerve.

Carpal tunnel syndrome is often linked to computer work, texting, or video gaming, but it can occur with low-tech activities too, such as painting and knitting. People who work in construction and use vibrating equipment, such as a jackhammer, are also at risk.

Additional risk factors include being born with a smaller carpal tunnel than average or one with less space for the nerve. (Both issues can run in families.) Having diabetes, an autoimmune disorder such as rheumatoid arthritis, or obesity also increases risk.

The Continuum of Symptoms

The earliest symptom of carpal tunnel syndrome is usually numbness or tingling in the affected hand at nighttime or when waking up in the morning. You'll feel these sensations in the fingers through which the median nerve courses, so not on the pinkie side of the ring finger or the pinkie. Symptoms there signal a different problem. Pain and a burning sensation are also common.

Sometimes, symptoms spontaneously resolve. But if they do not, and carpal tunnel syndrome progresses, you may experience

---

John Dowdle, MD, a board-certified orthopedic surgeon, assistant attending orthopedic surgeon at the Hospital for Special Surgery and at New York-Presbyterian Hospital in New York, director of hand and upper extremity surgery at Stamford Hospital in Connecticut, and assistant professor of orthopedic surgery at Weill Cornell Medical College.

symptoms throughout the day, especially when you're doing activities with repetitive motions. You may experience shock-like twinges that radiate across your first four fingers. Pain or tingling may run up your arm toward your shoulder. You may sense weakness in your hand and feel clumsy. You might have a hard time getting dressed or frequently drop things.

Over time, your symptoms can become constant. While your dominant hand is usually the first to be affected, many people develop carpal tunnel syndrome in both hands. If carpal tunnel is left untreated, you run the risk of permanent nerve damage, with loss of feeling as well as weakness. This is why it's so important to get an evaluation from a hand specialist, ideally a hand surgeon, for symptoms that last more than two to three days. The earlier the intervention, the better the prognosis.

Getting the Right Diagnosis

Your doctor will likely begin with a physical exam to look for sensory and motor signs that point to carpal tunnel syndrome while ruling out other conditions. One key sensory exam is called the carpal compression test. It simply involves applying pressure directly over the carpal tunnel for 30 seconds to see if this provokes symptoms.

For a definitive diagnosis, your doctor may do an electromyography and nerve conduction study to look for specific abnormalities that indicate carpal tunnel syndrome. This test can also rule out other conditions that can cause numbness and tingling, such as cervical radiculopathy (a pinched nerve in the neck), diabetic neuropathy, or nerve compression elsewhere in the arm. Test results also help determine whether your carpal tunnel syndrome is mild, moderate, or severe and the extent of any nerve damage.

Early Treatment

In the early stages, conservative steps may bring relief. The initial treatment is usually wearing a wrist splint at night for sleeping. The splint keeps your wrist in a neutral position to maximize the space within the carpal tunnel. Sleeping with the wrist in a flexed or extended position can put more pressure on the median nerve, producing symptoms. *Here are some additional strategies...*

• **Cut down or take a break from repetitive activities.**

• **Pay attention to how you position your hands** when you're at your computer keyboard or laptop or on your devices, both at work and at home. Keep your wrists in a neutral position. An occupational therapist can show you the best position for your keyboard, teach you how to minimize flexion and extension as you type, and suggest adjustments to make when you use your hands for hobbies.

• **Set up your desk for success.** Instructions for an ergonomic workstation are available at OSHA.gov/etools/computer workstations.

• **When working at a desk, take regular breaks every 30 to 45 minutes.**

• **If you have a health condition that may have factored in to your getting carpal tunnel syndrome,** getting it under control may help ease your carpal tunnel symptoms.

Walking a Leashed Dog Can Be Dangerous

About 422,659 adults sought treatment in U.S. emergency rooms for dog-walking injuries between 2001 and 2020...typically after being pulled by the dog or tripping over its leash.

Common injuries: Traumatic brain injuries, fractured fingers, and shoulder sprains and strains. Women and adults over age 65 were particularly susceptible to serious dog-walk injuries.

Study of U.S. Consumer Product Safety Commission data by researchers at Johns Hopkins University, published in *Medicine & Science in Sports & Exercise*.

Weight loss, if needed, and aerobic exercise can be beneficial for both conditions.

When Splinting Isn't Enough

Other treatment options include cortisone injections and surgery. Cortisone injections are usually helpful but typically provide only temporary improvement.

Carpal tunnel surgery, called carpal tunnel release, increases the size of the tunnel and relieves the nerve compression. It usually results in permanent improvement. Surgery is minimally invasive and performed on an outpatient basis, frequently under local anesthesia. Most people can use their hand immediately afterward. Carpal tunnel release is the best treatment option for severe or stubborn cases.

Approaches such as therapy, lasers, acupuncture, and manipulation have been tried, but frequently are not helpful and can even be harmful. Over-the-counter medications like nonsteroidal anti-inflammatory drugs (NSAIDs) often don't help enough. They might ease pain from inflammation, but not the tingling or burning. Working with a hand specialist remains the best approach to get a handle on carpal tunnel syndrome.

Are You Getting the Right Bone Density Test?

Robert H. Wagner, MD, director of nuclear medicine at the Loyola University Medical Center in Chicago and assistant professor of radiology.

Quick and painless, bone scans are essential screening tests for assessing bone health. They can uncover the start of bone loss, called osteopenia, or the more advanced osteoporosis, letting you know when you might need treatment.

Dual-energy X-ray absorptiometry, often referred to as a DXA or DEXA scan, has long been the gold standard screening test to measure bone mineral density (BMD). But, in recent years a different screening tool, called quantitative computed tomography (QCT), has replaced DXA in some states. Here's what you need to know about these tests and which one is appropriate for you.

DXA Details

DXA provides precise measurements of bone mineral density at important sites—

Preventing Carpal Tunnel Pain

If you do any kind of work or hobby that puts you at risk of carpal tunnel syndrome, from typing to knitting to working with power tools, try these strategies to reduce your risk...

- **Don't lean on your wrists or the heels of your hands.**
- **Keep your hands warm. Consider using gloves or fingerless gloves.**
- **Maintain a healthy weight.**
- **Relax your grip when holding tools.**
- **Reduce your force when typing, using a cash register, etc.**
- **Take frequent breaks.**
- **Try to keep your wrist in a neutral position.**
- **Use correct posture.**
- **Stretch your hands and wrists...**
  - Make a fist, and then fan out your fingers.
  - Rotate your wrist up and down to relieve stiffness.
  - Put your palms together over your head, move your hands downward as far as you can, and hold for five to 10 seconds.
  - Push your thumb back until you feel a gentle stretch.
  - Hold your left hand out, with the palm facing down. Use your right hand to pull the left back until you feel a stretch. Switch sides.

the spine, the hip and, when needed, the forearm—with minimal radiation. Results are most often given as T-scores, which show how your bone density compares to a 30-year-old.

The lower your T-score, the greater your fracture risk.

• **Normal bone mineral density** is a T-score between +1 and -1.

• **Low bone mass (osteopenia)** is a T-score between -1.1 and -2.4. Having lower-than-normal bone density puts you at a higher risk of developing osteoporosis. Your doctor may suggest adding calcium and vitamin D to your diet and doing weight-bearing exercise.

• **Osteoporosis** is a T-score lower than -2.5. Often this means you'll be prescribed medication. Along with T-scores, your FRAX (Fracture Risk Assessment Tool) score will help determine your 10-year risk for a major fracture. The FRAX assesses 12 factors, like your age, weight, and whether you smoke, drink alcohol, take steroids, and had a fracture or a parent who had a hip fracture.

In some cases, people under age 50 may also be given a Z-score that compares bone density to other people of the same age.

Questions About QCT

Quantitative computerized tomography is a type of CT scan that uses a 3D image that contrasts the outer cortical bone and the inner spongy trabecular bone (DXA is 2D).

It can be appropriate for people in very specific circumstances. For instance, it may offer more detail than DXA for people with a very low or very high BMI, with a severe degenerative disease of the spine, or when results of a DXA are inconsistent. That means it may be the right test for people with rheumatoid arthritis, scoliosis, or another disease that causes the body to put down more bone and artificially elevate the bone density calculation. (One clue this may be happening to you is if your spine shows an increase in calcium from a previous test, but your hip score is in the osteopenia range.)

According to the American College of Radiology, QCT can be used as a tool to diagnose and manage osteoporosis and other diseases that affect BMD because it can help assess how well you're responding to treatment. *While QCT has its place, it may not be the right BMD test for the general public for a few reasons...*

• **Radiation exposure.** QCT delivers between 1,000 and 3,000 times the radiation

---

Osteoporosis Is Underdiagnosed

Osteoporosis is underdiagnosed in the United States because people are missing out on BMD screenings in general. With osteoporosis, you don't have any symptoms until you break a bone, and that can have devastating consequences. Testing is the only way to know if you have bone loss before a break occurs.

Since the Deficit Reduction Act of 2007 cut reimbursement rates for DXA scans, there's been a sharp drop in the number of procedures being done. "Increasing Access to Osteoporosis Testing for Medicare Beneficiaries Act of 2021," a bill to improve DXA payments, had been in front of Congress for nearly two years. Unfortunately the bill did not pass.

In the meantime, talk to your healthcare provider about BMD testing, especially if you have a family history of osteopenia or osteoporosis, have any health condition that can cause estrogen deficiency, are frail, underweight, or a smoker. The recommendation to start osteoporosis screening is age 65 for women and age 70 for men, but based on health factors and family history, your doctor may suggest it sooner.

of DXA. Women having a scan of their hip are getting that radiation across the entire pelvis, including the ovaries and other sensitive structures. If you need to retest every two years, that extra radiation adds up.

• **Misinterpreted results.** Endocrinologists must not use the T-score to interpret QCT results. The QCT measures more of the spongy area of the bone, whereas DXA focuses on cortical bone. Looking at results the same way is like making an apples-to-orange comparison. If a T-score given by a DXA of the spine is -2.0, it's likely that the QCT T-score on the same person would be -2.7, showing more bone density loss than actually exists. The American College of Radiology recommends using an absolute value of <80 mg/cm^3, and not a T-score, when results are being evaluated.

If your doctor orders a QCT even though you're not in a situation that warrants it, and your results indicate osteoporosis, consider getting a second opinion and a DXA before going on any bone medications.

• **Cost.** QCT is much more expensive than DXA. That could be costly if you have a deductible or co-pay. QCTs can also be a strain on Medicare, which reimburses for the test at a much higher rate than it does for a DXA.

> **IMPORTANT:** Whenever you need a follow-up BMD study, try to do it at the same facility as the prior one. There are different models of DXA instruments, and the results are easier to compare if they have been taken on the same model.

enhanced fitness, or injury rehabilitation as their reason for practicing. But one goal you don't often hear is "stronger bones." Most people think of strength-training, walking, and other floor-pounding workouts when they hear "weight-bearing activity," but yoga also can make your bones stronger. It stimulates bone cells in a similar way and often with less injury risk. It also improves balance and flexibility and decreases stress, all of which protect bones.

Your Busy Bones

You might think that bones are fixed, unchangeable objects. The truth is that bones, just like skin and muscles, are alive and constantly evolving. From childhood through the mid-20s, our bones are busy growing stronger. In our 30s and 40s, the body engages in a process called bone remodeling, in which old bone tissue is broken down and replaced with equal amounts of new bone. It's even possible to gain bone mass during this time, albeit at a far slower pace than during your youth and only if you engage in regular weight-bearing exercise such as strength-training or jogging.

After age 50, as the rate of bone breakdown starts to outpace the rate of replacement, those bones that held you up for so long begin to weaken. And since estrogen is needed to help lay down new bone, this process speeds up even faster for women during menopause. The result often is a condition called osteopenia, which means your bones are thinner and less dense than normal. Osteopenia can progress to osteoporosis, a more severe form of bone loss. Approximately 54 million Americans

Yes...Yoga Can Make Your Bones Strong

Gabriella Espinosa, a yoga and somatic movement instructor, menopause mentor, and female sexuality educator based in Austin, Texas. She is founder of Women's Body Wisdom (GabriellaEspinosa.com). You can watch her "Yoga for Strong Bones" yoga class on Movement for Modern Life (MovementFor ModernLife.com) by searching for "Espinosa."

Yoga is becoming more popular every year. A recent survey showed that approximately 34 million Americans tried the 5,000-year-old practice at least once in the previous year. Most people cite stress relief,

> **12 BONE-CENTRIC YOGA POSES**
>
> Vriksasana (Tree pose)
> Trikonasana (Triangle pose)
> Virabhadrasana II (Warrior II pose)
> Parsvakonasana (Side-angle pose)
> Parivrtta Trikonasana (Twisted triangle pose)
> Salabhasana (Locust pose)
> Setu Bandhasana (Bridge pose)
> Supta Padangusthasana I (Supine hand-to-foot I pose)
> Supta Padangusthasana II (Supine hand-to-foot II pose)
> Marichyasana II (Straight-legged twist pose)
> Matsyendrasana (Bent-knee twist pose)
> Savasana (Corpse pose)

have osteopenia or osteoporosis, dramatically increasing their risk for one or more fractures.

Yoga: A Pillar of Bone Health

How yoga helps keep bones healthy...

•**Yoga makes bones stronger.** When you hold a yoga pose such as Seated Spinal Twist pose (Ardha Matsyendrasana) or Triangle pose (Trikonasana), your muscles pull on your bones. That pressure stimulates osteoblasts, the cells that build bone. It's similar to how weight-training strengthens bone—you lift a dumbbell or push against your own body weight in a lunge or a pushup, and the force of that weight pushes back and tugs on the bones, enhancing osteoblast activity. As muscles strengthen, they continue to exert more beneficial pressure on the bones, even when you're at rest.

Landmark research: Loren M. Fishman, MD, of Columbia College of Physicians and Surgeons in New York City has found that performing a daily 12-minute sequence of 12 yoga poses was sufficient to improve bone density in older adults' spines and femurs. Some of his study participants even reversed their osteopenia or upgraded from osteoporosis to osteopenia. To view the exercises, go to https://bit.ly/3MDZlCV.

•**Yoga improves balance and flexibility.** Consider a one-legged pose or even a two-legged pose with your feet staggered, such as Virabhadrasana II (Warrior II pose). You engage all your muscles to remain upright, so not only do you reap the weight-bearing benefit of standing up while pressing away from the floor (which stimulates osteoblasts), but you're cultivating balance by challenging your proprioceptive system—internal sense of where your body is in space and what it is doing at any given time. Also the stretching inherent in yoga builds flexibility.

•**Yoga alleviates mental stress.** When you're overstressed, your body increases production of the hormone *cortisol,* which, in excess quantities, breaks down bone by inhibiting osteoblasts. Slow, deep breathing, like the kind practiced in yoga, dials down the sympathetic ("fight-or-flight") nervous system, which reduces cortisol. Also, yoga poses cultivate an inner awareness of the body's abilities—you must be mindful of where you're placing your foot…where you're gazing…where you're holding your arms, all of which elevate mood. In this way, even a lying-down pose such as Savasana (Corpse pose) can benefit bones.

Poses for Bone Strength

Most yoga poses can help protect bones in some way. But when it comes to improving bone density, balance, and flexibility, the three best are Tree pose (Vriksasana)…

Warrior II pose (Virabhadrasana II)...and Downward-facing Dog pose (Adho mukha svanasana). All you need for these three poses is a standard yoga mat. It takes at least 10 seconds for bone-forming proteins to synthesize under pressure, so hold each pose for that length of time, eventually working your way up to 30 seconds.

Reminder: Talk to your health-care provider before starting an exercise plan, especially if you have been diagnosed with spinal osteoporosis. If so, you should avoid yoga moves that require you to roll up or down through the spine, such as Sun Salutations or backbend-type moves.

POSE #1: Tree pose. Stand with your feet hip-width apart and arms relaxed by your sides, weight balanced evenly between both feet. Spread your toes, and press your feet into the mat. Imagine your hip bones reaching up toward your lower ribs to gently lift your lower belly. Inhale deeply, lifting your chest, and exhale as you draw your shoulder blades down your back. Look straight ahead at a steady gazing spot. You are now in Tadasana (Mountain pose.)

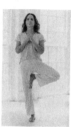

Next, place your hands on your hips and raise your right foot high, resting it on your left inner thigh...or keep it lower and rest it on your left calf or ankle. Avoid resting it on your left knee. Press the right foot and left leg into each other. Check that your pelvis is level and squared to the front.

When you feel steady, bring your palms together at the center of your chest or stretch your arms overhead like tree branches for an added challenge. You are in Tree pose. Hold for five to 10 breaths, then step back into Mountain pose, and repeat on the other side. Feel free to use a wall or chair to steady yourself. Lightly touching your hand to the wall or even standing near a wall can give you confidence in case you lose your balance.

POSE #2: Warrior II pose. Begin by facing the long side of your yoga mat with your arms extended straight out from your shoulders (left arm out to the left and right arm out to the right). Your feet should be parallel to each other in a wide stance with your ankles approximately beneath your wrists.

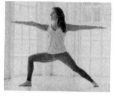

Keeping your upper body still, turn your right foot and knee to face one end of the mat. Angle your left toes slightly in toward the upper left corner of the mat. Now slowly turn your gaze in the same direction as your right foot. Bend your right knee, and position it over your right ankle, distributing your weight evenly between both legs. Press down through the outer edge of your back foot. Reach strongly through both arms toward the front and back of the mat as you look past your right fingertips. Hold for five to 10 breaths.

To emerge from the pose, exhale as you press down through your feet, then inhale and straighten your legs. Return your feet to parallel facing the long side of the mat. Repeat on the other side.

POSE #3: Downward-facing Dog pose. Begin on your hands and knees, knees beneath your hips, hands a bit in front of your shoulders and fingers spread. Pressing into your hands, raise your knees off the mat, taking your hips up and back to come into an upside down "V" shape.

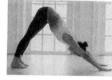

Keeping your knees softly bent, press through your hands and extend your spine, drawing your tailbone back and up. Firm your shoulder blades against your back... imagine drawing your ribs toward your thighs...keep your neck long and ears between your upper arms.

Engage your thigh muscles as you press your thighs back and stretch your heels toward the floor. (Legs should be straight but knees should not be locked.) If you feel your spine rounding, keep the knees bent. Hold for five to 10 breaths. To emerge from the pose, exhale and bring your knees to the floor.

Exercise photos courtesy of @yogaandphoto.

Beyond Calcium: Minerals That Protect Bone Density

Bahram H. Arjmandi, PhD, RDN, professor and director of the Center for Advanced Exercise and Nutrition Research on Aging, Department of Health, Nutrition, and Food Sciences at the College of Health and Human Sciences of Florida State University and coauthor of the study "Associations Between Major and Trace Minerals Intake and Bone Health in Postmenopausal Women with Osteopenia."

As estrogen declines after menopause, women become more vulnerable to osteoporosis. The focus usually is on major minerals, mostly calcium, to protect bone health. Trace minerals receive less attention, but a study from Florida State University found that certain trace minerals actually are vital for bone health.

Background: The major minerals are calcium, chloride, magnesium, phosphorus, potassium, sodium, and sulfur. Trace minerals that are important for good health but are needed in much smaller amounts: Chromium, copper, fluoride, iodine, iron, manganese, molybdenum, selenium, and zinc.

Study findings: This cross-sectional study included 132 healthy postmenopausal women who had osteopenia (when the body does not make new bone as quickly as it absorbs old bone) but were otherwise healthy and were not on hormone therapy or any medication aimed at improving bone strength. DEXA scans were used to assess bone-mineral density (BMD) as well as blood tests to measure bone turnover…and exercise levels and a seven-day food-frequency questionnaire were analyzed and evaluated.

Results: There is a link between some trace minerals and better BMD in key bones—L3, the third lumbar spine vertebra, was positively and significantly linked with iron, copper, zinc, fluorine and manganese as well as phosphorus…L4, the fourth lumbar spine vertebra, was positively and significantly linked with copper, zinc, fluorine, manganese and phosphorus…copper on its own was significantly linked with better BMD of the ultra-distal radius (part of the forearm, a good place to assess bone loss) and of the total body…zinc and copper were positively and significantly associated with better BMD in the upper and lower neck.

What this means: Increasing intake of certain minerals may be beneficial for bone health after menopause. While these trace minerals are vital, too much can be toxic so it is best to get them through food rather than relying on supplements. Food provides a balance of many diverse nutrients, including micronutrients that may be lacking in supplements.

What to do: Focus on eating a well-rounded diet of whole foods, including nuts, seeds, fruits and vegetables, as well as meat, fish, dairy, and grains to provide what you need for bone health. Of special note are dried fruits, because they have concentrated minerals in a single serving—prunes, which protect bone in the absence of estrogen, are at the top of the leaderboard. They not only help prevent bone loss but also have the potential to erase a loss after it has occurred.

7 Things You Are Doing Wrong When Exercising

Joel Harper, celebrity fitness trainer based in New York City. He is creator of the workout DVD series *Fit Pack*, the PBS programs *Slim & Fit* and *Firming After 50*, and of the workout chapters in *The New York Times* best-selling *YOU* book series and accompanying DVDs. He is author of *Mind Your Body*. JoelHarperFitness.com

"Just do it" is a prudent exercise philosophy…but only if you're doing it right. Execute an exercise improperly, and not only will your efforts fail to produce optimal fit-

Physical Injury and Bone Health

ness benefits, it could lead to back, neck, and leg injury.

When we experience post-exercise discomfort, we often conclude that exercising just isn't for us or that our bodies are too old for this much exertion. Not so, says celebrity trainer Joel Harper. A few minor modifications to the way we perform these exercises could result in pain-free fitness gains.

Here are the seven most common exercise mistakes—and how to do them correctly...

MISTAKE #1: **Uneven feet during standing exercises.** If you're doing any standing exercise where your feet are supposed to be even with each other, such as squats, then your feet must be precisely even—equally far forward and at matching angles.

Example: If one foot is pointed 20 degrees outward, the other should be angled 20 degrees outward, too. Subtle differences in foot positioning during standing exercises can throw the knees, hips and/or back out of alignment, which can lead to injury in those body parts, especially if this foot positioning becomes a habit.

To do it right: Before starting each set of standing exercises, visually confirm that your toes are equally far forward and that your feet are at comparable angles. It's fine to point the feet either directly forward or slightly outward when doing squats and many other standing exercises, as long as both feet are doing the same thing.

MISTAKE #2: **Uneven shoulder tension during pushups and other upper-body exercises.** Many of us carry a substantially different amount of tension in one shoulder than the other, likely because we use our dominant arm more often or we sleep on our side. But just as improperly aligned feet can lead to back and lower-body pain following standing exercises, uneven shoulder tension can lead to unnecessary neck tension following upper-body exercises.

To do it right: Before beginning any upper-body exercise, use "elbow circling" to balance the tension in your shoulders. Touch your fingertips to your shoulders, 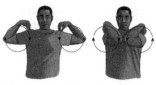 then rotate your elbows in five large circles—large enough that your elbows briefly touch in front of your chest during each circle. Then reverse the circles, and do five in the other direction as well. Look straight ahead, and keep your head in alignment the entire time.

MISTAKE #3: **Failing to stretch your feet before standing exercises.** Even people who always stretch before workouts neglect to stretch the muscles of their feet. But those forgotten foot muscles play a role in any standing exercise, and overlooking them can lead to pain not only in the feet but also in the Achilles tendon, calves, knees, or elsewhere in the lower body.

To do it right: Here's a great foot-muscle stretch to use before lower-body exercises—while barefoot and with your knees and feet together, come onto your knees and curl your toes under, with the soles of your feet facing backward. Make sure your heels remain straight up. Slowly sit back onto your airborne heels until you feel a stretch in your toes and the arches of your feet. For a deeper stretch, gently inch your knees closer to your toes causing a deeper bend in your toes. Place your fingertips on the floor in front of you to help with balance. Ultimately with time, you want your heels above the joints of your toes and your shoulders above your hips. Hold for five deep inhales.

MISTAKE #4: **Locking your elbows at the top of pushups.** Some people think it's cheating to stop a pushup before your arms are fully extended to where the elbows lock. But the goal of exercise is to put stress on muscles, and locking the elbows during pushups actually takes stress off the muscles and puts it on the elbow joints.

Result: A less effective workout and potential joint pain.

To do it right: End each pushup just short of locking your elbows. That way the muscles must work throughout the exercise, and the joints are never under significant strain. In fact, it's 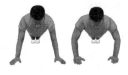 a good policy to stop just short of locking your elbows or knees with most exercises.

MISTAKE #5: **Straining your neck muscles while doing abdominal exercises.** The goal of crunches—those challenging cousins of sit-ups—is to exercise the abdominal muscles. But because the head is held at awkward angles during crunches, it's easy to stress the neck muscles, potentially resulting in neck pain.

To do it right: As you lie on your back preparing to do a set of crunches, cross your wrists to form an X behind your head. Set your head onto this X—think of the wrist X as a plate to support your head's weight, removing that responsibility from your neck muscles.

Also: Resist the urge to tuck your chin against your chest during crunches—imagine there's a tennis ball between your chin and chest.

Alternative: Skip the crunches entirely and choose a different ab exercise that doesn't risk neck strain.

One good option: Lie on your back with your knees bent and above your hips, lower legs parallel to the floor. Use your hands to push against your upper legs/quads...but offset this by using your legs to push back against your hands. The net result should be that your 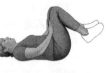 legs don't move. While you're doing this, imagine that you're pulling your belly button down through your back and into the floor so that your back does not arch. This exercise works the abs, the quads and the arms, all without risk of neck strain.

MISTAKE #6: **Arching your back while doing squats.** Many people lean slightly forward and arch their backs as they do squats, that well-known knee bend exercise. This subtle curve can feel like a natural way to balance the body's weight...but it also tightens the back muscles in a way that can lead to back discomfort.

To do it right: When doing squats, cross your arms in front of your body with your elbows up at approximately shoulder height. Also keep your chin up and eyes aimed forward. This arm and head position keeps both your spine perfectly straight and body weight properly positioned.

MISTAKE #7: **Grabbing the foot with the wrong hand when doing single-leg stretches.** It's among the most well-known and seemingly simplest of stretches—you sit with one leg extended and grab the extended foot with a hand. But many people—even some professional athletes—get it wrong. They use their right hand to reach for their right foot and vice versa. That puts the spine out of alignment and risks back pain, especially if one side is tighter than the other.

To do it right: Reach toward the toes with the opposite hand when doing single-leg stretches. If you cannot reach the toe, use the other hand behind you as leverage to gently push yourself forward. Think elongating your back, not just bending forward. The only 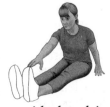 time to reach with the same-side hand is when doing "ballet stretches," which are uncommon.

Illustrations by Alayna Paquette

Prep Your Joints for Chilly Weather

Michael M. Kheir, MD, orthopedic surgeon, researcher and assistant clinical professor at University of Michigan Health System, Northville. UOFMhealth.org

It's not in your head—many people with arthritis, chronic joint pain or joint injuries experience increased pain in their hips, knees, spine, hands, and shoulders when the seasons transition.

Good news: You can prepare those joints for colder weather by strengthening them while the weather is still warm.

What causes seasonal pain: Colder weather causes an increase in humidity and a drop in atmospheric pressure. When the pressure drops, the soft tissue in your joints expands, causing pressure in your joint capsule and pain in already problematic joints. In winter, you also may notice joint pain not just when you wake up but also in the evening, when the pressure is the highest due to the dropping temperature. The tendency to exercise less when the weather's cold also works against you.

If you go into winter with added strength, you'll have less inflammation and pain...and your joints will warm up faster. Start prepping now, regardless of the temperature. *Here's how...*

•**Train, don't strain.** You don't need a special fitness program, just a consistent one with low-impact exercises that won't tax achy joints. Swimming is ideal—the buoyancy of the water cushions joints and takes away gravity, relieving the pressure you might feel with land-based workouts, plus it targets the muscles supporting upper-body joints. Aquatic exercises and therapy, such as treading water and doing short laps, also are good for cardiac health. Try walking from side to side in the pool—just being in the water will take pressure off your joints.

When to Get Guidance for Injuries

If you experience a minor injury and don't feel better after two weeks of DIY efforts or if you have a lot of daily aches and pains, consult a specialist to see if something serious is going on. For instance, a sprain that stays painful could be a sign of an avulsion fracture. Your doctor or an orthopedist can identify the source of your discomfort and prescribe the right course of action. Many physical therapists (PTs) specialize in areas from neurology to sports medicine, so you can find one with the expertise you need. If you're a weekend warrior, even if you feel fine in general, consider seeing a PT for a musculoskeletal evaluation—you'll get guidance on what areas to work on, how to avoid injury, and which cold/hot therapies meet your needs. Then you can transition to a personal trainer to help you work on goals. Visit ChoosePT.com to locate a PT near you.

Maura Daly Iversen, DPT, SD, MPH, a physical therapist and behavioral scientist/clinical epidemiologist with a primary focus in rheumatology, and the dean of the College of Health and Wellness at Johnson and Wales University in Providence, Rhode Island.

Other low-impact activities include biking, walking, yoga, and tai chi. The American Heart Association recommends 150 minutes of exercise a week in the form of five 30-minute chunks, but you can exercise in 10-minute chunks if that's more comfortable for you. Your joints eventually will feel better, and you will have more mobility and less stiffness.

Caution: You may feel a little discomfort when exercising, but significant pain is your body's way of telling you to slow down.

•**Work with a physical therapist for a plan tailored to your needs.** This could involve light weights or resistance bands, particularly for upper-body joints that don't get any stimulation from walking or biking. Find a therapist who is willing

Physical Injury and Bone Health

to motivate and push you. The point of physical therapy is to build up the muscle around the joints to stabilize them and restore normal biomechanics, as well as improve range of motion. *Stay motivated...*

•**Start slow.** Don't push yourself more than you can handle the first month.

•**Find an accountability partner or support group.** Doing things together sometimes can be more motivating.

•**Have a daily to-do list, and place "Exercise" at the top.** Make it part of your routine. Listen to podcasts, music, or news while you exercise.

Strengthening your joints now doesn't mean that you'll be completely free from pain later, but developing the habit can encourage you to continue year-round with modified versions that will keep pain at bay.

Reminder: When pain flares, try soothing remedies such as wearing extra clothing layers to keep joints warm and placing a heating pad around stiff joints when they need a boost.

Keep Yourself Safe: Top 10 Winter Hazards

Mitchel Faulkner, MD, emergency medicine doctor and visiting instructor at The University of Utah, Salt Lake City, where he is completing a fellowship in wilderness medicine. Utah.edu

Winter can be an especially dangerous season. But knowing about the common hazards can help you take precautions to protect yourself from a visit to the ER during the colder months...

1. Shoveling snow. Don't risk clearing a path or your driveway if you aren't used to heavy-duty cardio and especially if you have any kind of heart condition. This level of exertion can result in a heart attack.

2. Car accidents. When roads are wet, icy or snow-covered, keep extra distance between your vehicle and the one in front of yours to reduce risk for a collision. Significantly reduce your speed—cars can slip on hard-to-see black ice.

Even better: If you don't have to drive, don't. If you must drive, wait until conditions improve or the temperature rises enough to melt any ice.

3. Slips on icy paths. Any fall can lead to a serious injury from a broken wrist, ankle, or hip to head trauma.

Prepare in advance—before a storm, put down a dense layer of salt on any paths around your home. Check that handrails on outside stairs are secure. Upgrade footwear to boots with nonskid soles.

4. Falls from ladders. These falls can result in severe head trauma, even paralysis. When putting up holiday decorations, leave the second story and higher to trained professionals. If you must get on a ladder, make sure it's secure and that someone strong is holding the base. Be creative—instead of stringing lights, project them onto your house from the ground.

5. Falling icicles. They are pretty when they catch the light, but icicles can break off and cut you like a dagger. Never walk

---

Replace Old Fire Extinguishers—Even If Unused

A fire extinguisher's life span is 10 to 12 years, but many people keep them much longer, risking that they may not deploy properly when needed.

To find the date of manufacture: Look on the UL nameplate on the cannister.

Best: Get the largest extinguisher you can safely lift and use, generally about five to 10 pounds. For the best places in your home to place an extinguisher, check the guide at CR.org/extinguishermap.

Consumer Reports. ConsumerReports.org

under them and, as often as needed, use a broomstick to break them off overhangs.

6. Hypothermia. Prolonged exposure to low temperatures can cause your body temperature to drop to an unsafe level. At greatest risk are the very young and seniors whose bodies are less able to regulate their temperature.

First sign of hypothermia: Fast shaking as your muscles contract to generate heat. As it gets worse, the shaking stops—that is a sign that all body systems are affected. Confusion, exhaustion, and slurred speech may follow. Get indoors as soon as you can. If you (or a loved one) is experiencing signs of hypothermia, call 911. While waiting for help to arrive, wrap yourself in blankets and drink hot liquids.

7. Frostbite. This is a more localized reaction to exposure to very cold temperatures. Fingers, toes, ears, and nose are most at risk.

First signs: Painful sensation like pins and needles—those are your nerve fibers warning you to get someplace warmer. Then parts of your body will start to feel numb. Similar to a severe burn, frostbite needs emergency treatment.

If you must be out in frigid weather: Wear a hat, mittens, heavy socks and boots, and a scarf to cover your mouth and nose.

If you suspect frostbite: Get to the ER for evaluation right away.

8. House fires. Never leave candles or a wood-burning fireplace unattended. If there are children in the house, fireplaces should have fire-proof screens. Wood stoves should be professionally installed and bricked off. Never leave paper or other flammable materials anywhere near fireplaces or stoves. Don't burn open fires indoors because they will give off carbon monoxide.

If you must use a space heater: Keep it at least three feet away from anything flammable—furniture, curtains, and bedding, etc. Do not plug them into a power-strip or surge protector.

9. Carbon monoxide poisoning. Fireplaces, wood and gas stoves, and gas appliances that aren't properly maintained or vented can emit this odorless and deadly gas into your home.

Warning signs of carbon monoxide poisoning: Flu-like symptoms that include headache, weakness, nausea or vomiting, dizziness or confusion, and/or blurred vision. If a few people in your house start to experience the same symptoms, get out immediately and call 911 or your utility company to do an inspection.

Prevention: Place smoke detectors and battery-operated carbon monoxide detectors near these appliances. Have your chimneys and flues inspected and cleaned by a licensed chimney sweep every year. Never use an outdoor grill or stove to heat your home.

SUV, Pickup Truck Blind Spots Put Pedestrians at Risk

When making left turns, drivers of pickup trucks are 42 percent more likely than car drivers to hit pedestrians and SUVs are 23 percent more likely, according to recent research. Making right turns is not an issue. Pickups also are 80 percent more likely than cars to hit a pedestrian standing, walking, or running along a road away from an intersection…SUVs are 61 percent more likely… and minivans, 45 percent more likely.

Reasons: The pillars that hold up roofs of larger vehicles are thicker because safety standards require them to be stronger, which creates a blind spot in the front of the vehicle that may make it harder for drivers to see people walking near the vehicle's corners. Also, the high hoods of larger vehicles can obstruct drivers' views of pedestrians, especially for shorter drivers.

Research by Insurance Institute for Highway Safety, Arlington, Virginia. IIHS.org

10. Being stranded in your vehicle. Beside winterizing your car—filling up on antifreeze, checking wiper blades, and changing to snow tires if needed—keep emergency essentials in your trunk. Include extra jackets, gloves, hats, and socks...a first-aid kit...water and nonperishable snacks...an ice scraper and a bag of kitty litter to provide traction in case your vehicle gets stuck... and keep a spare phone charger in the glove compartment.

Choose the Best Footwear to Protect Against Winter Falls

Jamison Starbuck, ND, is a naturopathic physician in family practice in Missoula, Montana, and producer of Dr. Starbuck's Health Tips for Kids, a weekly program on Montana Public Radio, MTPR.org.

Many winter falls can be prevented by choosing the right footwear. Canadian researchers at the University of Toronto recently found that only nine out of 98 so-called winter boots actually worked to keep people stable on icy surfaces. If your boot soles get slick and slippery on a patch of ice, a fall is inevitable.

Ascertain how well your shoes and boots perform on ice. Consider buying a new pair that have a tested slip-resistant rating. You can also improve the safety of your current winter boots by using traction cleats designed for use in everyday winter chores. These rubber and wire devices slip on to most stout footwear. They work well and cost a fraction of the price of new boots.

Falls on ice are sudden and surprising. They can cause fractured ribs, separated shoulders, concussion, and even depression. If you hit your head, are in pain, or mentally confused after a fall, see your doctor immediately. If you're just a bit bruised, apply homeopathic Arnica gel to the bruised spots and take one Arnica 30 C homeopathic tablet under the tongue, away from meals, three times a day for one or two days.

TLC for Chronic Wounds

Robert Kirsner, MD, PhD, director of the University of Miami Hospital and Clinics Wound Center, and the University of Miami Wound Clinic, Chief of Dermatology at the University of Miami Hospitals and Jackson Memorial Hospital, and Chair and Harvey Blank Professor in the Dr. Phillip Frost Department of Dermatology & Cutaneous Surgery at the University of Miami Miller School of Medicine.

For 7 million Americans, chronic, hard-to-heal wounds are a big problem. Chronic wounds are those that haven't healed completely in four weeks, even with standard care. They're most common in seniors and people with circulatory disease, cancer, and spinal cord injuries. Americans with diabetes are particularly at risk because of poor circulation (bringing less blood and oxygen to the wound) and a weakened immune system (increasing the risk of infection, which stalls wound healing). One million people with diabetes develop a foot ulcer every year.

Unhealed wounds—including diabetic ulcers, vascular ulcers, pressure ulcers, radiation wounds, nonhealing surgical wounds, and the like—are a major problem. They're painful. They often drain and emit odors, and have unsightly dressings. They can lead to disability and amputation. They're even linked to dying. Having a chronic wound is more predictive of death over a five-year period than having breast or prostate cancer.

Care Can Be Hard to Access

If you have a chronic wound, you need the best care possible to stabilize and heal. But topnotch care isn't always easy to get. *Chronic wounds are a largely unrecognized and underserved problem for a few reasons...*

• **They disproportionately affect seniors and minorities,** neither of whom have a major voice to lobby for resources for wound care from the government, insurance companies, and other sources of funding.

• **They often affect areas that aren't typically seen,** like the foot and the buttocks. Out of sight, out of mind.

• **There is no medical specialty devoted to healing wounds.** Rather, they are treated by several categories of physicians (like dermatologists and vascular surgeons), podiatrists, nurses, and physical therapists. These health professionals approach chronic wounds without a nationally standardized curriculum of training or a consistent, consensus-driven pathway of care.

When a Wound Doesn't Heal

There are four phases of wound healing. If one or more of them are incomplete, you develop a chronic wound.

1. **Hemostasis.** After an injury, blood vessels constrict to reduce blood flow, and clotting factors like fibrin are released at the site.

2. **Inflammation.** Immune cells like phagocytes and white blood cells enter the site to kill bacteria, remove debris, and prepare the area for new tissue growth. With all the activity, the site becomes red, swollen, hot, and painful.

3. **Proliferation.** New blood vessels and tissue form to close up the site. Colla-

---

The Healing Power of Hyperbaric Oxygen Therapy

In hyperbaric oxygen therapy (HBOT), you sit in a chamber and breathe pure, pressurized oxygen. HBOT is best known as a treatment for scuba divers with decompression sickness, or "the bends"—the shortness of breath, dizziness, confusion, and other symptoms that can occur when a diver stays too long at depth or ascends too quickly, and toxic nitrogen bubbles form in the blood and other tissues. HBOT compresses those bubbles, they dissolve, and the symptoms usually disappear. But pure, pressurized oxygen is Medicare-approved for more than a dozen other health problems, including chronic wounds.

Right now, the oxygen content of the air you're breathing is about 21 percent. In a hyperbaric oxygen chamber, the air is 99 to 100 percent oxygen. And it's also pressurized at a level two to three times higher than oxygen at sea level. These two factors boost the level of oxygen in the blood 20-fold. And this hyperoxygenation improves circulation, allowing chronic wounds to heal.

Medicare has approved HBOT for several types of chronic wounds, including...

• **Diabetic foot osteomyelitis.** A chronic, unhealed foot ulcer in diabetes becomes infected, the infection spreads to the bone, and nothing is working to solve the problem. This condition (chronic refractory osteomyelitis) often leads to amputation. But in many cases, HBOT can help stop the infection—and prevent the patient from losing their foot.

• **Diabetic wounds of the lower extremities.** Fifteen percent of diabetics will develop a diabetic foot ulcer. And any type of diabetic wound of the lower extremity that hasn't healed with standard therapy is a candidate for HBOT. In a study in the *Journal of Vascular Surgery* in February 2020, people with a diabetic foot ulcer who didn't get HBOT were more than twice as likely to undergo amputation.

• **Radiation-induced skin injury.** The medical term for this condition is soft tissue radionecrosis. It typically occurs when radiation treatment for cancer kills skin tissue and the tissue doesn't regenerate. HBOT can turn the situation around.

• **Flesh-eating disease.** The medical term for this type of infection is necrotizing fasciitis—when bacteria quickly eat away at skin and underlying tissue. HBOT can help stop and reverse the process.

Joseph Cavorsi, MD, medical director, Carl Webber Center for Wound Care and Hyperbaric Medicine, White Plains Hospital, White Plains, New York.

gen, the protein that maintains the integrity of skin, is the main player.

4. Remodeling. The tissue becomes stronger and more flexible, and a scar forms.

Goals for Healing

There are several things you can do to make sure you and your chronic wound get the best possible care…

• **Find a wound care center.** Given the inconsistency of care for chronic wounds, it's best to see a health-care provider at a wound care center. Do an online search using the phrase (in quotes) "wound care center" and the name of your city or town.

• **Maximize the five steps of caring for a chronic wound.** The wound care center should systematically address your wound with five key steps—while also maximizing your ability and that of your family to deliver effective wound care.

1. Debridement. Debridement is the removal of dead tissue. Early, aggressive, and consistent (weekly) debridement is the cornerstone of wound care.

2. Infection control. Infections are the number-one reason why wounds don't heal. But figuring out what bacteria is infecting the wound (so the doctor can prescribe the appropriate antibiotic) is iffy, with only a 20 percent accuracy rate from taking a culture with a swab. DNA identification, on the other hand, is 100 percent accurate. And remember not to touch your own wound with bare hands. Always wear gloves, just like the health professionals.

3. Dressing management. Dressings protect, moisturize, reduce pain, improve appearance, compress (for better venous circulation), immobilize, and offload pressure.

There are many dressings to choose from based on your wound: Some add moisture, some improve drainage, some fill a space or cavity.

4. Grafting. One way to heal a chronic wound is by grafting tissue to the wound for rapid coverage. There are many types of grafts to choose from.

5. Pain management. A chronic wound is usually painful, and managing that pain is important for well-being. In fact, research shows that when pain is managed, wounds heal faster. Start with a nonsteroidal anti-inflammatory drug, such as ibuprofen. If that doesn't work, your physician may add an opioid, such as codeine or tramadol. If this combination doesn't work, your doctor may use a more potent oral narcotic.

• **Have a range of goals for healing.** It may not always be possible to achieve complete healing of a chronic wound. But you can stop the wound from becoming bigger. You can make it smaller. You can prevent infections. You can prevent an amputation. Those are good goals, too.

• **Eat a nutrient-rich diet and hydrate.** If you're not getting a recommended level of protein, vitamins, and minerals, your body can't maintain healthy tissue. For example, without adequate protein, vitamin A, vitamin C, and zinc, the body can't adequately synthesize collagen, the protein that supplies structural integrity to skin.

The Mediterranean-style diet—rich in poultry, fish, vegetables, fruit, beans, and whole grains—is a good diet for wound healing. In a study in the *Journal of Vascular Nursing,* published in September 2021, patients with skin ulcers had a better rate of healing if they adhered to the Mediterranean diet. They also healed faster if they drank more than one liter (34 ounces) of water daily.

• **Double-check your medications.** Several classes of medications can impair wound healing. They include anticoagulants, chemotherapeutic agents, corticosteroids, disease-modifying antirheumatic drugs (DMARDs) for rheumatoid arthritis, and immunosuppressants. If you're taking one or more of these classes of drugs, talk to your wound care professional about how to minimize their impact.

Chapter 14

RESPIRATORY HEALTH AND ALLERGIES

COPD Deaths Are Rising in Women

Chronic obstructive pulmonary disease (COPD), a progressive illness that can cause wheezing, coughing, excess phlegm, shortness of breath, and chest tightness is an umbrella term for two, often overlapping conditions: emphysema, which is the result of damage to the walls between many of the air sacs in the lungs, and chronic bronchitis, which is caused by repeated or constant irritation and inflammation in the lining of the airways. COPD primarily affects current or former smokers, but up to 30 percent of people with COPD never smoked.

In addition to smoking and secondhand smoke, exposure to air pollution, dust, chemicals, and smoke from home cooking or fireplaces can increase a person's risk of developing this irreversible illness. People who are born with alpha-1 antitrypsin (AAT) deficiency have an elevated risk, and those with asthma often develop COPD as well.

Sex Differences

COPD affects both men and women, but not in the same way. Women are more likely to develop the disease, to have more severe symptoms, and to experience more flares. While COPD deaths are declining in men, they're rising in women. Women with COPD report a lower ability to exercise and worse overall health-related quality of life compared with men with the condition. Women with COPD were often lighter smokers than their male counterparts. This may be because women's lungs and airways are often smaller than those of men, making cigarette smoking more dangerous. Secondhand smoke, wood fires, and even home cooking can increase the risk of COPD. Women may be exposed to more indoor air pollution from spending more time in the home, for example. And in many families, women do more household chores, such as cleaning, that can exacerbate COPD.

COPD doesn't affect only breathing. About half of people with COPD also have osteoporosis or weakening of the bones that can lead to fractures. Further, rates of anxiety and depression are elevated in people with COPD—especially women.

Jamie Garfield, MD, professor, thoracic medicine and surgery, Lewis Katz School of Medicine, Temple University, Philadelphia.

Treatment

When it comes to treatment, the most important measure for both men and women is to quit smoking. *From there, a doctor may recommend one or more of the following...*

•**Medications** to treat COPD symptoms include inhaled bronchodilators (which relax the muscles around your airways) and steroids (which reduce inflammation in the airways). There are evidence-based guidelines to help doctors choose the best medication for each patient's specific disease and triggers. If your COPD is mild, you may need only a short-acting bronchodilator that lasts for about four to six hours. If your COPD is moderate or severe, you may need long-acting bronchodilators that last about 12 hours or more. If your COPD is severe, you may need a combination of bronchodilators and an inhaled steroid. If your oxygen levels are low, you may also use portable oxygen. You can receive oxygen therapy from tubes resting in your nose, a face mask, or a tube placed in your trachea. There is a great deal of evidence to help doctors choose the best medications for your particular symptoms, but you may run into hiccups with insurance coverage. "Often, we have an optimal agent and we have to modify that based on what the patient's insurance will cover," Jamie Garfield, MD, professor of thoracic medicine at Temple University, told us.

•**Pulmonary rehabilitation** teaches you how to manage your COPD symptoms by learning to breathe better, how to conserve energy, and how to eat and exercise in ways that improve your symptoms.

•**Prevention and treatment of lung infections.** Certain vaccines, such as flu and pneumonia vaccines, are especially important for people with COPD.

•**Surgery.** If more conservative measures don't give you relief, your doctor may recommend surgery to remove air spaces that interfere with breathing (bullectomy), to remove damaged tissue (lung volume reduction surgery), to insert valves that keep air from re-entering a diseased part of the lung, or to replace a damaged lung with a healthy donor lung.

Reduce Triggers

You may notice your symptoms get worse (or flare) because of certain triggers, such as pollution, smells, or cold air. Taking steps to reduce triggers can help you feel better.

•**Fight allergies.** If you have allergies, consider taking allergy medicine or eliminating triggers. Replace carpets with hard flooring, keep pets out of the bedroom, and use mattress and pillow covers to keep dust mites out. Use air filters in your HVAC system to help clean the air, or use HEPA air filters.

•**Greener cleaning.** Several chemicals that are commonly used in cleaning products, including ammonia, hydrogen peroxide, chlorine bleach, and alcohol, can irritate the bronchial passages and make it harder to breathe. To stay safer while cleaning, skip these ingredients, as well as aerosolized products and those with fragrance. Instead, opt for soap and water, baking soda, and vinegar. Air fresheners, scented soaps, perfume, candles, and incense can irritate your lungs, as well.

Misdiagnosis of COPD in Women

Women with COPD may not be diagnosed until later in the disease, when treatment options are more limited. Dr. Garfield reports that she often sees women who were diagnosed with asthma, but not COPD, even when they had both conditions. If you suspect that you may have COPD, ask your doctor to perform a spirometry test, which measures how much air you exhale and how fast you do it. If your doctor is unable or unwilling to do this test, see a pulmonologist for a follow-up. It's OK to question your doctor. Don't be afraid to ask questions, expect clear answers, and, when needed, get a second opinion.

- **Watch out for wood smoke.** Fireplaces, wood-burning stoves, and firepits all emit tint particles that can damage your lungs. Avoid secondhand smoke (from other smokers), too.
- **Cooking.** If you use a gas stove, you can be exposed to elevated levels of nitrogen dioxide. Use either the above-stove fan or open a window and use a fan to blow air out that way instead. If you're ready for a new stove, consider switching to electric.
- **Monitor** air quality and stay indoors when the air quality is poor. Wear a scarf or mask to warm the air you breathe in cold weather.

A New Breathing Device Improves COPD Breathlessness

Muhammad Ahsan Zafar, MD, associate professor of internal medicine, University of Chicago.

For people with COPD, it takes longer to get inhaled air out of the lungs with each breath due to tighter air tubes. Air is retained in the lungs, causing breathlessness and lower oxygen levels. The PEP Buddy, a device that is the size of a whistle, counters this effect by generating a slight resistance to exhalation, creating what's called positive expiratory pressure, which slows breathing and prolongs exhalation. In a clinical trial, 72 percent of participants reported less shortness of breath and improved quality of life after using the device.

Beetroot Juice Beneficial for People with COPD

European Respiratory Journal.

Adults with chronic obstructive pulmonary disease and elevated blood pressure who drank beetroot juice every day for 12 weeks had significantly improved blood pressure, vascular function, and exercise capacity. The juice contained 400 milligrams of nitrate, which has been associated with lower cardiovascular risk. The beet juice was associated with a 4.5 mmHg reduction in systolic blood pressure and the ability to walk 30 meters more in six minutes.

Halt a Lingering Cough

Jonathan P. Parsons, MD, MSc, FCCP, professor of internal medicine at The Ohio State University College of Medicine and director of the Multidisciplinary Cough Clinic and the OSU Asthma Center at The Ohio State University Wexner Medical Center, all in Columbus. WexnerMedical.osu.edu

Upper-respiratory tract infections usually pass within a week or two—but the annoying coughing sometimes persists much longer.

Good news: That cough doesn't mean that you're still infectious, and it is unlikely to cause any long-term damage to your health. It's usually just a sign that your airways are still irritated from the infection that's now passed.

Still, a cough that won't go away can be uncomfortable and disruptive, making it difficult to sleep and exercise—consequences that themselves can have a negative impact on your health. A cough also can make everyone you encounter concerned that that you might be spreading germs. *What to do...*

- **See your doctor if you're still coughing six to eight weeks after a respiratory infection has passed.** When a cough lingers this long, your health-care provider might prescribe oral steroids to reduce inflammation of the airways or an albuterol inhaler to open up the airways. In the meantime, home remedies and over-the-counter products may provide some short-term relief from a persistent cough, including honey, cough medicine, lozenges, and hot showers.

•**See your doctor immediately if you cough up blood...run a persistent fever... experience chills or body aches...or any other symptoms accompany the lingering cough.** These symptoms could indicate an ongoing infection, not just a remnant of one that has passed.

Caution: A lingering cough that was not preceded by an upper-respiratory tract infection such as flu or COVID could be a symptom of asthma, allergies, gastroesophageal reflux disease, chronic obstructive pulmonary disease, or even lung cancer.

Also: Taking an ACE inhibitor—a medication often prescribed for high blood pressure—can cause a persistent cough.

New Strategy for Severe Asthma

Study titled "Reduction of Daily Maintenance Inhaled Corticosteroids in Patients with Severe Eosinophilic Asthma Treated with Benralizumab (SHAMAL): A Randomised, Multicentre, Open-Label, Phase 4 Study," led by researchers at Kings College London, published in *The Lancet*.

The chronic lung disease asthma can result in more than inconvenient wheezing. Close to 10 percent of adults with asthma have a severe, life-threatening type, known as eosinophilic asthma. For these individuals, asthma is frequent, unpredictable, and hard to control. Severe asthma often requires the use of steroid drugs through an inhaler or in pill form. The most common treatment is a high-dose inhaled corticosteroid (ICS). Even with these drugs on board, asthma can have a heavy physical and emotional impact on quality of life.

A new study from Kings College London, hailed as a landmark study, has shown that once a patient starts a biologic drug, they can safely reduce or even eliminate the need for steroids, along with the side effects steroids often bring such as osteoporosis, bone fractures, diabetes, and cataracts. The study was conducted at 22 sites in the United Kingdom, France, Germany, and Italy. The results are published in the prestigious British medical journal *The Lancet*.

Eosinophils with a Purpose

Eosinophils are white blood cells that play an important role in the body's immune system. They are meant to protect the lungs against foreign invaders such as viruses or bacteria, but in people with severe asthma, eosinophils attack normal tissues of the lung and cause inflammation. When a person's immune system overreacts and attacks normal body tissues it is called an autoimmune response or disease.

Benralizumab (Fasenra) is a biologic drug (or man-made antibody) that latches on to eosinophils and reduces their numbers and effects. Biologic drugs are a new type of drug that can dial back the autoimmune response. These drugs are called biologics because they are made from living cells and tissues.

A Biologic Beats Steroids

For the study, patients with severe eosinophilic asthma were started on at least three doses of benralizumab, given as an injection every four to eight weeks. The research team used a five-item Asthma Control Questionnaire to qualify the patient's asthma as severe. Participants began taking benralizumab before starting the study. When the study began, 208 patients were randomly assigned to continue their high dose ICS or to start tapering their steroid medication over 32 weeks, and then continue at that level of medication for another 16 weeks. *These were the key findings for the patients who were in the taper group as compared to those in the continue-steroid-meds group...*

•**Almost all patients** (92 percent) were able to significantly reduce steroid use and maintain control of their asthma.

- **Sixty percent of patients were able to stop all steroid use.**
- **Most patients did not experience flare-ups (exacerbations)** during the study period: 87 percent in the taper group and 88 percent in the full-strength ICS group.

The research team concludes that this study highlights the role of eosinophils in severe asthma, and that the biologic drug-controlled eosinophils curbs asthma safely and with minimal or no use of high-dose ICS. They hope their study and others will highlight the opportunity to shift away from high-dose steroids for severe asthma.

Poor Sleep May Increase the Risk of Asthma

BMJ Open Respiratory Research.

Researchers looked at the sleep habits of more than 450,000 people and found that those who reported poor sleep had a 55 percent higher risk of being diagnosed with asthma over a nine-year follow-up period. Indicators of poor sleep included getting less than seven to nine hours of sleep each night, experiencing insomnia, snoring, experiencing frequent daytime sleepiness, and having a late chronotype (being a "night owl"). That was higher than the risk for people with a genetic predisposition for asthma (47 percent). People with both a high genetic risk and poor sleep were 122 percent more likely to be diagnosed with asthma. Asthma can also cause disordered sleep.

CPAP Mask Comparison

Ann Augustine, MD, assistant professor of neurology, Duke University School of Medicine, Durham, North Carolina.

For many people with obstructive sleep apnea (OSA), the first sign that something is wrong is unrelenting daytime sleepiness. That's because OSA causes the airway to narrow or collapse until the person wakes up to take a breath—five to 30 or more times every hour. Once these exhausted patients are diagnosed, the standard treatment is continuous positive airway pressure (CPAP), a bedside device that sends a continuous stream of compressed air into the airway to hold it open.

While CPAP can return both breathing and sleep to normal levels—and slash the risk of heart attack and stroke in the process—one detail can make a significant difference in how well it works: what type of mask is used.

Researchers reported in *Chest* that when patients wear masks that cover both the nose and mouth, they often have less relief from their OSA and poorer adherence to the treatment than patients who choose nose-only interfaces.

"An oronasal mask required higher pressures and resulted in less control of apnea," says Ann Augustine, MD, assistant professor of neurology, Duke University School of Medicine.

Persistent Asthma May Increase Stroke Risk

Study participants with persistent asthma (symptoms occur at least more than two days a week) had nearly twice the risk of having plaque in carotid arteries, compared with people who did not have asthma. Chronic inflammation is known to contribute to arterial plaque, and both inflammation and arterial plaque are factors that can increase the risk for stroke and heart attack. If you have asthma, discuss with your doctor what you can do to reduce your cardiovascular risk.

Study of more than 5,000 adults by researchers at University of Wisconsin, Madison, published in *Journal of the American Heart Association.*

Nose vs. Mouth Breathing

To learn more about this difference, the researchers zeroed in on people with a history of breathing through their mouths some or all of the time. For each person, they used a process called titration to determine the optimal air pressure that would be tolerable to the patient and eliminate obstructive events with both a nasal and an oronasal mask. For patients who breathed through their noses, the researchers were able to find an air pressure that eliminated all apnea events with both masks. The oronasal mask, however, consistently required a higher air pressure to be effective. When using an oronasal mask, close to half of the people who breathed through their mouths at least 25 percent of the time could not be successfully titrated. Even at the highest levels of CPAP treatment, they had residual airway closures.

Take-Home Message

The researchers stressed the importance of using a nasal mask whenever possible. Many people can transition to nose breathing by using select strategies, but not everyone can. That is where oronasal masks take a starring role. They may not perform as well as nasal masks when people can choose between nose and mouth breathing, but they make CPAP treatment possible for those with chronically stuffy noses. Even nose breathers turn to them when allergies and colds hit. Many CPAP users keep both masks handy so they can choose the best care when they need it most.

"The best mask is the one that you can wear throughout the night, every time you sleep," Dr. Augustine concludes. "For many people, that is a nasal mask. It uses a lower effective pressure and has a smaller profile that covers less of the face, which can be more easily accommodated in side and stomach sleepers."

Airway Mechanics

The pressure transmitted when breathing through the mouth, the researchers explained, neutralizes the positive pressure applied through the nose. In a previous study published in *Sleep Breath*, researchers observed this effect with magnetic resonance imaging. They discovered that when a person using an oronasal mask breathes through the nose, higher air pressure causes the space between the hard palate and the inferior aspect of the soft palate (retropalatal space) to become progressively larger, as one would expect. But if that person breathes through his or her mouth instead, the retropalatal space becomes smaller as air pressure rises.

Mouth Exercises That Reduce Snoring

Geraldo Lorenzi Filho, PhD, director, Sleep Lab, Heart Institute, University of Sao Paulo, Brazil.

As long as sleep apnea has been ruled out, these exercises that strengthen the soft palate can help reduce snoring. Do three sets of 20 each day. *Tip of the tongue*—push your tongue against the roof of your mouth and slide it backward. *Whole tongue*—suck your tongue up against the roof of your mouth and hold it there. *Back of the tongue*—push your tongue against the floor of your mouth while keeping the tip in contact with your bottom front teeth. *Say "aaaay"*—raise the back of your mouth (you can feel this happen when you yawn) and the uvula (the little fleshy flap that dangles in the back of your throat) while making an "aaay" sound.

Bet You Know Someone Who Still Smokes

Daniel Dilling, MD, FACP, pulmonary and critical care physician and medical director of the Lung and Heart-Lung Transplant Programs at Loyola University Medical Center, Maywood, Illinois. He is a professor of medicine at Loyola University Chicago, Stritch School of Medicine and a member of the American Lung Association's local leadership board in Greater Chicago. LoyolaMedicine.org

Good news! Cigarette smoking among U.S. adults has dropped steadily over the last 50 years. And yet—you are likely to know someone who still smokes. About one in five people between ages 45 and 64 still use some form of tobacco. That's the same as a decade ago and higher than the national average of 14 percent. Even worse, many people who smoke don't acknowledge the toll it is taking on their bodies. Despite the evidence, research shows that adults age 65 and older are less likely to label cigarettes as very or extremely harmful than adults ages 18 to 24.

Fact: Tobacco is the number-one cause of preventable illness and death in the U.S., and it ends up killing half of its users.

Equal Opportunity Organ Destroyer

While the lungs are the most significantly affected, no organ or system in the body can escape the destruction that smoking causes, including…

• **Heart.** Smoking causes blood vessels to narrow and thicken, increasing blood pressure, quickening your heart rate and predisposing you to blood clots that can cause a heart attack, a blood clot to the lung (called a *pulmonary embolism*) or a stroke. Smokers face two to four times the heart disease risk of nonsmokers. Not even casual smokers are safe—smoking just one cigarette a day elevates heart disease and stroke risk to nearly half that of pack-a-day smokers.

• **Brain.** Smoking impairs day-to-day cognitive functioning, including memory, focus and the ability to process information. Dementia, including Alzheimer's disease, strikes smokers at a higher-than-average rate. Much of this increased risk is linked with smoking's detrimental effects on the heart—when blood flow is compromised, all the organs in the body are starved for oxygen, including the brain—but chemicals in tobacco smoke also accelerate the brain's natural aging process.

• **Bones and joints.** System-wide inflammation triggered by smoking hastens bone loss, predisposing smokers to low bone density and osteoporosis, including hip fractures. It also raises the risk for rheumatoid arthritis, which tends to strike smokers earlier and with greater severity.

• **Vision and hearing.** Smokers lose their hearing faster and earlier than nonsmokers…and they are more prone to cataracts, dry eye syndrome, glaucoma, and macular degeneration, the number-one cause of blindness in adults over 65.

• **Gums and mouth.** Bad breath and stained teeth are the least of smokers' oral health troubles. They develop more bacterial plaque on their teeth, a root cause of gum infections, often leading to gum disease, jaw deterioration, and tooth loss. Smoking also boosts the risk for complications after oral surgery and raises risk for oral cancer, including cancer of the throat and lips.

• **And more.** The fallout from smoking also includes, among other things, type 2 diabetes (along with an increased risk for complications such as limb loss)…erectile dysfunction…a compromised immune system…and slower wound healing.

And Then There's the Lungs

Interestingly, when it comes to smoking-induced lung damage, nicotine is not the culprit—the highly addictive chemical primarily just gets people hooked. It's a one-two punch of airway inflammation (caused by inhaling a cocktail of thousands of chemicals, of which nearly 100 are cancer-causing) and tar, a sticky black goo created by the combustion of those chemicals that occurs when a person lights up. When inhaled, tar coats the interior of the lungs with a poisonous film similar to the tar used to pave roads.

Smoke slowly obliterates the hundreds of millions of tiny air sacs in your lungs that help you breathe. It also toughens lung tissue, impeding its ability to expand. And it doesn't matter if you're smoking cigarettes, cigars, e-cigarettes, or marijuana...when you inhale something that doesn't belong in your lungs, your body is not happy.

Toxins in smoke damage cellular DNA, paving the way for tumors—so much so that smokers have a 20-fold increased risk for lung cancer versus nonsmokers. (Smokers also have higher rates of cancer of the nasal cavity, mouth, throat, voice box, breast, kidney, bladder, liver, pancreas, colon/rectum, and more.)

Smokers' lungs suffer in several other potentially life-threatening ways...

• **Chronic obstructive pulmonary disease (COPD).** A leading cause of death in the U.S., COPD is an umbrella term for two lung diseases—emphysema and chronic bronchitis—that often hit people who have smoked for decades.

With emphysema, lung damage reduces the amount of oxygen entering the blood, causing coughing and breathlessness that can render even bathing and dressing difficult. It usually affects people in their 50s, 60s, and 70s, many of whom end up needing supplemental oxygen.

With chronic bronchitis, lung damage causes excess mucus production, triggering shortness of breath, frequent coughing and, eventually, scar tissue buildup and pneumonia. This tends to hit smokers a bit earlier than emphysema...usually in their 40s, 50s, and 60s.

• **Pulmonary fibrosis.** This progressive scarring disease causes a gradual loss of lung function and several of the same symptoms as COPD. In fact, it often is misdiagnosed as COPD or even as heart disease. But doctors can differentiate pulmonary fibrosis from other diseases if they hear a crackling noise, almost like Velcro tearing apart, when they listen to the base of the lungs. The average patient develops pulmonary fibrosis in his/her 60s, 70s, or 80s.

Both pulmonary fibrosis and COPD are irreversible, but quitting smoking may slow the worsening of symptoms by adding less fuel to the fire.

The Challenge: How to Quit

There's no way to sugarcoat it—quitting smoking is difficult. Nicotine physically changes the way your brain cells work—within 10 seconds of inhalation, it reaches the brain, where it stimulates the release of *dopamine* and other feel-good chemicals. When you stop smoking, your brain feels deprived and prompts you to light up again to get that neurochemical hit. This not only drives smoking throughout the day but also is responsible for the intense cravings and withdrawal symptoms (irritability, insomnia, anxiousness, trouble concentrating, and hunger) that make quitting so difficult. *But there are tools to help you stop smoking...*

• **Don't quit cold turkey.** Research from Mayo Clinic shows that if 100 smokers try to quit this way, only three to five of them will make it past six months—meaning that 95 percent or more fail. *Your doctor can prescribe medication to help ease the with-*

Cannabis Concerns

Marijuana smoke contains many of the same cancer-causing agents as tobacco smoke. And because marijuana users tend to inhale deeply and hold the smoke in their lungs, smoking pot results in four times the amount of tar deposition versus cigarette smoke. Regular users have an elevated risk for emphysema, chronic bronchitis, heart attack, and stroke.

drawal symptoms and wean your brain off nicotine, including...

• Nicotine replacement therapy (NRT). Prescription nasal sprays and inhalers, as well as over-the-counter skin patches, lozenges, and gums, deliver small amounts of nicotine without the chemicals and toxins found in smoke. The amount of nicotine is reduced week by week, helping you slowly wean off smoking.

• *Bupropion.* Started one to two weeks before your quit date, this medicine works by curbing nicotine cravings. It does not contain nicotine and usually is taken for about 12 weeks. Bupropion and NRT may be used simultaneously.

• **Change your habits.** Medicine combined with a personalized behavior-modification program (avoiding places and situations where you used to smoke...being aware of the emotions that trigger you to reach for a cigarette...chewing sugarless gum or snacking on crunchy vegetables to satisfy the hand-to-mouth urge...using relaxation techniques) offers the best chance of success. Ask your doctor for help or...

• Call 1-800-LUNGUSA (1-800-586-4872, and press 2) to reach the American Lung Association Lung HelpLine and Tobacco QuitLine. You'll connect with certified tobacco treatment specialists, nurses, and respiratory therapists who can help you craft an evidence-based personalized cessation plan.

• Text QUIT to 47848 (or if you're a Veteran enrolled in VA health care, text VET to 47848) to receive daily motivational text messages from the National Cancer Institute's Smokefree.gov. Vets also can call the U.S. Department of Veterans Affairs tobacco quitline at 1-855-QUIT-VET (1-855-784-8838).

Can e-cigarettes help you quit? The short answer is no. These battery-operated devices deliver nicotine, chemicals, and flavors without creating smoke. They have been marketed as a way to avoid the perils of smoking and even facilitate quitting. But using e-cigarettes (known as "vaping") has not been shown to help smokers quit and still contributes to lung diseases such as COPD and lung cancer, heart disease, and more.

The Reward for Quitting

Even if you've been smoking for decades, it's never too late to stop. *Here are the benefits if you do...*

Two weeks to three months after quitting...

• **Heart attack risk begins to drop.**

• **Lung function begins to improve.**

One year after quitting...

• **Added risk for coronary heart disease is half that of a current smoker.**

Five to 15 years after quitting...

• **Stroke risk is reduced to that of a nonsmoker.**

• **Risk of getting cancer of the mouth, throat, or esophagus is half that of a current smoker.**

10 years after quitting...

• **Risk of dying from lung cancer is about half that of a current smoker.**

• **Risk for bladder, kidney, pancreatic, and cervical cancer drops.**

15 years after quitting...

• **Risk for coronary heart disease is the same as that of a nonsmoker.**

American Lung Association and University of Southern California's Keck Medicine.

DIY Ways to Quit Vaping

Amanda L. Graham, PhD, adjunct professor of medicine, Mayo Clinic College of Medicine and Science, Rochester, Minnesota, and chief of innovations at Truth Initiative, a nonprofit company focused on tobacco and nicotine cessation, Washington, DC. TruthInitiative.org

Quitting cold turkey is the least likely method to work—it makes you feel terrible and likely to go right back to nicotine.

Better: Challenge yourself to stretch the time between a craving and a hit. Try to cut your consumption in half over a week. Distract yourself—when you get a craving, squeeze a stress ball, do some jumping jacks, drink a glass of ice water, chew on a toothpick, or take a walk. Writing down why you want to quit also helps keep you focused on your goal.

Stuffy Air Can Give You Brain Fog

Esther Sternberg, MD, professor of medicine and psychology, College of Medicine, University of Arizona, Tucson, and author of *Well at Work: Creating Wellbeing in Any Workspace*. Medicine.Arizona.edu

In a poorly ventilated space, human breath can generate a buildup of carbon dioxide that, at high enough levels, can cut your cognitive performance in half. If you work in such a space, install a fan, open a window and/or keep meetings short.

You Probably Have "Screen Apnea"

Stephen Porges, PhD, professor of psychiatry, University of North Carolina at Chapel Hill. Med.UNC.edu...and James Nestor, author of *Breath: The New Science of a Lost Art*. MrJamesNestor.com.

Working on a laptop, computer or smartphone screen actually disrupts breathing—a phenomenon called screen apnea. The nervous system automatically checks all stimuli (i.e., a text message, an e-mail alert, an ad flashing up on a website) to decide whether there is a threat—and evaluating that decision requires mental effort that leads to shallower breathing. The more unexpected a stimulus is, the more likely the body will perceive it as a threat. While not harmful when infrequent, screen apnea can contribute to mental and physical exhaustion if the stimuli is nearly constant.

Self-defense: Create breathing-awareness alerts for yourself throughout the day...try larger screens, which are less mentally taxing than small ones...take relaxation breaks to listen to music or take a walk.

How to Prepare for Allergy Season

Leonard Bielory, MD, a professor of medicine, allergy, immunology and ophthalmology at the Hackensack Meridian School of Medicine, in New Jersey, and professor of allergy and immunology at the Thomas Jefferson University-Sidney Kimmel School of Medicine in Philadelphia. Dr. Bielory conducts research on the links between climate change and allergy.

When the air is heavy with mold spores or pollens from trees, grasses, or weeds, about 35 million Americans experience sneezing, stuffy or runny noses and itchy, watery eyes. For some, allergies can also trigger asthma symptoms.

Here's what you need to know about allergy timing, and how you can use that knowledge to feel better.

Seasonal Timing

For most seasonal allergy sufferers, winter brings welcome relief. That's because cold, dry air limits mold growth and most pollen-producing plants go quiet, at least for a while.

There are exceptions: Molds in Florida and grass pollens in California persist year-round. And mountain cedar trees spew pollen through most of the winter in central Texas and some other parts of the Southwest. Elsewhere, allergy season starts when trees resume growing and pollinating in the spring.

From an allergy standpoint, spring doesn't necessarily start in March or at the same time everywhere. Instead, a northward march of rising tree pollen levels starts in the South, usually in January, and reaches more northern climes, including the Northeast, Midwest, and Pacific Northwest, often between mid-February and mid-March. As different tree species awaken from their winter rest, new pollens join the mix, extending tree pollen season through June in some places.

Meanwhile, grass pollens emerge between April and June and are shortly joined by weed pollens, which typically peak in late summer. In some places, grasses peak again in the late summer as well.

The first frost, which varies depending on where you live, puts an end to pollen season in most of the United States.

Warmer Weather, More Allergies

If you have seasonal allergies, you may have noticed that pollen seasons seem to start earlier these days.

Studies confirm the change is real: Plants are releasing pollens earlier, starting with trees in the late winter and early spring. In the first decade of the 2000s, pollen seasons for trees, grasses, and weeds in the United States started an average of three days earlier than they did in the 1990s. A more recent study found that North American pollen seasons last an average of eight days longer than they did in the 1990s. The shift toward earlier, longer seasons is expected to continue.

Rising temperatures are to blame. Warmer weather in the winter and early spring jump start the growing seasons of pollinating plants, while later frosts in the autumn keep them going. Climate change also appears to be responsible for higher pollen levels in the air.

Taken together, the changes mean people are exposed to more allergy-causing substances for a longer time, something that may explain why seasonal allergies are becoming more common. Even older adults, once considered unlikely to develop

Watching Patterns

You can't control plant pollination or outdoor mold growth, but you can use your knowledge of seasonal patterns as a starting point to tackle allergy symptoms.

.Symptom patterns. If you sneeze and rub your eyes only in early spring, a tree pollen allergy is a good guess. If you have symptoms from early spring through fall, you may well have allergies to several plant species. Year-round symptoms suggest you may have allergies to indoor substances, such as dust mites, or that you have a nonallergic form of rhinitis.

The best way to confirm any hunches and get treatment advice: Get allergy skin testing from a board-certified allergist.

.Pollen counts. While your nose may seem to know when pollen counts are rising, a better indicator is a count from the nearest station of the National Allergy Bureau, a network maintained by the American Academy of Allergy, Asthma and Immunology. You can sign up online, at Pollen.aaaai.org, for alerts from your nearest station.

.Weather. Even during peak pollen season, some days are better or worse than others. Dry, windy days mean higher pollen counts. Hot, humid weather encourages mold growth. On a rainy, windless day, pollens fall to the ground and stay put, giving many allergy sufferers a break (at least until the fallen pollen starts drying out and blowing around). A windy thunderstorm, on the other hand, can blow a lot of extra pollen through the air and cause symptom flare-ups.

.Time of day. As a rule, pollen counts tend to be lightest during the morning, because, as sailors know, mornings are usually less windy than afternoons. So that can be a good time to get out for exercise or other outdoor activities.

new allergies, are becoming newly allergic at higher rates than in the past.

How to Feel Better

Use these tips to limit your exposure to pollens and molds when counts are high...

• **Keep your windows closed at night** and, if possible, use air conditioning to clean, cool, and dry the air.

• **Keep windows closed and air conditioning on when you travel by car.**

• **If you have severe symptoms but must be outside for long periods, wear a mask.** The N95 and KN95 masks that effectively filter out viruses can also reduce your exposure to airborne allergens.

• **If you can, avoid mowing lawns or raking leaves,** because those activities stir up pollen and mold spores.

• **If you do decide to do gardening or other lawn work,** avoid touching your eyes and other parts of your face while outside.

• **After a long outdoor exposure,** leave your shoes at the door and then take a shower, wash your hair, and put on fresh clothes.

• **In general, it's smart for allergy sufferers to take their showers at night,** so that they aren't going to sleep with pollen on their skin and hair.

• **Don't hang your sheets or clothes outside to dry.**

Treatment Timing

Talk to your doctor about a treatment plan. It may include medications in addition to limiting your exposure. One strategy may be to start some medications before pollen counts start to rise. For example, inhaled nasal steroids, a mainstay of treatment, take several days to start working, so it can be smart to begin using them a week or two before your symptoms typically start. If you have severe or long-lasting symptoms that are hard to control in other ways, you may be a candidate for allergy shots, which are injections that reduce your sensitivity.

That can be a great long-term strategy but not a path to instant relief: It can take several months to see results.

> Even older adults, once considered unlikely to develop new allergies, are becoming newly allergic at higher rates than in the past.

Don't Sleep with a Fan If You Have Allergies

For people who have allergies, asthma or other lung conditions, leaving a fan on overnight can exacerbate their health conditions. Fans pick up and circulate dust and other small particles in the room as well as from the fan blades themselves...and a fan in an open window can suck in pollen that can contribute to hay fever.

Self-defense: A humidifier near the bed adds moisture to the air and helps reduce the effects of dry air.

Reminder: Clean the room regularly to reduce dust and other irritants.

Xuan Han, MD, pulmonologist, Tufts Medical Center, Boston. TuftsMedicalCenter.org

---

Natural Ways to Beat Sinusitis

Jamison Starbuck, ND, a naturopathic physician in family practice in Missoula, Montana, and producer of *Dr. Starbuck's Health Tips for Kids*, a weekly program on Montana Public Radio, MTPR.org. She is a past president of the American Association of Naturopathic Physicians and a contributing editor to *The Alternative Advisor: The Complete Guide to Natural Therapies and Alternative Treatments*.

Spring with its rainy days, flowers blooming, pollen blowing, and gardeners everywhere tilling up decayed and rotting plant material creates the perfect setting for respiratory inflammation and a rip-roaring case of sinusitis.

Sinusitis is inflammation of the nasal sinuses, the normally air-filled cavities that lie beside and above the nose. Sinus cavities help filter and warm the air we breathe. They also provide a protective air cushion between the face and brain. When you have sinusitis, these cavities are inflamed, swollen, and filled with mucus. The face is usually painfully tender to any touch. You may also have a headache, ear pain, nasal congestion, and mucus dripping out of your sinuses and down the back of your throat.

Sinusitis can be acute (lasting up to 10 days) or chronic (lasting for several months without relief). And while any sort of upper respiratory infection, viral, bacterial, or fungal, can lead to a sinus infection, allergic reactivity is also a primary cause of sinus inflammation.

Several natural medicines are uniquely useful in treating sinusitis because they provide symptom relief while simultaneously strengthening the immune health of your sinus and respiratory tract systems. *Here are several of my favorites…*

•**N-acetylcysteine** is an antioxidant derived from the amino acid L-cysteine. It can help reduce mucus production while speeding the healing of inflamed mucus membranes.

Dosage: 500 milligrams (mg) three times a day. For chronic sinusitis, I recommend an ongoing dose of 1,000 mg daily.

•**Quercetin** is a flavonoid found in many fruits and vegetables. It's anti-inflammatory and a natural antihistamine. Onions and kale are great sources of quercetin. You can also find it as a supplement.

Dosage: For acute sinusitis, take 350 mg four times a day. For chronic sinusitis, take 700 mg daily.

•**Bromelain** is a proteolytic enzyme complex derived from pineapple. Bromelain helps your immune system break down mucus and fight inflammation. Eating pineapple, away from other food, is good medicine when you have sinusitis or any nasal congestion.

Double Check on a Penicillin Allergy

Think You're Allergic to Penicillin?

Maybe not. More than 90 percent of patients who report being allergic to penicillin are not. Avoiding penicillin means that these people do not get some of the common and effective antibiotics that treat chest, skin, and urinary tract infections and instead are given alternative antibiotics that may be less effective. Some patients who believe they are allergic experienced unpleasant side effects after taking penicillin at some point in the past, but not every side effect means that someone is allergic. Others once were allergic to penicillin but no longer are—penicillin allergies tend to disappear over time. Ask your doctor about having an allergist conduct a penicillin allergy skin test to confirm any allergy.

American Academy of Allergy, Asthma & Immunology. AAAAI.org

Easier Penicillin Allergy Testing

A skin test usually is the first step to determine if a person has an allergy to penicillin. If there is no reaction, penicillin is given orally in small, gradually increasing doses to diagnose an allergy or rule it out.

Recent finding: The oral test alone is enough to determine whether someone who has had a mild reaction attributed to penicillin is truly allergic to it. The oral approach can be done safely in a doctor's office. If you have had a mild reaction to penicillin, ask whether it is appropriate for you.

Study of 382 patients with reported low-risk penicillin allergies by researchers at Heidelberg Health, Victoria, Australia, published in *JAMA Internal Medicine.*

Respiratory Health and Allergies

Dosage: Supplement with bromelain 500 mg up to four times a day, away from food, for both acute and chronic sinusitis.

•**Nasal irrigation** is an excellent way to relieve acute sinus pain and inflammation. Studies show that rinsing your nose with a saltwater solution reduces mucus and swelling in the nose and sinuses, bringing symptom relief for up to six hours. I recommend patients use a *neti pot,* a small container specifically designed for medical nasal irrigation. It's best to use a sterile saline solution that you purchase at a pharmacy. If you must make your own, boil tap water first to make sure it is bacteria free, then add one teaspoon of sea salt per two cups of water.

•**Allergy testing.** Finally, if sinusitis is a recurrent problem for you, seek both food and inhalant allergy testing. In my experience, many people with sinus problems have allergies to dairy, wheat, and/or mold, dust mites, and pets. For food allergy testing, IgG blood testing is the best method. Skin scratch or blood testing can determine inhalant allergies.

Plants Improve Indoor Air Quality

Fraser Torpy, PhD, associate professor, University of Technology, Sydney, Australia.

Researchers found that a wall filled with a mix of indoor plants removed 97 percent of cancer-causing pollutants from the surrounding air in just eight hours. Previous studies have shown that house plants can remove a broad range of indoor air contaminants.

Chapter 15

SLEEP AND RESTORATIVE HEALTH

Countdown to Your Best Night's Sleep

Are you going to bed wrong? Maybe! The same scene plays out in homes all across America—while relaxing in your living room, you realize that you're struggling to keep your eyes open, so you get up from the sofa, floss, brush, wash your face, and climb into bed...only to discover that you are now wide awake.

What went wrong? The actual process of getting ready for bed, with all the activity and bright bathroom lights, can be sufficiently stimulating to stave off sleep. In fact, the minutes immediately before getting into bed are not the ideal time to get ready for bed...and that's just one mistake people make with their pre-bedtime schedule. *Here's a better getting-ready-for-bedtime plan...*

Eight Hours or More Before Bedtime

•**Stop consuming caffeine.** Caffeine can linger in the body much longer than people realize—half of its sleep-preventing power can remain a full six to eight hours after consumption. Eight hours before bedtime should be the absolute last-call for caffeine, if not earlier.

Three Hours Before Bedtime

•**Stop exercising.** Working out shortly before bed might seem sensible, since exercise tires us out, but it actually can inhibit sleep. Exercise causes body temperatures to climb and remain slightly elevated for several hours. That's precisely the opposite of the falling body temperatures that are conducive to sleep.

Two Hours Before Bedtime

•**Stop eating.** This will reduce the odds that your sleep will be disturbed by indigestion, GERD, or any other digestive issues.

90 Minutes Before Bedtime

•**Stop looking at electronic screens.** The wavelengths of light emitted by TVs, smart-

---

Michael J. Breus, PhD, clinical psychologist and a fellow of the American Academy of Sleep Medicine. He is author of *The Power of When: Discover Your Chronotype—and the Best Time to Eat Lunch, Ask for a Raise, Have Sex, Write a Novel, Take Your Meds, and More.* SleepDoctor.com

phones, tablets, and computer screens can interfere with circadian rhythms, making it difficult to fall asleep.

• **Take melatonin pills if appropriate.** Melatonin can help travelers overcome time-zone changes and night-shift workers adjust their circadian rhythms...or it can be taken if you have a melatonin deficiency. But taking these pills immediately before bedtime is far too late to be effective.

Exception: Melatonin in liquid form should be taken 20 to 25 minutes before bedtime.

Caution: Melatonin also can change the effectiveness of certain medications, in particular blood pressure medicine and antidepressants. Check with your doctor before taking melatonin.

• **Turn down the thermostat.** A room temperature of 68°F to 70°F is ideal.

60 Minutes Before Bedtime

• **Stop consuming liquids so that sleep won't be interrupted by the need to urinate.**

Exceptions: Do consume liquids less than an hour before bedtime if you need them to take medications...if you're dehydrated and/or if you have diabetes and the beverage will improve your blood sugar levels through the night.

What Is the Ideal Sleeping Temperature?

According to a small study, when adults aged 65 wore sleep monitors that measured sleep duration, efficiency, and restlessness, their best quality of sleep was when the room temperature was between 68°F and 77°F, with the real sweet spot between 70°F and 74°F.

Study of 50 adults by researchers at Harvard Medical School, Boston, published in *Science of the Total Environment.*

• **Prep for the following morning.** Think through your morning schedule and responsibilities...jot down plans for the following day...lay out your clothes...and prepare your breakfast. Tackling morning tasks in the evening can help your mind relax.

40 Minutes Before Bedtime

• **Take care of evening hygiene.** Floss, brush, and wash now—don't wait until right before bed. If your bathroom lights are bright, install a dimmer switch and turn these lights low in the evening.

Helpful: Take a hot bath—soak up to your neck in water above 100°F. When you get out of this hot bath, your body will rapidly cool—and those declining body temps are conducive to sleep. Hot showers work, too, though not quite as well.

20 Minutes Before Bedtime

• **Do something quiet and calm.** Meditate, pray, listen to relaxing music, or a podcast that isn't too exciting, or read an actual printed book—not a digital book on a screen. Whatever sedate activity you select for this final 20 minutes, do it in relatively low light.

Helpful: On evenings when you don't have enough time to follow this bedtime routine precisely, still spend at least the 10 minutes before bed in quiet, low-light relaxation.

Best Cooling Pillows

Health.com

Coop Home Goods Eden Memory Foam Pillow provides all-night cooling, and the fill can be adjusted by adding or removing shredded foam, $96 at Amazon.com. *Slumber Cloud Core Down Alternative Pillow* comes with a 60-night trial and free returns, $64 at SlumberCloud.com. *HIMOON Bed Pillows for Sleeping* are a comfortable height and easily refluff in the dryer...they are not cool to the touch but don't heat up during the night, $20 for a two-pack on Amazon.com. *Nest Easy Breather Pillow,* for sleepers with neck pain, allows easily adjustable filling and keeps its shape even after washing, $107 on NestBedding.com.

Some Like It Hot, Some Like It Cold

Maura Daly Iversen, DPT, SD, MPH, a physical therapist and behavioral scientist/clinical epidemiologist with a primary focus in rheumatology, and the dean of the College of Health and Wellness at Johnson and Wales University in Providence, Rhode Island.

Heating pads. Cold packs. Icy plunges. There's no shortage of modalities for hot and cold therapies. But when are the right times to use them, and when should you stop DIY efforts and get specialized care?

The General Guideline

Heat is a vasodilator, which means it increases blood flow. Heat helps once the acute phase of an injury has passed as well as when you want relief from chronic or longstanding aches and pains. It can help remove toxins, relax muscles, and help loosen connective tissue. That's how it eases stiffness, boosts healing and, in turn, lessens discomfort.

Cold is a vasoconstrictor, meaning it reduces blood flow. In general, cold therapy works best for acute injuries, like a sudden strain or sprain, and flares of inflammatory conditions like bursitis. If you have a swollen ankle, for example, applying cold can reduce swelling and lessen pain.

Feel the Heat

At-home heat therapy options deliver superficial heat, penetrating less than 1 centimeter (cm) deep. Deep heat treatment, which can reach between 3 and 5 cm, is typically administered by a physical therapist or another orthopedic professional. Heat treatments can be dry, like a sauna, or moist, like a steam room or a simple soak in a hot bath (or a hot tub). You may find you respond better to one than the other.

•**Heating pads and sleeves.** This heat-delivering mainstay has benefited from many advances, including gel technology. Many styles are made to envelop a joint—you wrap it over the area like a towel. There are also many different sizes available (some so large they will cover your entire back) as well as shaped "sleeves" for arms and legs. Some pads have settings for dry heat, moist heat, and even cold for ice therapy.

In a pinch, you can dampen a towel, zap it in the microwave for a few seconds to heat it up, and then place over the achy area—note that the towel shouldn't be too hot to handle.

Timing: 20 minutes on, repeat hourly as needed.

•**Paraffin baths.** Formerly available only in spas or nail salons, these small units can improve circulation in hands, feet, and elbows. The tub holds a special wax that melts and reaches between 125 to 129°F. By quickly and repeatedly (about 10 times) dipping your extremity in the wax, you create a warming glove that penetrates to the small muscles and then peels off. For other parts of the body, like a hip or thigh, you can use a brush to layer on the wax.

Timing: Wait 30 minutes before peeling off the wax. It's great to follow this up with any muscle exercises you've been given to improve function.

•**Saunas, steam rooms, and hot tubs.** If you have access to these facilities, you may find them very soothing.

Timing: 20 minutes. Set a timer if there's any risk of your falling asleep.

•**Deep heat modalities.** A number of modes of deep heat, including ultrasound, microwave, and diathermy radio and sound waves, are available to health-care professionals. The most commonly used is ultrasound, similar to a diagnostic ultrasound. A gel is swabbed over the area to be treated and then a soundhead rolls over it, usually in a continuous mode over soft tissue and in a pulsed mode over bony areas. Ultrasound also encourages healing, so it may be part of your recovery plan after an injury.

Timing: 5 to 10 minutes on each area, administered by a licensed health-care professional.

• **Weighted wraps.** Similar to the effects of a weighted blanket, a weighted wrap may offer some relief from the anxiety that can accompany pain. Some wraps are shaped for specific problem areas like the neck and shoulders or lower back. They may have a dual function so they can be heated in a microwave or chilled in the freezer.

Timing: 20 minutes on, repeat hourly as needed.

The Big Chill

Forms of cold therapy run the gamut from a simple ice pack to cryogenic chambers cooled to hundreds of degrees below zero.

• **Topicals.** These include sprays, gels, creams, and sticks that cool skin on contact. Some are made with botanicals like peppermint or its extract menthol, while others are formulated with chemicals, sometimes with an anesthetic like lidocaine. Sprays are popular, especially with runners, because they're easy to carry and use. It only takes a second to spray a problem area like the Achilles tendon or iliotibial band, the network of fibers that runs from the outer hip down the thigh to the tibia.

Timing: These products work instantly, but it helps to follow up a spray with very gentle stretches, especially if you're working through a contraction or spasm. Hold each stretch for 30 to 60 seconds if you can.

Important: If your skin develops a local irritation to any topical product, stop using it.

• **Cold packs and wraps.** These include single-use chemical packs that are activated when you snap or break them (good for on-the-go) and reusable options you store in the freezer. The reusables have come a long way from rigid rectangles. Some pads or wraps are so thin that they'll conform to any part of the body, even when frozen. Some come with Velcro straps to hold the pad in place. In a pinch, a bag of frozen vegetables like corn kernels or peas can mimic the effect of a cold wrap and can be reused (just place a thin towel between your skin and the bag, and label the bag so no one eats them by mistake).

Some heating pads now offer a cold therapy setting, giving you cold and hot options in one product.

Timing: 20 minutes on, repeat hourly as needed.

• **Ice cup.** Fill a small paper cup with water and freeze it, then give yourself an ice massage, making circles with the ice and peeling off the paper as you go.

Timing: 7 to 10 minutes, repeat hourly as needed. This is the only type of ice application where you don't need a towel between your skin and the ice.

• **Ice baths.** You might have seen photos of athletes submerged in tubs filled with ice water as part of their post-game routine. You can replicate this at home by taking the plunge in your own bathtub filled with cold water and ice cubes.

At some spas, you can use a strategy that has been popular in Scandinavian countries for centuries: plunging into a cold pool before entering a sauna or hot tub. It has the effect of pumping blood supply for enhanced circulation.

Timing: 30 seconds to 10 minutes, depending on what you can tolerate.

• **Cold-compression sleeves and wraps.** These are typically used in a clinic or hospital after a severe injury or a procedure like rotator cuff surgery. Cold water runs through a wearable device that also provides compression. Home versions are available, but their use should be guided by a physical therapist or other licensed health-care professional.

• **Cryotherapy chambers.** Available at specialized clinics, these are extremely cold environments that you sit in (as you would a sauna), but only for a few minutes at a time.

Timing: As indicated by your PT.

Precautions

Some health conditions make using hot, cold or both dangerous. If you're being treated for a serious illness, such as cancer, get clearance from your doctor. *Here are general guidelines...*

Don't use hot or cold if you...

• **Have any cognitive issues that prevent you from tracking time.**

• **Are on medication that makes you drowsy and could make you fall asleep.**

• **Have nerve damage that prevents you from correctly sensing hot or cold.**

• **Have any open wound or a burn in the treatment area.**

Don't use cold if you...

• **Have poor circulation because of a condition like Reynaud's disease.**

Don't use heat if you...

• **Have any infection in the area needing therapy.**

• **Have any vascular disease that affects circulation or any blood disorder.**

Don't use deep heat if you...

• **Have any metal implants like a hip replacement.** Its metal component will draw in too much heat. Consult with your physical therapist.

Proven! You Can Think Your Way to Better Health

Ellen Langer, PhD, professor of psychology at Harvard University. She has won both a Guggenheim Fellowship and the Liberty Science Genius Award and is author of *The Mindful Body: Thinking Our Way to Chronic Health.*

Early in her career, Harvard psychologist Ellen Langer, PhD, asked a group of men in their 70s to travel back in time. They spent five days on a retreat in New Hampshire, living as they would have lived two decades earlier—the TV shows they watched, the magazines they read, the clothes they wore, and the events they discussed all were from that earlier time.

Result: These men didn't just relive their younger lives...their bodies seemed to become younger and healthier in measurable ways—their manual dexterity, strength, hearing, and vision all improved. They even looked younger.

Sounds like an episode of *The Twilight Zone,* right? But the experiment was rooted in a scientifically established idea—that the mind and body are best understood as a single unit. So wherever you put the mind, you also are putting the body. Thus, changing how we think can influence our health and fitness in meaningful ways. Consider the placebo. It is well-established that placebos can have measurable effects on health even though a placebo itself doesn't provide any health advantage. The change is created by the mind of the patient who takes the placebo.

We asked Dr. Langer—whose new book is *The Mindful Body*—to share some research-backed ways in which we can put the mind-body connection to use to improve our own health and fitness...

• **Reframe your daily activity as "exercise."** We all know that exercising is good for our health. What's surprising, though, is that how much exercise we get isn't the only factor that matters. How much we believe we get can have a meaningful effect on our health, too.

In one of Dr. Langer's studies, researchers encouraged a group of hotel chambermaids to view their everyday work as exercise. The chambermaids were informed of the similarities between their workplace efforts and the workouts provided by exercise equipment.

Result: These chambermaids lost weight and experienced reduced blood pressure compared with chambermaids who were not instructed to think of their work as exercise. The chambermaids who reframed their jobs as exercise didn't work any longer or harder—the physical benefits apparently occurred because their minds believed they were exercising.

Additional research conducted at Stanford University corroborated these results and further found that people who don't perceive themselves as physically active have significantly higher mortality rates than those who do perceive themselves to be active—regardless of how active they actually are.

Takeaway: Whenever you do housework or yardwork...walk from your vehicle to a shop or up a set of stairs...or engage in any other daily activity that involves physical movement or effort, tell yourself, *This is exercise.*

• **Imagine yourself eating to lose weight.** Dieters often try to avoid thinking about food. But counterintuitively, if done properly, thinking about food can reduce the desire to eat. The key is to imagine yourself eating lots of the specific foods that most tempt you. Real and imagined eating can be surprisingly similar to the brain. In one study, researchers at Carnegie Mellon University asked participants to imagine eating cheese. Those who imagined eating the most cheese ate less actual cheese when it was offered to them—they already felt fairly full because of their imagined eating.

Takeaway: When you feel like snacking or eating an unhealthy food, try imagining yourself eating that food. Make these imaginary binges as detailed as possible—if you're tempted by pizza, for example, imagine not only the taste, but the smell, the warmth of the cheese, and the feel of the crust in your mouth.

Similar: When it isn't possible to exercise, imagine yourself exercising. Researchers at Cleveland Clinic's Lerner Research Institute found that people who regularly imagine themselves exercising a specific muscle experience improvements in the strength of that muscle, though not as much as if they had actually exercised it. Imaginary exercise could be useful when you're recovering from an illness or injury, for example.

• **Don't allow arbitrary health-related "borderlines" to endanger your health.** Say two people receive virtually identical results on a glycated hemoglobin test—also known as the A1C test, a measurement of blood sugar levels—during their physicals. One is measured at 5.6 percent...the other at 5.7 percent—a difference so small that it's medically meaningless. Yet the person who receives the 5.7 percent is more likely to develop diabetes in coming years than the person who got the 5.6 percent—in fact, much more so than that tiny difference would suggest.

Why? The line between "normal" and "prediabetic" is drawn here, so the person who is measured at 5.7 percent is told he/she is prediabetic, while the person measured at 5.6 percent is not. This blood sugar difference is medically inconsequential, but the difference between being labeled "prediabetic" or "normal" is meaningful psychologically. People told that they were "prediabetic" went on to become sick...those who were initially no different continued to be normal. This is called the *borderline effect*—patients who fall on opposite sides of somewhat arbitrary medical lines often have very different health outcomes due to the psychological impact of the diagnoses and labels.

Takeaway: When you receive a medical diagnosis, remind yourself that it's likely an expression of probability, not your destiny. Ask the doctor for further information about what the diagnosis means... what percentage of people who receive it avoid the fate that it seems to foretell... and what actions you can take to improve your odds of doing so.

• **Control chronic health conditions by being mindful of symptom variability.** When people have chronic health problems, they believe those problems are unrelenting. They might think, *I'm stressed all the time...*or *This back pain never lets up,* for example. But it's more likely that their symptoms rise and fall—they just notice them most when they're at their worst. Becoming aware of symptom variability can reduce overall suffering. One study by Harvard University and University of Haifa found that pregnant women had easier pregnancies if they became mindful of the variability of their morning sickness and other sensations. Harvard studies using this attention to symptom variability with chronic pain, Parkinson's, multiple sclerosis, and arthritis also had successful outcomes.

Takeaway: Set your smartphone to beep or vibrate several times each day during waking hours. When it does, jot down how much the chronic symptom is affecting you at that moment...what you're doing...what you've recently done...where you are...and who you're with. When the symptom is particularly good or bad, take extra time to consider what's different about your life at that moment. Patterns will begin to emerge—perhaps you feel worse when you've been inactive...just eaten a certain food...or are interacting with an unpleasant colleague. You might be able to use the patterns to make lifestyle and diet adjustments that minimize the symptoms...and even if you can't, your increased awareness that your symptoms are not terrible all the time likely will help you feel somewhat better.

• **Reshape long tasks to reduce the dangers of fatigue.** Fatigue is a common cause of highway accidents, workplace injuries, and other dangers. But fatigue is not primarily the result of reaching our physical limits. It is governed in large part by our mental perception of how far we have progressed with a lengthy task.

When Harvard researchers examined at what point during a long drive fatigue sets in, they found that it is almost always somewhere between the drive's one-half and three-quarter mark—regardless of the length of the drive. Someone driving four hours is likely to start to feel fatigued between the second and third hours...someone driving 10 hours won't feel fatigued until the fifth hour or later. Researchers found comparable results with studies of lengthy, dull mental and physical tasks—people tend to feel fatigue not after a certain amount of time, as they would if physical or mental limits were being reached...but after a certain percentage of the task has been completed—usually between half and three-quarters. That suggests that fatigue is related to our expectations—which means we might be able to overcome it by mentally reframing long tasks.

Takeaway: Convert long tasks into smaller sections, each featuring a different form of mental engagement.

Example: On a long drive, spend the first third listening to an engaging audio book...the second third playing a mental game with car mates...and the third singing along with the radio.

The Strangest Sleep Disorder: Sleep Paralysis

Brian Sharpless, PhD, a clinical psychologist who practices via telemedicine in multiple states across the U.S. He is a visiting research fellow at Goldsmiths, University of London, the coauthor of *Sleep Paralysis: Historical Psychological, and Medical Perspectives,* and the author of *Monsters on the Couch: The Real Psychological Disorders Behind your Favorite Horror Movies.* BrianSharpless.com.

You wake up in the middle of the night and realize that you can't move. You're frozen in place and feel a heavy weight upon you. Then you see a menacing figure sitting on your chest or approaching from across the room. There's no question that you're awake, but you're helpless as fear and dread envelop you.

This experience has been striking people throughout history, and the menacing figures have been given many names around the world: demon, maere, alptraum, night hag, pisadeira. Fortunately, as real as the experience feels, nothing supernatural is happening. It's just a strange and terrifying sleep disorder called sleep paralysis.

We spoke with Brian Sharpless, PhD, a licensed clinical psychologist and sleep paralysis expert, and author, to learn more.

How to Reduce Episodes

- **Sleep on your side.**
- **Establish a regular sleep schedule.** Aim for seven to nine hours of sleep.
- **Try to reduce stress.**
- **Manage other health conditions,** such as obstructive sleep apnea.
- **Avoid alcohol and caffeine before bed.**
- **If you have an episode, focus on moving one part of your body, like a finger, to wake up faster.**
- **Treatment options include psychotherapy** (e.g., cognitive-behavior therapy for isolated sleep paralysis developed by Dr. Sharpless or a meditation-based approach), use of certain antidepressants, and tools to train you to sleep on your side.

What's Happening

Sleep paralysis is a state between sleep and wakefulness. Even though you're conscious, your body is still in REM-sleep-induced atonia (paralysis) and some remnants of REM-like brain activity persist. Electroencephalograms of people experiencing sleep paralysis show that their brains look both awake and asleep. The experience often occurs in stages: You wake up and realize you can't move. Next, you may sense that something terrifying is in the room with you before you see whatever your imagination conjures up. The type of entity that people experience is influenced by time, place, and cultural norms. Some people feel the entity touching them, sitting on or choking them, or even sexually assaulting them. The whole episode lasts a few minutes.

Sleep paralysis can strike anyone, but it's much more common in people with narcolepsy, some psychological disorders, or a history of trauma. It's more likely to affect people with disrupted sleep and people who drink, use drugs, or take certain medications. There's a genetic component as well: It's associated with a mutation on the PER2 gene.

A Brief History

Whatever the cause, being awake, paralyzed, and seeing shadowy figures is often terrifying for those who experience it—like something out of a horror movie. In fact, researchers suspect that more than a few folk monsters were born of this surprising common experience. The word nightmare itself originally referred to paralysis, feelings of chest pressure, intense fear, and the perception of being attacked.

Researchers believe that reported encounters with demons, ghosts, vampires, and, more recently, alien abductions may all have come from episodes of sleep paralysis. During the Salem witch trials, multiple "witches" were convicted after reports of nightly visitations to their neighbors.

Sharpless reports that despite the current scientific understanding of this strange experience, about 7 percent of people firmly believe their experiences are supernatural. If you're in doubt, check out his rebuttal to this belief in his book, *Monsters on the Couch*. In the meantime, see the sidebar to the left for some practical tips on how to prevent or reduce these spooky experiences.

Yes...You Can Fix Your Genes

Michael F. Roizen, MD, chief wellness officer emeritus at Cleveland Clinic and chief of its Wellness Institute. Board-certified in internal medicine and anesthesiology, he has authored 195 peer-reviewed publications and served 16 years on FDA advisory committees. He is coauthor of *The Great Age Reboot: Cracking the Longevity Code for a Younger Tomorrow.* LongevityPlaybook.com

Do-it-yourself genetic fixes might sound like science fiction, but it turns out that we do have considerable control over our genes. We may not be able to rewrite our genetic code, but we can influence whether certain genes are switched on or off—in other words, whether or not they're producing proteins. In some cases, flipping these switches influences how quickly we age and how likely we are to develop life-altering health problems such as cancer, dementia, and heart disease.

What's the secret to flipping these switches? Not surprisingly, our lifestyle decisions including what we eat and whether we remain fit.

Example: When we exercise, it switches on a gene that makes the protein *irisin*... which induces production of the protein brain-derived neurotrophic factor...which has been linked to decreased risk for dementia.

We all know that it's healthy to get a good night's sleep, exercise, and cut back on red meat and added sugars, even if we don't realize that doing these things can affect our genes. *But researchers have discovered some less obvious gene-switching steps that are worth taking, including...*

- **Take a sauna.** People who sauna regularly outlive those who don't. A study by researchers at University of Eastern Finland compared middle-age men who took four to seven saunas per week with similar men who rarely or never took a sauna.

Results: Those who took saunas were a stunning 40 percent less likely to die during the 20+ years studied. Other research by the same researchers has found that people who use saunas may be as much as 66 percent less likely to develop dementia.

Why it works: The sauna's high temperatures likely turn on genes that release heat shock proteins, a type of protein that envelops other proteins and protects them from degradation. Avoiding protein degradation is among the keys to living a long healthy life.

If you don't have access to a sauna: Taking several hot baths—96°F or higher—a week might deliver similar benefits.

- **Improve your stress response by strengthening your diaphragm.** The saying, "Stress is a killer" isn't entirely accurate. It is not how much stress you endure but how well you handle it—that's what affects your genes.

Example: Your genes don't know that you're facing financial problems, but your fears about those problems trigger hormonal consequences in your body, and those consequences are the single most significant way to switch on genes associated with aging—even more than eating an unhealthy diet or failing to exercise.

Strategies for reducing the stress response and its genetic consequences include such tactics as spending time with friends...finding something that gives your life greater meaning and focusing on that during stressful stretches...and including enjoyable activities in your day.

Also: Taking slow, deep breaths is an effective stress-management strategy—it sends a message to the body that the stress response isn't needed. We can train ourselves to send this message effectively even when we are stressed.

To do this: Practice daily with an "inspiratory muscle trainer," a small device available for about $20 on Amazon.com that provides resistance when you inhale, strengthening the diaphragm. During these twice-a-day sessions of 10 breaths each, place a finger on your belly button and feel it move outward as you breathe in, confirming that the diaphragm is contributing to your breath. Then when you're in a stressful situation, place your finger on your belly button and confirm the same outward motion. This is especially helpful for older people—as we age, we tend to breathe increasingly from the chest.

Result: A weakened diaphragm muscle that is less able to tolerate lung infections and muscle and rib injuries.

- **Periodically put yourself on a "fasting-mimicking diet."** We all know that how much we eat can affect our health and longevity. What is surprising, though, is that you might be able to reap significant long-term benefits by occasionally implementing relatively short-term diet restrictions.

Fasting forces the body to burn stores of fat for energy—and that appears to flip the genetic switches that deliver health benefits. A study by researchers at University of Southern California found that participants who dramatically reduced caloric intake for one five-day stretch each month for three consecutive months experienced reduced markers and risk factors for aging and age-related diseases.

You don't have to stop eating entirely to obtain the benefits of fasting—in the USC study, participants had 1,000 calories on the first fast day and 750 calories per day for the four days that followed. That's a fraction of the typical American's caloric intake but a far cry from going completely without food. Any food consumed should be low protein and low simple carb. The study's authors have speculated that it might not even be necessary to follow this fasting regimen every month—once every three months might be sufficient.

•**Game your way to decreased dementia risk.** Playing mentally challenging games can keep our brains sharp as we age—but not all games provide the same benefit. Research, including a University of Cambridge meta-analysis of 16 earlier studies, suggests that games that force players to analyze situations quickly deliver especially impressive results. People in their early 70s who played games like these regularly were found to be more than 30 percent less likely to develop dementia during the following decade.

Examples: The fast-paced games used in these academic studies include Double Decision and Freeze Frame, available via subscription from BrainHQ.com.

Supplements Worth Taking

Some supplements including multivitamins, vitamin D, and omega-3 seem to flip genetic switches in ways that favor long and healthy lives. But there are some less well-known and little-used supplements that seem to influence genes in beneficial ways as well.

Reminder: Check with your healthcare provider before adding any new supplements to your regimen.

•**Avocado soybean unsaponifiables (ASU)** can slow the progression of arthritis and perhaps prevent it entirely. There's significant evidence to back this—ASU has been prescribed in Europe since the 1990s, and a study of 399 people by researchers at Saint-Antoine Hospital in Paris showed that ASU significantly slows the progression of hip osteoarthritis.

Recommended dosage: 300 mg/day.

•**Coenzyme Q10 (CoQ10)** plays a role in the "electron transport chain," a series of proteins that facilitate energy production. Recent studies, including one by researchers at Spain's University of Cordoba, have pointed to a wide range of potential benefits from taking CoQ10 supplements, including lower risk for diabetes, hypertension, heart attack, and stroke as well as a decline in all-cause mortality. Additional research is needed to confirm the benefits, but there's already solid evidence that CoQ10 supplements have no dangerous side effects.

Recommended dosage: 200 mg/day.

•**Phospho-creatine** is used by bodybuilders hoping to pack on muscle, but it could be even more useful for older adults. It might not only help them add much needed muscle, but several studies have suggested that it also can boost cognitive function. One study by researchers at the UK's University of Chichester found that

Go to the Beach for Your Health

People who live near or visit the ocean report better health, according to a survey of people across 15 countries. The benefits may come from reduced exposure to air pollution, more physical activity, and views of the ocean, which are associated with lower psychological distress.

University of Vienna, Vienna, Austria.

elderly people experienced improved recall and memory performance after taking phospho-creatine for a week.

Caution: Phospho-creatine can increase blood creatine levels in ways that might mask kidney problems or lead to misinterpretation of blood test results, so check with your doctors before taking it.

Recommended dosage: 20 grams/day for the first week, followed by a maintenance dose of 2.25 to 10 grams/day.

• **Low-dose aspirin.** Until recently, taking one or two baby aspirin a day was long recommended for people age 50 and older to reduce the odds of first heart attack, stroke, blood clots, and many cancers.

But: The U.S. Preventive Services Task Force recently recommended against this because daily low-dose aspirin also increases risk for digestive tract bleeding. Now we know that the bleeding risk can be dramatically reduced if the aspirin is taken with warm water…and that the Task Force relied on flawed research that underestimated aspirin's benefits. On balance, daily low-dose aspirin is beneficial for most people age 50 and older, but ask your doctor.

Recommended dosage: Take one non-coated low-dose (81-mg) aspirin every morning and evening. Drink one-half glass of warm water before each aspirin, and finish the glass after taking the aspirin.

Living in Harmony with the Seasons

Dallas Hartwig, PT, cofounder of the Whole30 program, an elimination diet that has helped millions of people learn about their ideal personal food plan, and coauthor of *The New York Times* best-sellers *It Starts With Food* and *The Whole30*. A functional medicine practitioner, he has been featured on *Today, Good Morning America, The View,* and more. His latest book is *The 4 Season Solution*. DallasHartwig.com

Many disorders of modern life—from insomnia to unhealthy weight gain to anxiety to chronic stress and burnout—are in some way the result of our disconnect from natural, seasonal rhythms. Throughout most of human history, people lived in synchrony with nature's cycles and adjusted their behavior to the seasons—increasing their activity in spring and summer…and hunkering down in fall and winter to conserve and restore their energy. They shifted their sleep schedules based on the changing times of sunrise and sunset…ate foods available in season…and took part in physical and social activities adapted to the weather and available light.

But our increasingly technology-mediated way of life has separated us from those rhythms. We spend our days indoors in artificial light…and go to bed long past sunset and skimp on sleep. We import tropical fruits and eat them in the middle of winter…and we follow the same exercise routine year-round.

Instead of balancing summer's long days and short nights with extended periods of calm and restoration during winter, we act as though we are living in perpetual summer and giving ourselves no opportunity to recharge. We override the body's natural drives for alternating periods of intensity and rest. Our always-on way of life leaves us stretched thin, exhausted and unrecovered.

We spoke with functional medicine practitioner Dallas Hartwig, PT, author of *The 4 Season Solution*, about how synchronizing our lives with nature's cycles can improve our health, energy, and well-being year-round.

Seasonal Themes

• **Spring and summer are times of expansion.** In spring, the snow melts and new growth starts to appear. Fresh, fast-growing vegetables and leafy greens are abundant. As the weather gets warmer, we are attracted to physical activity, meeting new people, exploring new places and indulging our curiosity. As the days lengthen into summer, we spend more time outdoors, and the drive for activity becomes more pronounced. To fuel all this stimulation, our bodies crave foods that are light but energy-dense, such as cherries, berries, nectarines, and other high-sugar fruit.

•**Fall and winter are seasons of contraction.** Summer's variety of fresh produce is gradually replaced by starchier fruits and vegetables, such as apples, carrots, and potatoes. Our appetites shift toward stews, roasts, and other higher-fat, protein-rich foods. Vigorous physical activity becomes less appealing. The more superficial, widespread, and busy social connections of the warmer months give way to the motivation to deeply connect with people who matter most to us.

Where to Start

To reconnect with the body's seasonal wisdom, start with the season you are in. Consider making small shifts in key areas of daily life—sleeping, eating, physical exercise, and social connection. Each has an impact on the others, so it may not be difficult to make small shifts in all four areas at once.

Bring a spirit of experimentation to the venture. There is no one-size-fits-all prescription for seasonal living. Even if you focus on one of the four areas, you likely will see improvements in your energy, mood, and mental focus in just a few months, and that will motivate you to make changes in other areas as well.

Experiment with seasonal shifts...

•**Sleeping.** Sunrise and sunset have a profound influence on our body's daily and seasonal rhythms, which are highly responsive to light. Gradually shift your waking time closer to sunrise and your bedtime closer to sunset as those times change throughout the year. This will help you fall asleep more easily, sleep more soundly and wake up more refreshed.

You don't have to go to bed at sundown—a 5:00 p.m. bedtime in winter would not be practical for most people. But make adjustments after sunset to support the body's natural inclination to wind down and prepare for rest.

Examples: After dark, avoid stressful situations such as intense exercise, reading work-related e-mails, or having difficult conversations with family members. Dim the lights. Let yourself enjoy the sensation of settling into a safe place.

Reminder: Avoid looking at your phone and other electronic devices in the evening. The blue light emitted by screens suppresses the body's production of the sleep-promoting hormone melatonin.

During summer, indulge your impulse to stay up late and pack more activities into the daylight hours. Don't force yourself to go to bed early if you aren't sleepy. Humans can have long days without negative health consequences for a few months—as long as they spend extended time in restorative mode during winter.

To help your body adjust to seasonal sleep rhythms: Spend a few minutes outdoors in morning light soon after you get up. Receptors in the eyes are especially sensitive to this bright morning light, and exposing yourself to it in the morning activates hormonal responses that help you feel more alert during the day and sleepy at night. Between 10 and 30 minutes of exposure to natural light calibrates your body's internal state to the natural environment.

•**Eating.** Become familiar with seasonal foods by shopping at local farmers' markets. By eating mostly what is in season, you will eat far fewer highly processed foods, which tend to be high in calories but low in nutrients.

The Western diet is heavily weighted toward carbohydrates all year long. But our bodies are better suited to seasonal variations in the proportions of carbohydrate, fat and protein. In summer, with so many fresh fruits and vegetables available, it's easy and healthy to eat more carbohydrates relative to fat and protein. During colder months, eat more root vegetables and indulge the natural desire for hearty foods higher in fat and protein, such as meat, poultry, and nuts.

Bonus: Eating more minimally processed food causes your digestive system to work harder, breaking food down slowly, and increasing the sensation of satiety.

• **Movement.** Many people alternate between exercise extremes. They spend most of the day sitting. Then, when they do move, they push themselves hard at one or two types of exercise, overworking some muscles and joints and neglecting others. The key to seasonal movement is to vary intensity and duration.

During summer, we are naturally drawn to low-intensity activities that go on for extended periods—leisurely walks and hikes, swimming, gardening, playing catch with the children or grandchildren. In winter, when it's natural to spend more time indoors, shorter bouts of movement such as high-intensity interval training are appropriate.

Enjoy seasonal activities such as skating, skiing, and snowshoeing in winter... and rowing and mountain biking in summer. This variety will ensure that you work different muscle groups. Throughout the year, build core strength with yoga, calisthenics, and/or weight training.

• **Connection.** The expansiveness of spring and summer encourages novelty and entertainment in our socializing. We travel and meet new people, go to barbecues and concerts, and spend time with groups with whom we have fairly superficial connections.

Fall and winter encourage us to slow down and deepen our connections to the circle of people who matter most to us. More physical proximity creates opportunities for unhurried conversation. In addition to building relationships with others, we can deepen our connection to ourselves and our spiritual yearnings through contemplative activities such as reading, meditating, and journaling.

The Time of Your Life

Satchin Panda, PhD, a professor at the Salk Institute for Biological Studies in La Jolla, California, a founding executive member of the Center for Circadian Biology at the University of California, San Diego, and author of *The Circadian Code* and *The Circadian Diabetes Code.* MyCircadianClock.org

You probably look at clocks throughout the day to check the time—whether it's the alarm clock by your bed, the watch on your wrist, or the clock on your smartphone. But you're also looking at a clock when you look in the mirror.

Scientists have learned that your body is essentially a clock—that there are internal, 24-hour timetables that determine when every gene in your genome, every reaction-sparking enzyme, every hormone, and every chemical in your brain turns on and off.

Circadian Rhythms

These timetables are called circadian rhythms. They are the master programs that instruct what time of day or night the body carries out its daily tasks, like getting energy from food, defending itself against threats like viruses, and repairing and rejuvenating cells.

Scientists used to think that the body's circadian rhythms were controlled *externally,* by the day-night cycle of light and dark. But that's only half the story. Now, it's understood that the body's circadian rhythms are also regulated *internally,* by hundreds of cell-specific and organ-specific "clock genes" that optimize the body's ability to carry out its many tasks and functions.

When these gene-regulated clocks are working well—when you're living in sync with the natural rhythms of sleeping, eating, and being active—you're likely to be healthy. But when your circadian clocks are disrupted, you're more likely to feel lousy.

Out of Sync

Short-term—like when you have jet lag—you can suffer from insomnia, fatigue, headaches, irritability and moodiness, indigestion, constipation, susceptibility to infection, and muscle aches and pains. Long-term—because of an erratic sleep schedule, eating late at night, or being sedentary—you're at greater risk for nearly every chronic disease and condition, including heart disease, diabetes, obesity, fatty liver disease, gut diseases, immune problems, depression and anxiety, Alzheimer's disease, and various cancers.

Bottom line: Maintaining or restoring circadian rhythms is arguably the most important factor in maintaining or restoring good health.

The Rhythmic Lifestyle

There are simple guidelines to fix your circadian clock, nurture your circadian rhythms, and prevent, manage, and even reverse disease.

GUIDELINE #1: **Set a bedtime and be consistent with it.** Your day begins the night before, with how you slept. The best way to ensure sufficient, restful sleep is to have a regular (in other words, rhythmic) bedtime. Whatever time you choose—with 10 p.m. to 11 p.m. being the physiological sweet spot—try to be in bed for at least eight consecutive hours, in order to get 6.5 to 7.5 hours of sleep, which science shows is just right for rest and rejuvenation.

GUIDELINE #2: **Reduce blue light at night.** Another crucial circadian factor in getting a good night's sleep is to reduce your exposure to light at night in the hours before bedtime. You particularly want to reduce blue light at night. During the daytime, this wavelength of light boosts attention, reaction time, and mood. But at night, blue light reduces production of melatonin, the sleep-inducing hormone. The main source of blue light at night is screens: your smartphone, tablet, laptop, computer, gaming console, and TV.

The best strategy is to minimize or eliminate all use of screens two hours before your set bedtime. But for most of us, that's not realistic. An easy fix is to wear blue-light filtering glasses at night. Put them on right after dinner. Within 10 to 15 minutes, you'll notice your eyes relax, you'll experience less eyestrain, and your brain will adjust to the color.

You can also use an app on your smartphone that reduces blue light two hours before your preset bedtime, such as the Nightshift feature on the iPhone. Most new tablets and laptops also come with a function to reduce the brightness of the screen at a set time. After dinner, use the dimmer switch for LED lights in your home, which emit blue light.

GUIDELINE #3: **After waking up, wait one hour to eat breakfast.** After you wake up, wait at least one hour before eating any calorie-containing food. (Two hours is even better.) Within one hour of waking up, your level of the stress hormone cortisol reaches its peak, and your level of sleep-inducing melatonin hasn't returned to baseline. High cortisol and residual melatonin interfere with the regulation of glucose (blood sugar), and a steady level of glucose is crucial to maintaining your metabolic health. Favor noncaloric drinks during this time, like warm water, lemon water, or black coffee. (Noncalor-

SCN: The Master Clock

The *suprachiasmatic nucleus* (SCN) is the body's master clock. It receives information about light from the outside world through the retina and resets all the other clocks, including organ-specific clocks like the heart clock, the liver clock, and the gut clock. External light, the SCN, the organ clocks, and the genetic clocks form the three major rhythms that are key to health: sleep, nutrition, and activity.

ic sweeteners are also okay.) People with heartburn should stick to plain water.

GUIDELINE #4: **Eat all your daily calories within a 12-hour time period.** This approach is called *time-restricted eating*—and it works wonders to harmonize your circadian rhythms. (You also can choose a smaller window of eating opportunity, like eight, nine, 10, or 11 hours.) Most of us eat for 15 hours or more every day, but a shorter "feeding period" provides the digestive system the right amount of time to process food, uninterrupted by a new influx of nutrients. It also provides the gastrointestinal tract enough time to repair and rejuvenate, supporting the healthy bacteria that are the foundation of good digestion.

Research in animals and people shows that time-restricted eating stabilizes blood pressure, blood sugar, and blood fats, and helps prevent metabolic diseases like obesity, diabetes, heart disease, and stroke. To implement time-restricted eating, first set a breakfast time and stick with it. If breakfast begins at 8 a.m., dinner must end by 8 p.m. An earlier breakfast is better—because if you start early, you end early, before melatonin levels begin to rise, leading you toward sleep. Plus, once your body recognizes that no more food is coming in, it transitions to repair-and-rejuvenation mode. Alcohol is considered food too. If you like a drink or two in the evening, have it either before dinner or with dinner.

GUIDELINE #5: **Don't eat late at night.** It's the worst choice you can make. It disrupts the digestive clock, waking up the body when it is meant to be slowing down.

GUIDELINE #6: **Spend at least 30 minutes outdoors every day.** This doesn't mean only on sunny days. Spending time outdoors even on a cloudy day provides 4,000 to 5,000 lux, the standard measure of brightness. If you can't get outside, spend time next to a large window, perhaps when you're eating breakfast or lunch.

GUIDELINE #7: **If you can, combine light exposure with exercise.** Exercise is healthy no matter when and where you do

> **App to Find Rainbows!**
>
> The *RainbowChase* app shows users when nearby conditions are favorable for rainbow viewing and makes it easy to take rainbow photos. Developed by scientists in Hawaii, where geography, weather patterns, and clean air make rainbow sightings frequent—and spectacular—the app provides current and upcoming weather information, views of Doppler radar data, and satellite images of rain and clouds.
>
> Note: Currently the app is limited to weather conditions in Hawaii, the West Coast of the U.S., Idaho, Nevada, and Utah…the rest of North America is coming soon. Free at Google Play and Apple.
>
> *Steven Businger, PhD, professor, department of atmospheric sciences, University of Hawaii at Mānoa, and Paul Cynn, CFO, RainbowChase, codevelopers of RainbowChase app.*

it. It builds muscle mass and strength, builds bone, burns fat, and tones your metabolism, strengthens your heart, and enlivens your brain. But exercising outdoors helps you meet two guidelines simultaneously.

Plus, most people who exercise outdoors walk—and walking is the most common physical activity for people who maintain a habit of physical activity.

If you're prediabetic or diabetic, walking in the late afternoon or early evening is best to regulate blood sugar.

Secrets to Slowing Down the Clock

Marc Wittmann, PhD, research fellow at Institute for Frontier Areas of Psychology and Mental Health, Freiburg, Germany, and author of Felt Time: The Science of How We Experience Time. *IGPP.de*

Does it feel like time is moving faster as you get older? When you were a kid, a summer day lasted forever. Now, you look up and another month or year has passed and perhaps with little to show for it.

Good news: Neuropsychologist Marc Wittmann, PhD, says there is a lot you can do to change that fleeting feeling and slow down time. "Clock time" moves forward at a steady pace. So does your body's internal clock, which synchronizes and coordinates circadian rhythms and autonomous functions. But Dr. Wittmann has found that the way our brain perceives time is highly subjective.

Example: 30 minutes stuck in traffic feels much longer than 30 minutes playing with your grandchild. This is not random. It is influenced by a few predictable mechanisms such as the amount of novelty in your daily activities, your emotional state and your memory.

We asked Dr. Wittmann to explain how you can use these mechanisms to alter your perception of time…

How We Perceive Time

Every waking second of every day, you take in raw data about the world. Your mind continuously edits this information before presenting to you a version of what's transpiring out there. At the same time, your brain filters how fast or slow those events seem to happen.

Example: Several years ago, I was driving down a rain-slickened road. I turned a corner and lost control of my car. As the car spun, everything seemed to slow to a crawl. It took me no more than a fraction of a second to get the car on track again, but it felt much longer.

Why this happened: Danger that threatens your survival causes your brain's internal processes to run faster, and that heightened awareness creates the impression that events are unfolding slowly. Several other mechanisms also cause you to experience present time as moving faster or slower than it does. They include…

•**Novelty.** When you are bored or impatient and lack meaningful thoughts to engage your brain, you are more attuned to the actual passage of time. Conversely when you are busy or involved in new or challenging situations, you become so focused that you lose your sense of self and don't think about time at all.

•**Heightened emotion.** When you are experiencing anxiety, loneliness, or physical or emotional pain, you are constantly aware of time. But time accelerates when you engage in activities that create positive emotions such as a conversation with a close friend or when you get in the flow while playing music or reading a riveting novel.

Why Time Flies as You Age

How your brain handles retrospective time—when you are looking back at events in the past—works very differently than when your brain is processing in real time. Retrospective time is driven mostly by memory. The richer, more diverse and numerous your memories of a past event or period in your life, the slower you recall time passing. The less vivid your memories, the faster time will seem to have passed.

That's why many people regard childhood as such a drawn-out period. When you are young, you have a steady stream of brand-new experiences. The first time your brain encounters something, it encodes the memories in detail. But when you reach adulthood, you fall into routines (for example, the daily work commute), so the brain has to respond to much less surprising or new information. When you look back, nothing sticks out as very significant, so the duration of time you associate with that period shrinks. By the time you are elderly or retired, you may have very rigid lifestyle patterns. In your memory, the days merge into one another and become indistinguishable.

Example: During the pandemic, many older folks' lives were defined by forced isolation (not to mention the constant fear that every sniffle might mean they had caught COVID). When studying older people's recent experiences of time, they typically report that the days felt insufferably slow, and yet two years might have flown by.

Strategies for Slowing Down Time

My research suggests that making certain adjustments to your daily and regular behavior can change your sense of retrospective time. The more you can push yourself out of your comfort zone and create different, interesting experiences, the denser your memories...and the slower the months and years will seem to pass. Try the following strategies...

• **Get out of autopilot mode.** Performing the same routines every day may feel comforting, but it means learning and awareness aren't taking place, and there will be no outstanding memories to retrieve. Even minor changes can shake up your neural networks and enhance your perception of those experiences.

Examples: Drive a different way home from work for a month...wear your watch on the opposite wrist for a week...change up your exercise routine.

• **Give away your time to others.** Volunteering in a way that is very meaningful to you or puts you in a challenging situation leaves a powerful impression. While you have less time for yourself in the present, looking back at your efforts will make the time period seem fuller.

• **Have projects that require sustained effort and quantifiable goals.** Many of us reach the end of the year and realize that everything is still the same. You haven't dropped those 10 pounds or cracked the pile of books on your nightstand. Achieving satisfying and challenging objectives serve as powerful memory anchors. Making and recognizing progress not only builds up intrinsic motivation but also prevents you from slipping into automatic, forgettable routines.

Important: When you achieve a goal, recognize it in a memorable way. Announce it on Facebook, or reward yourself so you cement it in your mind as a milestone.

• **Seek a little novelty during the holidays.** If you have the same tree-decorating and dessert party every Christmas, your memories start to feel sparse.

Solution: Alter your holidays in special ways so each one stands out more. Make an unusual or exotic dessert...or invite a surprise guest to your party.

• **Plan special activities on the first and last full days of vacations.** Does it ever feel like your vacations are over in a heartbeat?

Reason: Even though we may have new and exciting experiences during a vacation, we tend to remember beginnings and ends most clearly. Those particular days often are forgettable, filled with mundane activities such as adjusting to the time zone, staying close to the hotel until you get your bearings and prepping for the return trip home.

Better: Schedule memorable events on transition days—splurge at a pricey restaurant or purchase a piece of artwork that you can display prominently in your house—so that these days stand out the most after you get home.

The Best Times... to Exercise...Nap... Take Medication... and More

Sara C. Mednick, PhD, cognitive neuroscientist and professor of psychology in the department of cognitive sciences at University of California, Irvine, and author of *The Power of the Downstate: Recharge Your Life Using Your Body's Own Restorative Systems* and *Take a Nap! Change Your Life*. She is director of the UC Irvine Sleep and Cognition (SaC) Lab. SaraMednick.com

Deep within the brain lives a collection of neurons called the suprachiasmatic nucleus, or SCN for short. The SCN is like a clock, helping every system, organ and cell in your body run on an optimal schedule. This master clock takes its cues from the 24-hour cycle of the sun and moon. Over millions of years, this constant cycling of light and dark has established a rhythm designed to optimize sleep, appetite, metabolism, mood, and more.

The SCN isn't the only clock in town, though. There are similar clocks in your heart, gut, nervous system, muscles, and more, constantly turning to the SCN for guidance. The master clock tells organs when to churn out hormones or kick-start crucial behavioral chains at the right time of day or night.

Example: As the sun begins to rise, its bluish early-morning rays travel through your eyes (even when they're closed) and trigger the SCN to rev things up. The pineal gland in the brain slows production of the sleep hormone melatonin...the adrenal glands churn out energizing cortisol and epinephrine...and your body temperature rises after dropping a degree or two overnight.

These sorts of 24-hour cycles, during which the brain and body undergo critical changes in biology, are known as the circadian rhythm.

It's About More Than Sleep

The circadian rhythm often is associated with sleep, weight loss, and metabolic health. It is the reason that intermittent fasting and other forms of time-restricted eating are successful—they involve eating when your organs are prepared to process nutrients, fats and sugars...and not eating when your organs are programmed to rest and rejuvenate. Eating at times that complement your circadian rhythm gives your body clocks what they need to thrive, resulting in better blood sugar regulation, enhanced weight maintenance, and more.

Here are four more ways to tap into your natural rhythm...

•**Best time to build strength.** *Afternoon through early evening.* Muscles live by their own circadian rhythm and are programmed for peak strength between 4 p.m. and 8 p.m. This helps explain why more strength-based world records are broken during evening competitions...why tennis serves tend to be faster later in the day...and why swim strokes are more powerful. These sorts of moves rely heavily on fast-twitch muscle fibers, which are more responsive to circadian rhythms than slow-twitch muscle fibers. Slow-twitch muscle fibers rely on aerobic respiration, and so are used for long, endurance sports such as marathons. Generally speaking, a regular 6 p.m. strength-training routine will lead to bigger gains in muscle mass versus the same routine performed in the mornings. The new words "chrono-exercise" and "chrono-activity" refer to the practice of adjusting your workout routine to mesh with your body clocks.

This doesn't mean you should skip morning workouts if that's the only time of day you can fit them in. But if you're looking for optimal results, save your push-ups, squats, and lunges for later in the day.

Reminder: Stop exercising at least three hours before bed—otherwise, your heart rate and body temperature may remain too elevated for sleep.

Bonus: If you have type 2 diabetes, afternoon strength workouts may be even more advantageous. Muscles use glucose, so any gains in strength benefit blood sugar control. If afternoon workouts help you gain even a little more muscle, that bodes well for blood-sugar management.

•**Best time for cardio.** *Between 8 a.m. and 11 a.m. (for women only).* In a study in *European Journal of Preventive Cardiology*, researchers from the Netherlands followed nearly 87,000 adults between the ages of 42 and 78 for six years. They found that women who exercised mainly in the morning had the lowest risk for heart attack and stroke. Compared with women who fit in most of their physical activity later in the day, early-morning exercisers (between 8 a.m. and 9 a.m.) and late-morning exercisers (between 10 a.m.

and 11 a.m.) had a 22 to 24 percent lower risk for heart disease, respectively.

Morning cardio's benefit likely stems from several sources, one of which involves the sympathetic nervous system—the "fight-or-flight" branch of the autonomic nervous system responsible for all the thinking and doing that happen during the day and that kicks into high gear during moments of stress. Your sympathetic nervous system's circadian rhythm maximizes its power during morning hours, so your run at 8 a.m., swim at 9 a.m., or spin class at 10 a.m. revs the engine at the optimal time. Cardio exercise later in the afternoon, when the heart has been go-go-going for hours and hours, might cause extra strain that hampers its functioning.

Note: These study results were not as pronounced for men, though the researchers aren't sure why.

Are You Sleepy...or Tired?

Signs that you're sleepy: You start yawning, your eyelids droop, and you find yourself nodding off. Given the right conditions, such as a dark room and a comfortable bed or couch, you are likely to quickly fall asleep and stay asleep.

Signs that you're tired: You don't necessarily need sleep. Tiredness can stem from depleted physical or mental energy...physical inactivity...dehydration or hunger...boredom...being emotionally drained...depression...or crashing after a caffeine rush. You are more likely to perk up by doing some physical activity, such as taking a brisk walk outside...having an engaging conversation with a friend...or hydrating with a drink of water and/or restoring depleted calories with a snack.

Jade Wu, PhD, behavioral sleep medicine specialist and researcher, Duke University School of Medicine, Durham, North Carolina, and author of *Hello Sleep: The Science and Art of Overcoming Insomnia Without Medications.* DrJadeWu.com

• **Best time to nap.** *Between 1 p.m. and 3 p.m.* Prime napping time strikes six to eight hours after you've woken up. This is one of the two time periods during which circadian rhythms cause humans to be the sleepiest (the other is just after midnight). A 90-minute nap initiated between 1 p.m. and 3 p.m. is what neuroscientists call the "perfect nap"—it's long enough to let your brain move through an entire cycle of sleep (including light sleep, slow-wave sleep and REM sleep). You'll also spend similar amounts of time in each sleep stage as you would during nocturnal sleep, but in a fraction of the time. A 90-minute snooze at this time might yield benefits similar to a seven-hour sleep at night...and you will wake up feeling refreshed because you'll have cycled through all the stages of sleep. Avoid naps between 30 and 60 minutes long, which put you into a deep sleep that can be hard to wake up from.

Don't have 90 minutes? Try a 10- to 20-minute nap within the same early-afternoon time frame. That's enough sleep to boost energy and alertness but you won't nap long enough to reach the deep stages of sleep, so you'll wake up ready to hit the ground running.

• **Best time to take heart medication.** *At bedtime.* Chronotherapy or chronomedicine is an approach to disease management that incorporates circadian rhythms into treatment of illnesses and chronic health conditions such as heart disease, arthritis, allergies, migraines, and cancer. Many of these conditions observe their own circadian rhythm, with symptoms intensifying at certain times of day or night...or the disease itself being more receptive to treatment.

Case in point: With the cardiovascular system, chief processes such as heart rate, blood pressure, and blood clotting undergo changes in the morning that increase risk for heart attack and stroke.

Recent finding: You are 50 percent more likely to have a stroke between 6 a.m. and noon versus the rest of the day, per a 2023 meta-analysis by researchers from Rush Medical College and Rush–Presbyterian–St Luke's Medical Center. You're two to three times more likely to experience a heart attack in the morning than at night, and morning heart attacks tend to be more severe.

Likely reasons: Circadian rhythms increase activity of clotting factors in the blood during the morning hours, and strokes and heart attacks occur when blood clots become dangerously lodged in the brain or heart.

For decades, doctors have prescribed short-acting statins (cholesterol-lowering drugs) such as *simvastatin* (Zocor) and *lovastatin* to be taken at night because the cholesterol-producing liver enzyme *HMG-CoA reductase* is active in the evening so the medication has a greater impact. Several studies also indicate that antihypertensive medication (for high blood pressure) is more effective when taken at night, though a large British study suggested no difference between morning and evening administration. But even if evening antihypertensive dosing isn't more effective than morning dosing, it's still just as effective, plus it reduces the intensity of some negative side effects such as lightheadedness or leg swelling.

Cannabis Might Not Improve Sleep

Study of 235,000 adults by researchers at Oregon Health and Sciences University, Portland, published in *Sleep Health*.

Previous research has linked cannabis products to better sleep.

Recent finding: Daily cannabis users had higher risk for sleep-duration problems—getting too little or too much sleep. "Daily use" is identified as at least 16 uses per month. Other research has suggested that cannabis is associated with diminished REM sleep and daytime sleepiness.

Chapter 16

VERY PERSONAL

Breast Reduction Surgery Helps More Than Appearance

Breast reduction surgery is usually considered a cosmetic procedure, but a recent study from the Department of Plastic and Reconstructive Surgery at Flinders Medical Centre and College of Medicine and Public Health at Flinders University in Australia finds that breast reduction has important health benefits for women, especially when it comes to meeting exercise guidelines.

Very large breasts, called *macromastia,* occurs in about five percent of women. Macromastia can be measured by breast cup size but is also defined by the symptoms it causes, which may include neck, back, and shoulder pain. Bra strap grooves, shortness of breath, headaches, embarrassment, reduced self-confidence, and depression are also possible. One less-obvious problem is reduced willingness and ability to participate in exercise.

More Comfort Means More Exercise

Prior research has found that due to embarrassment from excess breast movement as well as discomfort and pain, large breast size is the fourth most significant barrier to physical activity for women. Failure to meet World Health Organization (WHO) physical activity guidelines has been associated with a significantly increased risk of obesity and heart disease. According to the WHO, over 30 percent of women worldwide are not meeting these guidelines.

To understand how breast size affects physical activity for women, the research team from Flinders University surveyed nearly 2,000 women age 18 or older about their breast size, exercise history, and overall satisfaction with their breasts. Among this group were 56 women who had breast reduction surgery for very large breasts. The study is published in the *International Journal of Surgical Re-*

Study titled "Self-Reported Breast Size, Exercise Habits and BREAST-Q Data—an International Cross-Sectional Study of Community Runners," led by researchers at Flinders University, Adelaide, Australia, published in *JPRAS Open.*

Very Personal

construction JPRAS. *These were among the key findings…*

- **Women with smaller breast cup sizes (DD or less)** made up 75 percent of the women in the study who reached WHO physical activity guidelines.
- **Over half of the women with breast cup size DD or larger** believed that breast reduction would increase their willingness to exercise and improve their exercise performance.
- **Women who had breast reduction surgery** reported that after surgery, their willingness, frequency, and exercise endurance increased significantly, and they were more likely to try high-impact exercise.
- **Women who had breast reduction surgery** scored higher on breast satisfaction, life satisfaction, and overall happiness than women with cup size greater than E.

Smaller breast cup sizes were AA, A, B, C, and D. Larger sizes started at DD and increased to E, F, G, H, or larger. WHO guidelines for physical activity are at least 150 minutes of moderate-intensity physical activity throughout the week, or 75 minutes of vigorous-intensity physical activity.

Breast Reduction Surgery Is Low Priority

This study is supported by previous research on benefits of breast reduction surgery that include improved physical and mental health, weight loss, and physical fitness. A 2018 study from the U.S. Army found that female soldiers improved their physical fitness scores by 63 percent after breast reduction surgery.

In Australia, approval of this surgery often requires meeting pain or BMI guidelines, and women approved for reduction surgery are placed on a low-priority list with long wait times. In the United States, this surgery is often considered cosmetic and not covered by insurance. The authors of the study conclude that women, the public, healthcare providers, and policymakers need to be more aware of the important benefits of breast reduction surgery.

For Many Women, Pain During Sex Is Treatable

Northwestern University Feinberg School of Medicine.

Between 13 and 84 percent of postmenopausal women experience dyspareunia—vaginal pain during sex—but the condition is rarely evaluated or treated despite the availability of safe and effective therapies.

Postmenopausal vaginal pain is often due to lack of estrogen, but there are other, usually undetected and untreated causes, including post-hysterectomy problems, cancer treatments (chemotherapy, radiation, surgery), lichen sclerosus (patchy, discolored, thin skin) and other vulvar conditions, pelvic-floor tension, arthritis and other musculoskeletal problems, pelvic organ prolapse, and sexually transmitted infections.

Possible treatments include silicone lubricants, moisturizers, vaginal estrogen, ospemifene, dehydroepiandrosterone, local testosterone therapy, cannabidiol, fractional CO_2 laser treatments, and physical therapy.

"Sexuality in women after the age of 50 years is marginalized, and gynecologic care is not prioritized," Lauren Streicher, MD, clinical professor of obstetrics and gynecology at Northwestern University Feinberg School of Medicine, said in a statement, but "postmenopausal women shouldn't accept painful sex as their new norm."

Even Older Adults Can Get STIs

Matthew Hamill, MD, PhD, MPH, assistant professor of medicine at Johns Hopkins University School of Medicine, Baltimore, and a specialist and researcher in the areas of STIs and HIV/AIDS. HopkinsMedicine.org

There's an epidemic in the U.S., but doctors and patients often fail to discuss it—sexually transmitted infections (STIs).

There are 20 million new cases of STIs each year...and people under age 25 represent only half of that number. *How to protect yourself...*

•**Know the most common STIs in older adults**—trichomoniasis (especially prevalent in women over 40), syphilis, chlamydia, HIV, and gonorrhea. Most have no obvious symptoms, but you may notice a rash (especially with syphilis and possibly with HIV)...yellow or greenish discharge (chlamydia, gonorrhea) or bad-smelling discharge (trichomoniasis)...oozing from the penis...painful sex...or nonmenstrual bleeding. Some signs can be dismissed or incorrectly treated as menstrual pain, a yeast infection, or a urinary tract infection.

Also: An infection can take hold via any part of body that has been sexually exposed, including through oral and anal sex.

•**Return to safe-sex practices of your youth.** Ask your partner about other partners. Proceed with caution until you reach a comfortable level of trust.

•**Get tested regularly.** Ideally, you and a new partner should be tested before you engage in sexual activity. Get regular screenings for STIs—don't be embarrassed to discuss your sexual health with your doctor. Testing can reveal an asymptomatic infection, and early treatment can prevent complications.

Alternative: You can be tested without a doctor's order at a local STI testing site—Quest Diagnostics offers this. There also are reputable online services where you can order a test kit and mail your swabbed sample to a lab.

One free option: I Want the Kit. (IWantTheKit.org), based at Johns Hopkins.

Important: Human papillomavirus (HPV) infects nearly everyone, usually in their teens or early 20s. It can drive head and neck, penile, cervical, vulvar, and anal cancers later in life. Talk to your doctor about cancer screenings, especially if the HPV vaccine, first introduced in 2006, wasn't available when you were younger.

> **How to Discuss STI Testing with a New Partner**
>
> Not all sexually transmitted infections (STIs) have visible symptoms, so testing is the best way to protect yourself against genital herpes, hepatitis, chlamydia, gonorrhea, syphilis, pubic lice, HPV, and HIV/AIDS.
>
> **Best approach:** Have the discussion during a nonsexual moment, and present it as a way to protect the health of both parties...suggest getting tested together at a doctor's office, urgent-care center, or a pharmacy-based or community health clinic...or getting tested separately and sharing the results.
>
> *Harvard Women's Health Watch. Health.Harvard.edu*

Ask your dentist to check for signs of oral cancer at every cleaning. Check yourself for red or white patches or lesions on your tongue, gums, or lips.

Cannabis Might Improve Sex

Joseph Feuerstein, MD, assistant professor of clinical medicine, Columbia University, New York City, and coauthor of *The Cannabinoid Cookbook*.

Multiple studies suggest that for men and women, using cannabis before sex can improve libido, sensitivity, and orgasm.

But: A small number of people report that it makes sex less satisfactory...and for some men, it can lead to less motivation for sex, erectile dysfunction, trouble reaching orgasm, or premature ejaculation.

If you choose to experiment: If cannabis is legal where you live, try a tiny amount, perhaps just one milligram, in an extract taken orally (tincture) rather than smoking a joint or using an oil vape pen, both of which can harm lungs...use only with

Very Personal

a trusted partner or experiment alone first to see how your body and mind react.

Reading Erotica Can Rekindle Romance

Sharon Bober, PhD, director, Sexual Health Program, Dana-Farber Cancer Institute, Boston, reported in *Harvard Men's Health Watch*. Dana-Farber.org

Unlike pornography, which is mainly visual, erotica is more verbal, allowing both mental and emotional participation… and provides a safe environment in which to explore desires and fantasies. Many novels, short stories, and websites focus on erotica for older adults and can be found through an Internet search. Try reading a short story together, taking turns reading out loud or reading to yourselves and sharing your responses—or listen together to an erotic audiobook or podcast. Be patient—it may take time to find something you both enjoy.

Sex Before Bed Works as Well as Sleeping Pills

Study of 53 adults by researchers at Atrium Health, Charlotte, North Carolina, presented at the annual SLEEP meeting of the American Academy of Sleep Medicine and the Sleep Research Society. AtriumHealth.org

Having sex with or without orgasm before bedtime was perceived by participants in a recent study as helping them to fall and stay asleep. For those who report that sex helps with sleep, 40 percent characterize the benefit as "moderate"…33 percent use orgasm, with or without a partner, to help them sleep on a weekly basis…and nearly two-thirds say sex is as effective or better than a pill.

Intimacy and Relationship Status

Couples Who Share Daily Housework Have More Sex

According to recent research, when both partners in a heterosexual couple share daily household chores equally, the couples report greater satisfaction with the relationship—and higher frequency and quality of sex—compared with couples where the woman is expected to do the bulk of household chores.

Study led by researchers at Cornell University, Ithaca, New York, published in *Journal of Marriage and Family*.

Intimacy Killer—the "Bristle Reaction"

When partners in long-term relationships touch only to initiate sex, it can make every touch feel as if it has a sexual expectation attached. Rather than a turn-on, touching becomes a turn-off—and the touched partner may react by unconsciously cringing, or "bristling."

Better: Develop new habits to de-program touching from just sex. Practice non-sexual touching, such as holding hands or gently reaching for each other in passing. Pay attention to your partner's reactions to touch—change your touching tactics if how you touch is misinterpreted or seems to cause anxiety. Talk to your partner about when and how to initiate sex.

The New York Times. NYTimes.com

Skin Lightening Products Can Be Dangerous

Northwestern University.

Doctors prescribe skin lighteners for some skin conditions, such as melasma, and the products can be safely used under physician guidance. Most people who use skin lighteners, however, buy them over the counter (OTC) without physician guidance. These OTC products are often adulterated with steroids, mercury, and other toxins that can damage the skin.

In 2020, the U.S. Food and Drug Administration received reports of serious side effects from the use of skin-lightening products containing *hydroquinone*, including skin rashes, facial swelling, and skin discoloration. The FDA advised consumers not to use these products due to the potential harm they may cause.

Researchers from Northwestern Medicine surveyed 455 people of color and found that 21.3 percent of respondents used skin-lightening products. Three-quarters of those used them to treat a skin condition such as acne, melasma, or hyperpigmentation. The others were using the agents for general skin lightening. The people who were using them for skin lightening perceived stronger colorism in their lives than those who did not use the products. Colorism refers to "the belief is that having lighter skin is tied to personal and professional success."

"The most surprising finding was the lack of awareness of ingredients in products being purchased over the counter and their potential detrimental effects," said lead investigator Roopal Kundu, MD, founder and director of the Northwestern Medicine Center for Ethnic Skin and Hair. "These products do not undergo the same type of regulation as prescriptions."

Battling Bloat

Janice Oh, MD, a resident physician within the Division of General Internal Medicine at Cedars-Sinai, Los Angeles.

One in seven Americans experience an uncomfortably swollen, tight feeling in the abdomen at least once a week—and most of them never mention it to their physicians. But if they did, they could likely find relief for this common symptom, called bloating. Bloating occurs when a person's gastrointestinal tract fills with air or gas. It can be caused by diet or an underlying condition, such as irritable bowel syndrome, carbohydrate enzyme deficiency, chronic constipation, or small intestine bacterial overgrowth. It's much more common in women, but men can also experience it.

How to Treat It

There are several strategies you can try at home to reduce discomfort...

• **Exercise.** A study published in the *Journal of Gastrointestinal and Liver Diseases* found that moderate-intensity aerobic exercise (such as jogging or brisk walking) reduced symptoms of bloating in people with irritable bowel syndrome. A study published in the journal *Gastroenterology* found that yoga may also provide relief. Finally, strengthening the muscles of the core can increase circulation, improve bowel regularity, and promote healthy digestion, which may reduce bloating.

• **Make dietary changes.** Keep a food diary to see which foods trigger your symptoms.

If it's unclear, try cutting out the common culprits: dairy, gluten, and a group of foods called FODMAPs (fermentable oligosaccharides, disaccharides, monosaccharides, and polyols). These are difficult-to-digest sugars found in some fruits, vegetables, grains, dairy products, and sweeteners (see sidebar on page 312).

In some people, the carbohydrates in high-FODMAP foods don't get digested in the small intestine. They advance to the large intestine, where bacteria feast on them, causing cramping and gas.

• **Treat constipation.** If you're not having regular bowel movements, eat more high-fiber foods (fruits, vegetables, whole grains, and legumes—look for low FODMAP options). Drink plenty of water to soften stools, and get some exercise, which

Very Personal

> ### FODMAPs to Avoid
>
> While not an exhaustive list, the following foods are particularly high in bloat-triggering FODMAPs.
>
> *Fruits:* apples, pears, mangoes, cherries, figs, pears, watermelon, dried fruit, apples, blackberries, peaches, and plums.
>
> *Vegetables:* artichoke, garlic, leek, onion, spring onion, mushrooms, cauliflower, and snow peas.
>
> *Grains:* whole-meal bread, rye bread, muesli containing wheat, wheat pasta, and rye crispbread.
>
> *Legumes and pulses:* red kidney beans, split peas, and baked beans.
>
> *High-lactose dairy:* soft cheeses, milk, and yogurt.
>
> *Sweeteners:* sorbitol, xylitol, erythritol, honey, and high-fructose corn syrup.

stimulates the muscles in the digestive system and promotes bowel movements.

- **Listen to your gut.** Some, but not all, studies have found that certain strains of probiotics may be effective in reducing symptoms of bloating. Probiotics contain live bacteria that may help to regulate the balance of bacteria in the gut. They may improve the digestion and absorption of nutrients in the gut, which can reduce the buildup of gas and other byproducts that contribute to bloating. Some strains of probiotics may have anti-inflammatory properties, and they may help to regulate the contractions of the muscles in the digestive system, which can promote more efficient movement of food and waste through the intestines.

To get more probiotics in your diet, try yogurt (look for nondairy options to lower FODMAPS); miso; kombucha, a fermented tea; and fermented vegetables, such as sauerkraut, kimchi, and pickles.

If you follow these suggestions and still have symptoms, talk to your primary care doctor, who can suggest medications as a next step.

A Vibrating Capsule Can Treat Constipation Without Drugs

Satish S.C. Rao, MD, PhD, director of neurogastroenterology/motility at the Medical College of Georgia, Augusta.

In a recent study, 300 people swallowed a device enclosed in a capsule that was programmed to stimulate the colon with a series of vibrations. People who used the capsule for five days per week for eight weeks had about twice the number of complete spontaneous bowel movements as those taking a placebo, researchers reported in *Gastroenterology*. Those using the vibrating capsule also had significant improvement in classic problems such as straining, stool consistency, and general quality of life. No significant side effects were reported, but some participants reported experiencing a mild vibrating sensation. The device directly affects the colon—where constipation occurs—without damaging the gut microbiome. The pill was approved by the U.S. Food and Drug Administration in August 2022 and is now available for physicians to prescribe.

Natural Ways to Treat Irritable Bowel Syndrome

Jamison Starbuck, ND, a naturopathic physician in family practice in Missoula, Montana.

Irritable bowel syndrome (IBS) is a chronic condition of the lower gastrointestinal tract. It's the most common diagnosis made by general practice gastroenterologists. Approximately 15 percent of adults worldwide have IBS symptoms, which include abdominal pain, distention, gas, indigestion, and stool variation including diarrhea and constipation.

IBS is considered a neurologic disorder because it's the *function* of the bowel—controlled by the nervous system—that is disordered. The actual bowel tissue of patients with IBS is completely normal. Having IBS does not increase your risk for bowel cancer or for the development of inflammatory bowel diseases like Crohn's or ulcerative colitis. IBS does not shorten life span, but it is considered a chronic condition because the symptoms often last for decades.

Only recently have researchers begun to seriously explore the links between the nervous system, the brain and bowel function. In that exploration, they've discovered that the primary cause of IBS is dysregulated messaging from the brain and nervous system to the bowel.

This does not mean that IBS is all in your head. What is does mean is if you've got IBS, you've got to look beyond bowel function to find successful treatment.

Finding Answers

Before you spend a lot of money on specialists, testing, or medications like pain relievers, digestive aids or gas reducers, start by checking in with several of your nervous system parameters. How is your sleep? Your mood? Your vitality and physical mobility? Ill or unbalanced health in any one of these areas could cause a nervous system disruption that affects bowel function. When we are stressed, tired, angry, depressed, or physically inactive, our digestive system does not work well. I've seen many patients recover from IBS by way of improved sleep, stress reduction, counseling, or gentle exercise like yoga or walking.

• **Consider using nervine herbs.** These are plant medicines that specifically treat the nervous system. Most nervine herbs also treat gastrointestinal symptoms common to IBS.

Among the best nervines for IBS: chamomile, peppermint, lemon balm, and catnip. Use them in tea form. Choose a single herb or combine several. Cover 2 teaspoons of dried herb or mixed herbs with 8 ounces of boiling water. Cover the pot and steep for 5 minutes. Drink 3 cups daily, away from food, until your symptoms improve. Add a pinch of lavender flowers or dried orange peel to enhance the relaxing effect of your tea. The scents of the volatile oils in flowers and citrus peels have a calming effect on the nervous system.

Note: if you have thyroid disease, avoid the regular use of lemon balm.

• **Apply topical castor oil packs to reduce pain and promote relaxation.** Saturate a soft cotton cloth with organic castor oil and lay it over your lower abdomen. Cover it with a dry towel and a heating pad or hot water bottle. Leave it in place for 20 to 60 minutes, and then remove the cloth. Massage your abdomen in a clockwise fashion—determined by imagining a clock placed at your navel, facing outward. Topical castor oil promotes blood flow to the area where it's applied. Apply castor oil packs as needed to reduce spasm, pain, and distention. Applying them at bedtime can also promote a good night's sleep.

• **Disordered bowel flora can aggravate IBS symptoms.** That's because the hundreds of microorganisms in the gut actually communicate with the cells of our digestive tract wall as they work to help—or hinder—immune and digestive activities in the bowel. While simply supplementing with a probiotic is rarely a cure for IBS, it is essential to do all you can to make sure your digestive tract is loaded up with lots of healthy microorganisms, beneficial bacteria that promote good gut health. Do this by eating fresh foods, especially fruit and vegetables, and foods naturally rich in enzymes and good bacteria—things like yogurt, kefir, miso, tempeh, and sauerkraut. Avoid excess sugar, as it can promote the growth of irritating microorganisms in your bowel, and consider supplementing with a probiotic supplement daily. Most IBS sufferers don't need a big dose. I typically prescribe 5 to 10 billion colony-forming units daily for my IBS patients.

Laxative Shortage Tied to Hybrid Work

Wendi LeBrett, MD, gastroenterologist and clinical fellow, UCLA Health, Los Angeles. UCLAHealth.org

Our digestive systems can be thrown off by changes to the body's daily routine—eating different foods and at different times…sleeping different hours…even using different toilets on a different schedule. Prime culprits for disruptions to daily routine are the increase in hybrid work and travel…along with social-media postings urging laxative use for weight loss.

Result: Many stores are finding it hard to keep laxatives in stock.

Safer alternative: Adding fiber to your diet by eating more fruits and vegetables often helps within a few days. You also can try a teaspoon a day of psyllium husk. If you must use a laxative, try an osmotic type, such as MiraLAX, which brings more water into the bowel. Avoid stimulant laxatives that cause intestinal muscles to contract.

When Varicose Veins Cause Pain…

Bottom Line Health.

If varicose veins are causing you pain and discomfort, you should consider some surgical options to remove them. These include sclerotherapy, in which the veins are injected with a solution that causes the vein walls to swell and stick together and the blood to coagulate. The vein then collapses and is no longer visible. Radiofrequency and laser ablation are two other minimally invasive methods. These procedures use a catheter inserted into the affected vein through a small incision, which, when withdrawn, causes the vein to collapse. Both methods take about an hour, require a local anesthetic, and are performed under ultrasound guidance. Another procedure is phlebectomy, which involves having a small incision made over the vein; the vein is then removed with a small crochet hook-like instrument. To prevent recurrence, exercise regularly to promote blood circulation, and if you can, elevate your feet for 10 to 15 minutes several times a day, which will boost circulation in your legs.

INDEX

A
AARP's CarFit, 12
Abdominal exercises and stretches, 246, 266
Abdominal fat. *See* Belly fat
Abdominal pain, 159, 219, 223, 251, 313
Absence seizures, 48–49
Accelerometers, 138, 179
Acceptance and commitment therapy (ACT), 239
Acetaminophen, 200, 201, 239, 256
Acetate, 222
Acid reflux and PPIs, 168–70
Acne, 125, 311
Acoustical panels, 22
Acupuncture, 97, 243, 259
Addictions
    medical trauma and, 108
    opioids, 239, 243
    sibling relationships and, 92
ADHD (attention-deficit/hyperactivity disorder), 27–28
Adhesive capsulitis, 86
Aducanumab (Aduhelm), 31–32
Adverse drug events, 160–61, 168
Aflibercept (Eylea), 16
African-American women. *See* Race
Age bias and ailments, 143
Aged garlic extract (AGE), 227, 228
Ageism, 24
Age-related macular degeneration (ARMD), 14–17, 19
Aging, 1–30
    genetic fixes, 294–97
    positive beliefs about, 46
Air pollution
    brain health and, 53
    breast cancer risk, 58–59
Air purifiers, 53
Alcohol
    brain health and, 34, 36, 45, 52
    CKD and, 214
    hypertension and, 186, 187
    insomnia and sleep, 184–85, 294, 301
    longevity and, 2
    motion sickness and, 211
    PVCs and, 176
    red wine, 2, 187, 232
    sibling relationships and, 93
    stomach pain and, 249
    suicide risk and, 97
    tinnitus and, 52
    triglycerides and, 177, 178
Alcoholics Anonymous, 100
Alirocumab (Praluent), 174
Allergies, 236, 274
    bee pollen for, 236
    dysbiosis and, 221
    eliminating triggers, 274
    food dyes and, 251
    penicillin, 285
    preparing for seasonal, 282–84
Allergy testing, 283, 285, 286
Alliums, 234–35
Allodynia, 240
Almonds, 2, 121
Alpha-1 antitrypsin (AAT) deficiency, 273
Altered mental status, 47–49
Alternating Leg Extensions, 246
Alzheimer's disease, 31–34
    belly fat and, 36
    cholesterol and, 189
    COVID-19 risk and, 33
    DTC blood test, 39–40
    exercise for, 34, 35–36, 43, 45
    eye exams and, 40
    gum disease and, 23
    hormone therapy for, 33
    infections and, 211
    medications for, 31–32, 36, 42, 43–44, 46
    microplastics and, 27
    risk factors, 33, 34, 36, 37
    saunas for, 46
    smoking and, 279
    supplements for, 44–46
    vaccinations for, 37
    warning signs, 36
Amphetamines, 176
Amyloid, 35–36, 37, 39, 40, 46, 233
Anastrozole (Arimidex), 61
Anemia, 125, 176, 223
Anesthesia, 159, 182, 259
Angina. *See* Chest pains
Angiotensin-converting enzyme inhibitors (ACEs), 187–88, 276
Angiotensin receptor blockers (ARBs), 187–88
Animal-object phobias, 103
Anise, 208
Ankle Circles, 254
Ankles, swollen, 289
Ankylosing spondylitis, 247
Antacids, 163, 170
Anthocyanins, 78, 119
Anti-aging serums, 3–4
Antiarrhythmics, 176
Antibiotics
    overuse, 160–61
    for pneumonia, 201
    side effects, 164
Antibiotic resistance, 160, 216–17
Anticoagulants. *See* Blood thinners
Antidepressants
    aripiprazole add-on, 93
    for chronic pain, 243
    drug-drug interactions, 163
    melatonin and, 235, 288
    omega-3s and, 112
    pharmacogenomics, 154, 155
    placebos and, 94
    prescribing, 99
    side effects, 14
Antifungals, 205, 206
Antimicrobial resistance, 206
Anti-nausea medications, 209, 211
Anti-obesity medications (AOMs), 121–22, 157–59, 189
Antioxidants, 4, 15, 17, 44, 118–20, 227, 232, 236
Antipsychotics, 14
Anti-seizure medications, 243
Anti-VEGF injections, 16
Anxiety
    cyclic sighing for, 106
    depression and, 20, 96, 98, 99
    freezing up, 48
    gardening for, 92, 94
    loneliness and, 101
    long COVID and, 203
    medical-test, 106–7
    pain and, 239, 240
    phobias, 102–4
    PVCs and, 175
    sibling relationships and, 93
A1C test, 76, 292
Aphasia, 41, 48, 196
Apolipoprotein B-100 (ApoB), 174
Apple Watch ECGs, 51–152
Apps
    blue light, 301
    calorie counters, 113
    decibel, 22
    drug shortages, 156
    to find rainbows, 301
    thermometers, 153
    weight loss, 113–14
    white noise, 51
Arachnophobia, 102, 104
AREDS, 15–16

Index

Aripiprazole (Abilify), 93
Arnica gel, 270
Aromatase inhibitors (AIs), 60–61
Arrhythmias, 152, 181–82
Arthritis. *See also* Osteoarthritis; Rheumatoid arthritis
    back pain and, 247
    cold weather and, 267
    exercise for, 251–53
    gender differences, 237
    gum disease and, 23
    hands and, 9–10
    knee, 256
    stress and, 238
Artificial intelligence (AI) and cancer, 59, 74
Artificial sweeteners, 117
    cancer risk, 62, 69–70
    diabetes and, 83–84
Ashwagandha, 231
Asian women, 80, 154, 237
Aspartame, 62, 83, 117
Aspirin, 164, 240, 242, 250, 297
Asthma, 276–77
    dysbiosis and, 221
    onion poultice for, 234
    pulse oximeters for, 151
    sleep and, 277
    steroid medications, 167
    strokes and, 277
Atherosclerosis, 21, 228
Atherosclerotic cardiovascular disease (CVD), 173–74
Athlete's foot, 205
Atogepant (Qulipta), 240–41
Atrial fibrillations (A-fibs)
    Apple Watch ECGs, 151–52
    cognitive health and, 197
    heart shape and, 181
    PVCs and, 176
    stress and insomnia, 175
Augmented Depression Therapy (ADepT), 100–101
Autoimmune diseases, 237–56. *See also specific diseases*
    Alzheimer's disease and, 32–33
Autophagy, 7
Autopilot mode, 303
Avacincaptad pegol intravitreal solution (Izervay), 16
Avocados, 78, 127, 186, 222
Avocado soybean unsaponifiables (ASU), 297

B

Babesiosis, 210, 212
Babysitting, 29
Back pain
    causes of, 247
    exercise for, 244–45, 246
    5 strategies for, 245–47
    gender gap, 237
    mental health and, 97
    spinal cord stimulation, 245
Back surgery, 247–49
Backward Walking, 137–38
Bacopa monnieri, 44, 45
Baking, 95
Bakuchiol, 4
Balance (balance issues)
    cannabis and, 28
    exercise for, 136–38
    tests, 12
    yoga for, 262
Bananas, 120–21
Bariatric surgery, 64, 85, 218, 241
Barrett's esophagus, 170, 233
Basal cell carcinoma (BCC), 67–69
Basic Jumping Jack, 131
Baths (bathing). *See* Hot baths; Ice baths; Paraffin baths
BDNF, 35
Beach, 296
Beans and legumes, 2, 76, 111, 119, 232, 272, 312
Bedtime routine, 287–88, 300
Bee pollen, 236
Bees, 236
Beetroot juice, 275
Behavioral-variant frontotemporal dementia, 41
Bell peppers, 120
Bellyaches, 249
Belly fat, 36, 87, 192, 218
Bempedoic acid, 174, 189
Bent Knee Raises, 246
Beta-amyloid, 31–33
Beta-blockers, 14, 167
Beta-carotene, 120
Bevacizumab (Avastin), 16
Bifidobacteria, 222–23
Binge-eating, 41, 292
Biofeedback, 241
Biologic therapy, 191
Biomarkers, 6, 70–71
Bipolar disorder, 41, 163
Birth control, 216
Black pepper, 118, 162
Blepharoptosis, 13–14
Bloat (bloating), 311–12
Blood clots
    aspirin for, 297
    circadian rhythms and, 306
    exercise, 134
    heart and, 174, 176, 198
    hospital risks, 148
    smoking and, 279
    supplements for, 227, 229
    vitamin D for, 229
Blood-injection-injury phobias, 103
Blood pressure, 185–88
    high. *See* Hypertension
    kidney disease and, 185, 214
Blood sugar, 17, 39, 73, 111, 292–93
    diet for, 3, 75–76, 78–80, 214, 233, 236, 301
    exercise for, 35, 76–77, 85–86, 128
    insulin resistance and, 82
Blood thinners (anticoagulants), 17, 19, 142, 148, 272
Blue light, 81, 239, 298, 301
Blue Zones, 1–3
Body mass index (BMI), 36, 37, 64, 114, 130, 158, 192, 198
Body temperature and aging, 28–29
Bone density test, 259–60
Bone health, 257–72
    exercise for, 130
    minerals for, 264
    smoking and, 279
    supplements for, 227
    yoga for, 261–64
Bone-mineral density (BMD), 264
Brain fog, 20, 124, 202, 203
    stuffy air and, 282
Brain games, 296
Brain health, 31–54. *See also* Alzheimer's disease; Dementia
    diet for, 38, 39, 43, 44–45, 47, 49–50
    exercise for, 34, 35–36, 43, 45
    heart health and, 37–39
    supplements for, 44–46
BRAT diet, 211
BRCA gene, 56, 71
Breast cancer, 55–56, 59–63, 232
    AI and chemotherapy, 59
    air pollution and, 58–59
    biomarkers, 71–72
    incidence risk, 55
    prevention and medications, 60–61
    screening, 59–60, 62. *See also* Mammograms
    survival rates, 61–63
    treatment, 70–71
Breast reduction surgery, 307–8
Breath, shortness of, 139, 151, 152, 175, 201, 202, 203, 234, 250, 271, 273, 280
    heart attacks, 177, 180
Breathing, 295
    cyclic sighing, 106
    hypoxic techniques, 8
"Bristle reaction," 310
Bromelain, 285–86
Bronchitis, 160, 167, 207, 234, 273, 280
Bronzed Chicken Breasts Over Red, Green, and Brown Rice, 78–79
Bullectomies, 274
Bupropion, 281
Butyrate, 121, 222

C

Cadmium, 127, 128
Caffeine. *See* Coffee
Calcitonin gene-related peptide (CGRP) antagonists, 240–41
Calcium, 227, 230, 260, 264
Calluses, 255
Cancer, 55–74. *See also specific forms of cancer*
    AI and, 59, 74
    anti-obesity medications and, 159
    artificial intelligence and, 59, 74
    diabetes and, 86
    diet and, 63, 64, 69–70, 123
    drug side effects, 163
    exercise for, 128, 134, 135, 139
    incidence risk, 55
    personalized treatment, 70–71
    pharmacogenomics, 154
    procyanidins for, 232–33
    second opinions, 63
    suicide risk and, 97
    targeted therapy, 62, 65, 70–71
Candida auris, 205–7
Cannabidiol (CBD)
    safety concerns, 159–60
    seniors and, 28
    for tinnitus, 51
Cannabis
    lung cancer and, 280
    seniors and, 28
    sex and, 309–10
    sleep and, 306
Cannabis-use disorder, 109
Carbon dioxide, 212, 282
Carbon monoxide poisoning, 269
Cardiac arrest, 177, 183–84
    CPR, 183, 184
Cardiac implantable electronic devices (CIED), 181
Cardiac stents, 193–94

Index

Cardiomyopathy, 176, 181–82
Cardiopulmonary resuscitation (CPR), 145, 183, 184
Cardiovascular disease. *See* Heart disease
Caregivers, finding, 24
Carotenoids, 120
Carpal tunnel release, 259
Carpal tunnel syndrome, 257–59
Cars and driving
    aging and, 12, 27–28
    blind spots, 269
    ER visits, 146
    winter weather, 268, 270
Castor oil packs, 313
Cataracts, 17, 19, 167, 276, 279
Cataract surgery, 17, 141–42
Catheter ablation, 176, 194, 244, 255
Catheter infections, 148, 205
Cats, 103, 224–26
Cefdinir, 160
Celery, 119–20
Celiac disease, 124–25, 251
Cereals, 236, 251
Cerebral spinal fluid flow, 53
Chair Rises, 137
Chair Squats, 134, 135
ChatGPT, 74
Checkpoint inhibitors, 65, 68–69, 71
Cherry bark, 208
Chest pains, 145, 152, 175, 177, 179, 185
  cardiac stents for, 193–94
Chitin, 126
Chlorothiazide (Diuril), 188
Chocolate, 5, 111, 127–28, 232, 249
Cholecystectomies, 220
Cholesterol
    dementia risk and, 189
    gallstones, 218
    heart disease and, 177, 198
    heart health and, 173, 174, 177–78, 180–81
    keto diet and, 75, 177
    phototherapy for, 192
    statins for. *See* Statins
    tests, 192
Chronic fatigue syndrome, 202
Chronic kidney disease (CKD), 213–15
  PPIs and, 169
Chronic obstructive pulmonary disease (COPD), 273–75
    long COVID and, 203
    mental health and, 97
    PEP Buddy, 275
    pulse oximeters, 151
    sex differences, 273
    smoking and, 280
    treatment, 274
    triggers, 274–75
Chronic pain syndrome, 242–43
Chronic wounds, 270–70
Chronotherapy, 305
Circadian rhythms, 129–30, 239, 299–301, 304
Cirrhosis, 158, 219
Climate change, 283
"Clock time," 302–3
Clostridium difficile (C. diff), 160, 169–70, 221
Cocaine, 176
Cocoa, 127–28, 231–32, 233
Coenzyme Q10 (CoQ10), 297

Coffee (caffeine)
    diabetes and, 77, 85
    hypertension and, 187
    longevity and, 2
    PVCs and, 175, 176
    sleep and, 77, 287, 294
    stomach pain and, 249
    tinnitus and, 52
Cognition
    A-fib and, 197
    aging and pets, 29
    cannabis and, 28
    drug side effects, 163
    exercise for, 34, 35–36, 43, 45
    learning multiple new skills, 8–9
    noise and, 21
    positive thinking for, 46
    scents for, 40
    smoking and, 279
    test, 39
Cognitive behavioral therapy (CBT), 97, 100, 101, 239, 241
Cognitive behavioral therapy for insomnia (CBT-I), 236, 294
Cognitive decline. *See also* Alzheimer's disease
    after bypass surgery, 194
    heart disease and, 37–39
    infections and, 211
    pets and, 224
    procyanidins for, 233
    tips to avoid, 34–36
    warning signs, 36
Cognitive processing therapy (CPT) 108
Colchicine, 175
Cold packs and wraps, 10, 289, 290
"Cold-pressed" oils, 126–27
Cold showers, 7–8
Cold sweats, 180
Cold therapy, 290–91
Cold weather, 267–70
    joints and, 267
    safety, 268–70
Colleges, free tuition for older students, 27
Cologuard, 72
Colonoscopies, 57–58, 152, 153
    alternatives to, 72
Colorectal cancer, 57–58, 73–74
    biomarkers, 72
    incidence, 55, 73
    obesity and, 63–65, 73–74
Colostomies, 108
Complex carbohydrates, 2, 111
Compression gloves, 10
Concussions, 18–21
    recovery road map, 20–21
    when to seek attention, 19–20
Congestive heart failure, 97, 171
Constipation, 30, 44, 158, 159, 171, 223, 251, 300
    bloat and, 311–12
    vibrating capsule for, 312
Contact lenses, 13, 206
Cooking, 95, 275
Cooling pillows, 288–89
COPD. *See* Chronic obstructive pulmonary disease
Copper peptides, 4
Core strengthening, 246
Coronary stents, 179
Coronavirus. *See* COVID-19
Correlated diffusion imaging (CDI), 59
Corticobasal syndrome, 41

Corticosteroids, 163, 256, 272, 276–77
Cortisol, 128, 129, 222, 224, 225, 231, 262, 301, 304
Costco, medical care, 166
Coughs (coughing), 275–76
Coumarin, 119–20
Couples therapy, 91
COVID-19, 202–4, 302
    Alzheimer's disease, 33
    cancer and, 55
    contagiousness, guidelines, 208
    diabetes and, 86
    lifestyle and, 203
    loneliness problem, 101–2
    long, 202–4
    negative long haulers, 202–3
    pulse oximeters, 151
    sleep for, 203–4
COVID-19 vaccinations, 200
CPAP (continuous positive airway pressure), 277–78
Cramping, 223, 311
Cranberry juice, 216, 228
Craniosacral therapy, 231
C-reactive protein (CRP), 36, 87
Credit cards, medical, 166
Criss-Cross Jumping Jacks, 132
Crohn's disease, 30, 167, 195, 251, 313
Cross-Country Skiing (exercise), 132
Cruises, health, 209
Crying, 106
Cryotherapy chambers, 290–91
Curcumin, 45
Cyclic sighing, 106
Cynophobia, 103
CYP2C19 gene, 154
Cytokines, 16, 232

D

Dairy, 2, 63, 122–23
    MyPlate guidelines, 117–18
Dancing, 34
Danuglipron, 158
Dark chocolate, 127–28, 233
DASH diet, 45, 115, 187
Debridement, 272
Decompression surgery, 248
Deep heat treatments, 289–90
Deep tissue massage, 231
Deep vein thrombosis (DVT), 148, 229
De-escalation, 74
Defibrillators, 182, 183, 184
Deli meats, 125
Dementia. *See also* Alzheimer's disease
    brain games for, 296
    cholesterol and, 189
    diagnosis, coping with, 42–44
    frontotemporal (FTD), 40–42
    heart health and, 37–39
    Internet use and, 54
    laxatives and, 44
    stress and, 7
    tips to avoid, 34–36
Dense breasts and diagnosis, 56, 60
Dental care, braces, 23–24
Dental coverage, 26
Dental infections, 32
Depression, 94–101
    ADepT for, 100–101
    aging and, 6
    brain health and, 45
    drug side effects, 163
    exercise for, 128–29
    long COVID and, 203

Index

medications and, 93, 97–98, 163
non-drug DIY treatments, 94–96
pain and, 239, 240
reminiscence therapy for, 108–9
sense of purpose, 5, 98
seven habits to fight, 94
sleep and, 21
stress and, 7
suicide, 96–99
Dermatochalasis, 13–14
Dermatophytes, 205
Diabetes, 75–88
  carpal tunnel and, 257
  colon cancer and drugs, 73–74
  diet for, 75–80, 118–20, 123
  exercise for, 76–77, 85–86, 128, 134, 139, 304
  gallstones and, 219
  heart disease and, 198
  long COVID and, 203
  procyanidins for, 233
  sleep and, 21, 77, 81–82
  stress and, 7
  vitamin D for, 229
Diabetic neuropathy, 85, 87
Diabetic retinopathy, 17
Dialysis, 213, 214–15
Diaphragms, 216
Diarrhea, 68, 85, 111, 121, 124, 145, 146, 154, 158, 160, 169, 201, 217, 221, 223, 249, 313
  vitamin C and, 207
Diclofenac gel (Voltaren), 243
Diet, 113–28. *See also* Recipes
  after stomach virus, 211
  for aging well, 1–3, 5, 9
  for arthritis, 252
  for bloat, 311–12
  for bone health, 264
  for brain health, 38, 39, 43, 44–45, 47, 49–50
  cancer and, 63, 64, 69–70, 123
  for constipation, 251
  DASH, 45, 115, 187
  for depression, 95
  for diabetes, 75–80, 118–20, 123
  for eyesight, 15
  for gallbladder, 218
  for hand health, 9
  for heartburn, 168
  for heart health, 115, 118–23, 178, 180–81
  for hypertension, 186–87
  IBS and, 313–14
  for kidney disease and, 214
  mood and, 111–12
  prebiotics, 221–23
  procyanidins, 231–34
  seasonal shifts, 298
  sleep and, 287, 301–2
  time-restricted eating, 301–2, 304
  for wounds, 272
Dietary fiber. *See* Fiber
Dietary supplements. *See* Supplements; *and specific supplements*
Digestive diseases. *See specific diseases*
Digestive health, aging and loneliness, 29–30
Dihydroergotamine mesylate (Trudhesa), 241
Dimenhydrinate (Dramamine), 211
Diphenhydramine (Benadryl), 43, 211
Discectomies, 248–49

Disease-modifying antirheumatic drugs (DMARDs), 272
Diuretics, 163, 164, 167, 187, 188
Dizziness, 8, 19, 20, 48, 167, 269, 271
  heart health and, 176, 181, 185, 187, 191
Doctors
  depersonalized care, 141–42
  dilemmas facing, 165
  finding, 142
  medical gaslighting, 142–44
  second opinions. *See* Second opinions
  specialists, 149
Dogs, 224–26
  dangers of walking leashed, 258
  pet therapy, 110, 224–26
  phobia, 103
  preparing for, 225
Donanemab, 46
Dopamine, 112, 128, 226, 280
Downward-Facing Dog Pose, 263–64
Dried fruits, 84, 264, 312
Drinking water. *See* Hydration
Drinks, toxic metals in, 123–24
Droopy eyelids, 13–14
Drug-drug interaction (DDI), 161–63
Drugs. *See* Medications
Dry eyes, 18, 279
Dual-energy X-ray absorptiometry (DXA), 259–61
Duloxetine (Cymbalta), 243
Dupuytren's contracture, 10
Dysbiosis, 221, 222, 223
Dyspareunia, 308

E

"Early birds," 80–81
Earplugs, 22, 23
E-cigarettes, 281–82
Eco-friendly straws, 122
EGFR gene, 65, 67, 71
Eggs, 2, 120, 180, 227, 229
  substitutes, 126
Ehrlichiosis, 210
Elecampane, 208
Electrocardiograms (ECGs), 151–52
Emergency bypass, 108
Emergency rooms (ER), 144–46
  gender bias in, 143
  urgent-care centers vs., 147
Emotional rescue, 89–112. *See also* Depression; Stress
Empathy, 91, 110
Endogenous opioids, 243
Endometriosis, 237, 238
Endorphins, 18, 128, 241, 246
Endothelium, 232
Energy, exercises for, 133–35
Enteric nervous system (ENS), 111
Eosinophils, 276
Epicatechin, 47
Erotica, 310
Erythritol, 83, 120, 312
Escherichia coli (*E. coli*), 126, 209, 210, 215–16, 217
Esophageal cancers, 69, 168, 233
Essential oil facial packs, 208
Estimated glomerular filtration rate (eGFR), 213–14
Estrogen receptors, 58–59, 60, 62, 71
Ethanol, 232
Evolocumab (Repatha), 174
Exemestane (Aromasin), 61

Exercise, 128–40
  aging and fitness tests, 11–12
  for aging well, 7, 13, 17
  for Alzheimer's disease, 34, 35–36, 43, 45
  for arthritis, 251–53
  for back pain, 244–45, 246
  best time for, 85–86, 304–5
  for bloat, 311
  for brain health, 34, 35–36, 43, 45
  breast size and, 307–8
  for cognition, 34, 35–36, 43, 45
  for depression, 96
  for diabetes, 76–77, 85–86, 128, 134, 139, 304
  11 minutes lowering disease risk, 135
  for eyes, 17
  fungal infections and gyms, 206
  gender differences, 139–40
  genes and, 295
  for hand mobility, 10–11
  for heart disease, 179, 180
  for heart health, 178, 179, 180
  heart health for, 128, 133–36, 139, 178, 179, 180
  hormetic stress and, 7
  for hypertension, 187
  for joints, 267
  for kidney disease and, 214
  mistakes, 264–26
  for pain relief, 238, 244–45, 246, 254, 256
  post-stroke, 195–96
  seasonal shifts, 299
  short bursts of activity, 13, 179
  sleep and, 287, 301
  for snoring, 278
  water, 130–33
Exposure therapy, 104
Eye diseases, 17
Eye exams and Alzheimer's disease, 40
Eyelids, droopy, 13–14
Eyesight. *See* Vision
Eye surgeries. *See* Cataract surgery

F

Facebook, 43, 303
Falls (falling), 268
  at hospitals, 148, 149
False-positive mammograms, 59–60
Family medical history, 170–71
Faricimab (Vabysmo), 16
"Fasting-mimicking diet," 296
Fasting plasma glucose, 76
Fatty liver disease, 158, 300
Fecal immunochemical test (FIT), 57–58, 72
Fermented foods, 116, 121–22, 223, 312
Ferulic acid, 4
Fezolinetant (Veozah), 4
Fiber, 2, 5, 111–12, 121–22, 314
Fibromyalgia, 203, 237, 238, 242, 243
Fire extinguishers, 268
First-aid basics, 210
Fish, 2, 44, 78, 95, 111, 112, 201, 218, 229, 264, 272
Fish oil. *See* Omega-3 fatty acids
Fitness. *See* Exercise
Fitness trackers, 13, 138
Flavanols, 47, 120–21, 127–28
Flavonoids, 231–32, 234
Flesh-eating disease, 271
Fluoxetine (Prozac), 14, 112

Index

Flu vaccinations, 37, 200
FODMAPs, 124–25, 311–12
Food. *See* Diet; Recipes
Food allergies, 125
Food dyes, 251
Food Guide Pyramid, 117–18
Food packaging, 70, 86
Food poisoning, 249–50
Foot Alphabet, 254
Foot osteomyelitis, 271
Foot pain, 253–55
    shoes for, 129, 253–54
Footwear, 129, 253–54, 270
Forest fires, 53
Four-stage balance tests, 12
Fractures, 140, 167, 230, 260, 273, 276, 279
FRAX (Fracture Risk Assessment Tool), 260
Freezing up, 47–49
Friendships
    caregiving, 24
    dementia support group, 43
Frontotemporal dementia (FTD), 40–42
Frontotemporal lobar degeneration (FTLD), 40–42
Frostbite, 269
Frozen shoulder, 86
Fruits and vegetables. *See also specific fruits and vegetables*
    for aging well, 1–3
    for brain health, 47
    for depression, 95
    for diabetes, 75–76, 78
    diabetes and, 83–84
    for gallbladder, 218
    for heart health, 180–81
    MyPlate guidelines, 117–18
Fungal infections, 205–7

G

Gabapentin (Neurontin), 243
Gallbladder, 217–20, 251
Gallstones, 218–20, 251
Gardening, 92, 94–95, 206
Garlic, 119, 227, 228, 234
Gastroesophageal reflux disease (GERD), 30, 250, 276, 287
Gastrointestinal bleeding, 154, 162, 243
Gender bias and women's ailments, 143
Genetic fixes, 294–97
Genetic tests
    ARMD, 16
    cancer, 66
    medications and, 153–55
    weight loss and, 114
Gepotidacin, 217
GFAP (glial fibrillary acidic protein), 27
Ginger, 116, 211, 223
    for immune system, 224, 252
Ginkgo biloba, 44
Ginseng, 231
Glasgow Coma Scale (GCS), 19
Glaucoma, 17, 167, 221, 279
Global assessment of functioning (GAF), 47–48
GLP-1 (glucagon-like peptide 1)
    agonists, 114–15, 157–59
    cancer and, 73–74
    fiber and, 121–22
    liver and, 219
Glucosamine, 188
Glucose. *See* Blood sugar
Gluten-free diet, 124–25
Glycolic acid, 4

Goal setting, 98–99, 113–14, 303
Goji berries, 15
Gout, 160, 189, 253
Grapefruit juice, 162
Grapes, 15
Gratitude, 6
Gray hair
    stem cells and, 18
    stress and, 109–10
Grooming, 95, 97
Gum disease
    braces, 23–24
    smoking and, 279
Gut-brain axis, 83, 111
Gut dysbiosis, 221, 222, 223
Gut health and microbiome, 221
    artificial sugars and, 83
    bloat and, 312
    diabetes and, 78
    depression and, 96
    diet for, 111–12, 221–23
    IBS and, 313–14
    prebiotics, 221–23
    supplements for, 228

H

Hamstring Curls, 244–45
Hands, 9–11
    exercises for mobility, 10–11
    grips, 9–10
    treatments for, 10
Hand washing, 200, 204–9
Happiness, 100, 110, 128–29, 226. *See also* Positivity
Hay fever, 284
HDL ("good") cholesterol. *See* Cholesterol
Headaches. *See* Migraines
Head injuries, concussions, 18–20
Head pain, 53
Headphones, 23
Health-care financing, 166
Health-care worker dilemmas, 165
Health insurance. *See* Insurance; Medicare
Health screening tests, 152–53
Hearing loss, 21, 34, 50
    drug side effects, 163–64
    noise pollution and, 21–23, 50
    smoking and, 279
Heart attacks, 173–75
    causes for, 173
    coronary stents after, 179
    diet and, 84, 122–23
    ER visits, 146
    gender differences, 175, 179–80
    medications, 174, 305–6
    noise and, 21
    obesity and drugs, 157
    shingles and, 189–90
    sleep and, 21
    stomach pain and, 250
    VEGF and, 16
Heartburn, 159, 169, 249, 301
    lifestyle changes, 168
    PPIs and, 168–70
    stomach pain and, 249, 250
Heart bypass surgery, 194
Heart (cardiovascular) disease, 173–80. *See also* Heart attacks; Strokes
    beyond pacemakers, 181–83
    dairy and, 122–23
    diet for, 122–24
    exercise for, 179, 180
    gender differences, 175, 179–80

Life's Simple 7, 37–39
    long COVID and, 203
    noise and, 21
    psoriasis and, 191–93
    reducing risk, 198
    shape of heart and risk, 181
    smoking and, 279
    stable angina and cardiac stents, 193–94
Heart health, 173–94
    brain health and, 37–39
    diet for, 115, 118–23, 173–74, 180–81
    exercise for, 128, 133–36, 139, 178, 179, 180
    gratitude and, 6
    partners and, 179–80
    pets for, 225
    semaglutide for, 189
    short bursts of activity for, 13, 179
    supplements for, 227
    vitamin D for, 227, 229–30
    weight loss, 116
Heart monitors, smartwatch, 151–52
Heart palpitations, 175–77
Heart shape, 181
Heating pads, 10, 267, 289
Heat stroke, 209
Heavy lifting, 9, 246, 247
Heel Lifts, 134–35
Heel-to-Toe Inline Walking, 137
Helicobacter pylori (H. pylori), 170, 250
Hemostasis, 270–71
Hemp seeds, 119
HER2 gene, 62, 70–71
Herniated disks, 242, 244, 247, 248
High blood pressure. *See* Hypertension
High-intensity interval training (HIIT), 7, 133–35
    before surgery, 164
High Knees Marching, 135
Hip Extensions, 245
Hip fractures, 260, 279
Hip pain, 237
Hippocampus, 33, 34, 47
Hip replacements, 165, 291
Histamine 2-receptor antagonists (H2RAs), 170
HIV/AIDS, 97, 205, 309
Hodgkin's lymphoma, 71, 74
Home medical essentials, 150–52
Honey, 84, 234–35, 236, 312
Hormetic stress, 7–8
Hormone therapy (HT), 3, 4, 33, 264
Horticulture therapy. *See* Gardening
Hospital-acquired infections, 149, 204–5
Hospitals. *See also* Emergency rooms
    medical complications, 148
    micro, 149–50
    patient-advocacy office, 144
    rejections, 165
    risks associated with, 146–49
    staffing policies, 148–49
Hot baths, 288, 289, 295
Hot flashes, 61
    fezolinetant for, 4
    prebiotics for, 223
House fires, 269
Housework, 292, 310
HPV (human papillomavirus), 74, 309
Huperzine, 44, 45
Hyaluronic acid, 4, 256
Hydration (drinking water), 2, 116
    diabetes and, 85

Index

drinking water outside U.S., 210
pneumonia, 201
for wounds, 272
Hydroquinone, 311
Hydroxychloroquine, 164
Hyperalgesia, 164
Hyperarousal, 107–8
Hyperbaric oxygen therapy, 109, 271
Hyperkyphosis, 130
Hypertension (high blood pressure), 184–88
    Alzheimer's disease and, 34
    drug-drug interactions, 162–63
    heart disease and, 198
    insomnia and, 184–85
    long COVID and, 203
    medications, 14, 162–63, 187–88
    noise and, 21, 186
    pets for, 225
    procyanidins for, 232
    salt and, 185, 186, 188
    self-care, 186–87
    when lying down, 188
Hyperthyroidism, 176
Hypothermia, 269
Hypothyroidism, 158
Hypoxic breathing, 8

I

Ibuprofen, 52, 154, 162, 164, 214, 242, 243, 250, 272
Ice baths, 290
Ice cups, 290
Icosapent ethyl (Vascepa), 174, 178
Ikigai, 4–5
Immune system (immunity)
    ginger for, 224, 252
    supplements for, 227
    vitamin D for, 227, 229
Immunotherapies, 65–66, 68–69, 71
Implantable cardioverter defibrillators (ICDs), 182
Inclisiran (Leqvio), 174
Index Abduction, 11
Indigestion, 218, 251, 300, 313
    bedtime routine, 287
    stomach pain and, 249
Indocyanine green imaging, 15
Infectious disease (infections), 199–212. *See also* COVID-19
    cognition and, 211
    diet and stomach viruses, 211
    fungal, 205–7
    in hospitals, 149, 204–5
    painkillers and infections, 201–2
    pneumonia, 199–201
    RSV, 207–8
    shingles vaccine and dementia, 201–2
    strep throat, 208
    vitamin D for, 230
    when traveling, 209–10
Inflammasome, 232
Inflammation
    diet for, 122
    lowering for heart health, 174–75
    stress and, 87–88
    wounds and, 271
Inflammatory bowel disease (IBD), 30, 195, 251, 313
Influenza vaccinations, 37, 200

Insects
    eating, 126
    first aid, 210
Insect repellent, 210, 212
Insomnia. *See* Sleep problems
Insulin resistance, 36, 76, 77, 82–83
Insurance. *See also* Medicare
    anti-obesity medications, 159
    emergencies, 145, 146
    health-care practices and, 143
    Medigap, 24–26
    mental health coverage, 99
    palliative care, 172
    surgeon or hospital rejections and, 165
Intensivists, 149
Interstitial cystitis, 237
Irritable bowel syndrome (IBS)
    bloating and, 311
    chronic pain and, 242
    food dyes and, 251
    natural remedies for, 312–14
    pain disparities, 237
    prebiotics for, 223
    social isolation and, 30

J

Jet lag, 300
Jock itch, 205
Jumping Jacks, 131–32
Junk food, 47, 95

K

Ketchup, 120
Keto (ketogenic) diet, 75, 177
Kidney beans, 121
Kidney cancer, 122
Kidney disease, 172, 213–15
    blood pressure, 185, 214
    PPIs and, 169
    sleep and, 21, 214
Kidney transplants, 213, 215
Knee arthritis, 256
Knee pain, 237, 256
KRAS gene, 65–66, 71

L

Lactobacillus, 3, 222
Laminectomies, 248–49
Language therapy, 42
Laryngltis, 160
Laser treatments, 4, 17, 259, 308
Lateness, 109
Lawn work, 22, 284
Laxatives
    dementia and, 44
    shortage, 314
Lecanemab (Leqembi), 31–32, 36
Lecithin, 218
Ledderhose disease, 10
Left ventricular assist devices (LVADs), 182–83
Levodopa, 14
Life purpose, 4–5, 98
Light exposure and sundowning, 54
Lipoprotein(a), 174
Liquid biopsy, 57, 65
Lithium, 163
Liver cancer, 219
Liver disease, 82, 158, 168, 219, 300
Loneliness, 101–2
    digestive health and, 29–30
    relationships and, 91, 93

Long COVID, 202–4
Longevity diet, 1–3, 5
Low-dose computed tomography (LDCT), 57, 66
Lung cancer, 65–67
    artificial intelligence and, 59
    biomarkers, 71
    early diagnosis, 66
    incidence risk, 55
    radon and, 196–97
    screening, 57, 66
    smokers and smoking, 57, 171, 196, 280, 281
    survival rate, 66–67
    treatment, 65–66
Lung disease, 134, 200, 276, 280, 281
Lungs and smoking, 279–80
Lupus, 164, 202, 223, 252
Lutein, 15, 17
Lycopene, 118, 120

M

Macromastia, 307
Macular degeneration, 14–17, 19, 279
Magnesium, 47
Major depressive disorder (MDD), 96
Malaria, 210, 212
Mammograms, 55–56, 62, 153
    false-positive, 59–60
Mannitol, 85
Marijuana. *See* Cannabis
Marriages
    science of better, 89–91
    sex and intimacy, 310
Massages, 5–6, 231
Meal skipping, 116
Meclizine (Bonine), 211
Medical billing scams, 166
Medical care, 141–72. *See also* Emergency rooms; Hospitals
    antibiotic overuse, 160–61
    depersonalized health care, 141–42
    family medical history, 170–71
    genetic testing and medications, 153–55
    health screening tests, 152–53
    home essentials, 150–52
    palliative care, 171–72, 215
    polypharmacy, 161–63
    private equity and adverse events, 149
    rejection by hospitals or surgeons, 165
    short supply of medications, 155–57
    special financing for, 166
    unsafe supplements, 159–60
Medical credit cards, 166
Medical gaslighting, 142–44
Medical history, creating family, 170–71
Medical insurance. *See* Insurance
Medical malpractice, 147
Medical records
    monitoring, 142
    stolen, 166
Medical specialists, 149
Medical-test anxiety, 106–7
Medical trauma, mental health after, 107–9
Medicare
    drug negotiations, 167
    lecanemab, 31
    surgical success rates and, 165

Index

Medicare Advantage, 25, 99
  misleading ads, 26–27
Medications. *See also specific medications*
  for Alzheimer's disease, 31–32, 36, 42, 43–44, 46
  for COPD, 274
  expired, 157
  eyelid drooping, 14
  genetic testing and, 153–55
  hospital errors, 147
  polypharmacy, 161–63
  shortages, 155–57
  side effects and hearing loss, 163–64
  for weight loss, 114–15, 157–59, 189
  when traveling, 209
Medigap, 25–26
Meditation
  cyclic sighing, 106
  for diabetes, 77
  for pain, 238, 239
  for sleep, 288, 294
  for stress, 187
MediterAsian diet, 115–16
Mediterranean diet, 45, 47, 49–50, 95, 115, 173–74
Mediterranean Steak with Minted Couscous, 79
Medjool dates, 119
Melanocyte stem cells, 18
Melanomas, 67–69
Melatonin, 235–36, 288
Memory. *See also* Alzheimer's disease; Brain fog; Cognitive decline
  after bypass surgery, 194
  cannabis and, 28
  depression and, 6
  drug side effects, 163
  multivitamins for, 38
  pets and, 224
  scents for, 40
  sleep and inhaling fragrances, 236
Menopause, 216
  obesity and, 3, 56
Menstrual migraines, 240
Mental dullness. *See* Brain fog
Mental health
  after medical emergency, 107–9
  finding help, 99–100
  sibling relationships and, 92
Metabolic syndrome, 87–88, 122, 192, 223
Metformin, 25, 73, 115
Methadone, 109
Micro hospitals, 149–50
Microplastics, 27
Microvascular lesions (MVLs), 37–39
Migraines, 239–41
  chronic pain and, 242
  long COVID and, 203
  nasal spray for, 239
  suicide risk and, 97
  treatments, 240–41
Mild cognitive impairment (MCI), 28, 34–35, 46, 233
Mind-body practices, 241, 291–92
Mindfulness, 291–93
Miscarriages, 108
Mitochondria, 32, 52
Moderate-to-vigorous physical activity (MVPA), 138–39
Monoclonal antibodies, 65, 71, 240–41

Mood
  breath work, 106
  colorful environments for, 112
  food and, 111–12
"Morton's neuroma," 255
Mosquitoes, 210, 212
Motion sickness, 209, 211
Mouth breathing, 278
Mouth exercises, for snoring, 278
Multi-cancer early detection tests (MCED), 57, 65
Multiple sclerosis, 293
  COVID-19 and, 202, 203
  diet for, 49–50
Multipurpose supplements, 227
Multivitamins, 38, 227
Muscle relaxants, 14
Mushroom Pesto Pasta with Pimento Pepper Salad, 79–80
Music, for pain relief, 253
Mycosis, 205–7
Myocardial infarction with nonobstructive coronary arteries (MINOCA), 175
Myofascial release, 231
MyPlate guidelines, 117–18

N

N-acetylcysteine (NAC), 17, 285
Nail-gel dryers and cancer risk, 67
Naps (napping), 305
Nasal irrigation, 286
Nasal sprays, 14, 281
  for migraines, 239
Natural remedies, 221–36. *See also specific remedies*
Nausea, 53, 114, 124, 146, 158, 159, 171, 180, 185, 201, 211, 212, 219, 239, 249, 250, 251, 269
Nearsightedness, 18
Negativity, 89, 97, 100, 101, 104
Neoadjuvant chemotherapy, 59
Nervine herbs, 313
NETosis, 252
Nicotine replacement therapy (NRT), 281
"Night owls" and diabetes risk, 80–81
Night sweats, 4, 238, 239
NLRP3, 232
N-Nitrosodimethylamine (NDMA), 168
Noise pollution, 21–23, 50, 186
  reducing, 22–23
Non-alcoholic fatty liver disease (NAFLD), 158
Non-small cell lung cancer (NSCLC), 65–67
Norovirus, 208, 209, 250
Nose breathing, 278
NSAIDs (nonsteroidal anti-inflammatory drugs), 52, 154, 162, 163, 164, 201, 214, 239, 240, 243, 250, 256, 259
Nutrition. *See* Diet
Nutritional supplements. *See* Supplements; *and specific supplements*
Nuts and seeds, 2, 47, 76, 78, 111, 112, 121, 222, 232, 236, 264

O

Obesity
  cancer and, 57, 59, 63–65, 73–74
  cancer risk and, 63–64
  carpal tunnel and, 257
  medications for, 114–15, 157–59, 189
  menopause and, 3, 56
  pets and, 224
  prediabetes, 75–76

  sleep and, 21, 77, 82, 116–17
  stress and, 7
  weight loss. *See* Weight loss
Obstructive sleep apnea (OSA), 277–78, 294
Oils, cold-pressed or refined, 126–27
Oligosaccharides, 122, 124, 221–22, 311
Olive oil, 2, 126–27
Omega-3 fatty acids, 44, 112, 227, 229
Onions, 119, 234–35, 285
Online medications, 157
Online scams, 107
Online therapy services, 100
Online weight-loss programs, 114–15
Onychomycosis, 205
Ophthalmic medications, 14
Opioids (opioid addiction), 239, 243
  hyperbaric oxygen therapy, 109
  safety warning, 164
Optical coherent tomography (OCT) angiography, 15
Optimism. *See* Positivity
Oral glucose tolerance test, 76
Orforglipron, 158
Organic foods, 63
Osha (herb), 208
Osimertinib (Tagrisso), 65–67
Osteoarthritis
  acetaminophen for, 239
  chronic pain and, 242, 243
  gender differences, 237
  glucosamine for, 188
  hands, 9–10
  knees, 256
  runners and, 140
  SNRIs for, 243
  spinal stenosis and, 247
Osteopenia, 260, 261–62, 264
Osteoporosis
  aromatase inhibitors and, 61
  back pain and, 245, 247
  bone density and, 260
  gum disease and, 23
  hyperkyphosis, 130
  steroid side effects, 167
  supplements, 160
Ovarian cancer, biomarkers, 71
Overweight. *See* Obesity
Oxybutynin chloride, 43
Oxycodone (OxyContin), 243
Oxygen machines, 152
Oxytocin, 225
Ozempic, 73–74, 114–15, 121–22, 157–59, 159, 189, 219, 241
Ozempic butt, 159
Ozempic face, 159

P

Pacemakers, 181–82
Pain. *See also specific types of pain*
  gender differences, 237–39
Pain medications, 240–41, 272. *See also specific medications*
  gender differences, 239
  infections and pneumonia, 201
  pharmacogenomics, 154
Pain relief, 237–56
  aging well and, 6
  for arthritis. *See* Arthritis
  for back. *See* Back pain
  for carpal tunnel, 259
  for chronic pain, 241–44
  exercise for, 238, 244–45, 246, 254, 256

321

Index

for feet, 253–255
for headaches. *See* Migraines
music for, 253
tummy troubles, 249–51
for wounds, 272
Pain reprocessing therapy (PRT), 244
Palliative care, 171–72, 215
Pancreatic cancer, 74, 86
Pantothenic acid, 207–8
Paraffin baths, 289
Parental favoritism, 92
Parkinson's disease, 48, 293
   air pollution and, 53
   driver rehabilitation, 12
   medications, 14
   mitochondria link, 52
   prebiotics for, 223
   ultrasound for, 52
Paroxetine (Paxil), 162
Patient advocates, 144
PCSK9 inhibitor, 174
Peanut butter, 76, 119, 120
Peas, 76, 118–19, 290, 312
Pegcetacoplan (Syfovre), 16
Pelacarsen, 174–75
Pemafibrate, 177–78
Penicillin allergy, 285
PEP Buddy, 275
Pepcid, 168, 170, 218
Percutaneous coronary intervention (PCI), 193–94
Perfectionism, 106
Pesticides, 63, 84
Pets
   aging and cognition, 29
   emergency care, 226
   health benefits of, 110, 224–26
   preparing for, 225
Phagocytes, 271
Pharmacodynamics, 163
Pharmacogenomics, 153–55
Pharmacokinetics, 163
Pharyngitis, 160
Phishing, 107
Phobias, 102–4
Phosphatidylserine, 44, 45
Phospho-creatine, 297
Photodynamic therapy (PDT), 16
Phthalates, 80, 86
Physical therapy, 42, 194, 195, 267
   for pain relief, 246, 247, 249, 255, 267
Phytohaemagglutinin (PHA), 121
Pickup truck blind spots, 269
Pigment gallstones, 218
Pillows, 288–89
Piperine, 118, 162
Placebo effect, 52, 291–92
Planks, 246
Plantar fasciitis, 129, 255
Platelet-rich plasma (PRP) therapy, 244
Plate method, 76
Pneumonia, 199–201
Pneumonia vaccine, 199–200, 207–8
Podiatrists, 254–55
Polio vaccinations, 210
Political differences and siblings, 92
Pollution. *See also* Air pollution
   noise, 21–23, 50
Polyfluoroalkyl substances (PFAS), 70, 122
Polypharmacy, 161–63
Polyphenol oxidase (PPO), 120–21
Polyphenols, 221–22
Pornography, 310

Portable oxygen concentrators (POCs), 152
Positive expiratory pressure, 275
Positivity (positive mindset), 4–5, 46, 98, 100, 110, 180
Postherpetic neuralgia (PHN), 191
Post-prandial walking, 128
Post-traumatic stress disorder (PTSD), 107–8, 224, 239
Posture
   balance and, 137
   exercise for, 130
   sitting, 94, 130
Potassium, 186–87
   sources of, 119, 126, 127
Prebiotics, 221–23
Prediabetes, 75–76
Pregabalin (Lyrica), 243
Premature ventricular contraction (PVC), 175–77
Prescription drugs. *See* Medications
Primary progressive aphasia, 41
Private equity and hospital adverse events, 149
Probiotics, 96, 313–14
Processed foods, 69–70, 84, 111, 125, 214, 222, 298
Procyanidins, 231–34
Prolactin, 106
Propionate, 222
Proprioception, 136
Prostate cancer, 56–57
Prostate-specific antigen (PSA) tests, 56–57, 71, 152–53
Protein, MyPlate guidelines, 117–18
Proteinases, 174–75
Proton pump inhibitors (PPIs), 154, 168–70
Pseudogout, 253
Psoriasis, 167, 191–93
Psychic numbing, 107–8
Psychology clinics, 100
Psychotherapy, 94, 294
Ptosis, 13–14
Pulmonary fibrosis, 280
Pulmonary rehabilitation, 274
Pulsatile tinnitus, 50–51
Pulse oximeters, 151
Pushups, 7, 265–66

Q

Quantitative computed tomography (QCT), 259–61
Quercetin, 285

R

Race
   chronic wounds and, 270
   pain disparities, 237, 242
Radiofrequency catheter ablation, 176, 194, 244, 255
Radon, 196–97
Rainbow app, 301
Rain-computer interface, 53–54
Ranibizumab (Lucentis), 16
Ranitidine, 167
Recipes
   Bronzed Chicken Breasts Over Red, Green, and Brown Rice, 78–79
   Mediterranean Steak with Minted Couscous, 79
   Mushroom Pesto Pasta with Pimento Pepper Salad, 79–80

Recurrent UTIs, 216
Red meat, 1–2, 63
Red wine, 2, 187, 232
Refrigerating foods, 120
Regenerative medicine, 244
Relationships. *See also* Friendships; Marriages; Socializing
   depression and, 101
   heart health and, 180
   marriages, 89–91
   sibling, 91–93
   support network, 105–6
Religion (religious faith), 43, 95, 100–102
Reminiscence therapy, 108–9
Renal disease, 97, 183
Respiratory health, 273–86
   allergy season, 282–84
   asthma. *See* Asthma
   COPD. *See* Chronic obstructive pulmonary disease
   CPAP comparison, 277–78
   lingering cough, 275–76
   mouth exercises for snoring, 278
   plants and indoor air quality, 286
   "screen apnea," 282
   sinusitis, 160, 234, 284–86
   smokers and, 279–82
   stuffy air and brain fog, 282
Respiratory strength training, 187
Respiratory syncytial virus (RSV), 207–8
   vaccine, 200, 207
Respiratory tract infections, 275–76
Restorative health, 287–306
Restylane, 4
Retatrutide, 158
Retinol, 3–4
Reynaud's disease, 291
Rheumatoid arthritis
   carpal tunnel and, 257
   COVID-19 and, 202
   DMARDs for, 272
   DXA scan, 260
   exercise for, 251–53
   gender differences, 237
   gum disease and, 23
   hands and, 9–10
   NSAIDs for, 239
   smoking and, 279
   SNRIs for, 243
   vitamin D for, 229
Rhodiola rosea, 231
Ringworm, 205
Rocking Horse, 132
Rocky Mountain Spotted Fever, 210
Rotavirus, 210, 250
Running (runners), 104, 129, 140
Rybelsus, 73–74, 158

S

Saccharin, 83, 117
St. John's Wort, 162
Salt, 9, 119
   CKD and, 215
   hypertension and, 185, 186, 188
   substitutes, 119
SARSCoV-2, 200, 202
Saturated fats, 123, 125, 126, 218, 252
Sauerkraut, 312, 314
Saunas, 8, 46, 289, 290–91, 295
Schizophrenia, 93, 109, 223
Sciatica, 247, 248
Scotomas, 15, 19
Scrambler therapy, 244
"Screen apnea," 282

Screen time
　bedtime routine, 287–88
　eye problems, 18
Seasonal rhythms, 297–99
Second opinions, 142, 144
　back surgery, 248
　cancer, 63
　osteoporosis, 261
　palliative care, 172
Sedentary time, 5, 57, 138–39. *See also* Sitting
Seizures, 48–49
Selective mutism, 48
Semaglutide, 157–59, 189. *See also* Ozempic
Sense of purpose, 4–5, 5, 98
Serotonin, 111, 112, 128, 243, 251
Serotonin and norepinephrine reuptake inhibitors (SNRIs), 243
Serotonin reuptake inhibitors (SSRIs), 14, 155, 162
Sertraline (Zoloft), 162
Setbacks and mistakes, 105
Sex
　before bed, 310
　cannabis and, 309–10
　intimacy and relationships, 310
　pain during, 308
Sexually transmitted infections (STIs), 308–9
Shingles, 189–91
Shingles vaccination, 37, 189–91, 201–2
Short-chain fatty acids, 221–22
Siberian ginseng, 231
Sibling relationships, 91–93
Sideways Walking, 137
Sinusitis, 160, 234, 284–86
Sitting
　exercise and, 138–39
　posture, 94, 130
Sit-to-stand tests, 12
Situational-environmental phobias, 103
Skin cancer, 67–69
　biomarkers, 72
Skin care, anti-aging serums, 3–4
Skin lightening products, 310–11
Sleep, 287–91
　asthma and, 277
　bedtime routine, 287–88, 300
　for brain health, 45
　cannabis and, 306
　circadian rhythms, 129–30, 239, 299–301
　for concussions, 20–21
　cooling pillows, 288–89
　for COVID-19, 203–4
　for depression, 94, 95–96
　diabetes and, 77, 81–82
　exercise for, 129–30
　gratitude and, 6
　for heartburn, 168
　for heart health, 180
　hypertension and, 184–85
　ideal temperature, 288
　inhaling fragrances during, 236
　melatonin and, 235–36, 288
　pain and, 238
　PVCs and, 176
　seasonal shifts, 297–98
　sex before bed, 310
　signs of sleepiness, 305
　weight loss and, 116–17
Sleep apnea, 21, 152, 159, 203, 277–78, 294
Sleep paralysis, 293–94

Sleep problems (insomnia)
　A-fib and, 175
　alcohol and, 184–85, 294, 301
　diabetes and, 77
　hypertension and, 184–85
　obesity and, 21, 77, 82, 116–17
　pain and, 238
　stroke risk, 195
　suicide risk and, 97
Small vessel disease (SVD), 37–39
Smartphones. *See also* Apps
　temperature check, 153
Smartwatches, heart monitors, 151–52
Smoking, 279–81
　Alzheimer's disease and, 34
　brain health and, 45
　heart disease and, 198
　how to quit, 280–81
　kidney disease and, 214
　lung cancer and, 57, 171, 196, 280, 281
　pain and, 246
　pneumonia and, 200
　PVCs and, 176
Smoothies, 120–21, 211
Snacks (snacking), 2, 76, 81, 118, 234, 281, 292
Snoring, 277
　mouth exercises for, 278
Snow shoveling, 268
Socializing (social support), 101–2
　aging and, 29–30
　for dementia, 43
　for depression, 94, 95, 97, 98
　eating together, 116
　post-stroke, 196
　seasonal shifts, 299
Social learning, 103
Social media, 165
Sorbitol, 85, 312
Sore throats, 146, 207, 234–35, 250
Sourdough, 3
Spicy foods, 211, 250
Spinal cord stimulation, 245
Spinal fusion, 248–49
Spinal stenosis, 247, 248
Squamous cell carcinoma (SCC), 67–69
Squats, 134, 135, 265, 266
SSRIs (serotonin reuptake inhibitors), 14, 155, 162
Stair climbing, 178
Standing desks, 138
State Health Insurance Program (SHIP), 26
Statins, 174, 178, 306
　alternatives, 189
Stem cells
　gray hair and, 18
　procyanidins and, 232
Steroid drugs, 276
　safety, 167
Stomach pain, 249–51
　drug side effects, 158
Stomach paralysis, 159
Stomach viruses, 211, 249–50
Strength training, 11, 133–35, 140, 187, 244, 246, 262
Strep throat, 208
Stress
　A-fib and, 175
　aging and, 6, 7–8, 26
　exercise for, 128–29
　genes and, 295
　from gray hair, 109–10
　heart health and, 180

　herbs for, 231
　hypertension and, 187
　medical trauma, 107–9
　metabolic syndrome and, 87–88
　noise and, 22
　online scams and, 107
　pain and, 238–39
　pets and, 224
　prebiotics for, 223
　PTSD, 107–8, 224, 239
　sense of purpose, 5
　supplements for, 228
　tinnitus and, 52
　to-do lists and, 106
Strokes, 194–98
　asthma and, 277
　blood pressure, 185
　diet and, 84, 122–23
　ER visits, 146
　noise and, 21
　obesity and drugs, 157
　plateau myth, 196
　post-stroke recovery, 194–96
　radon exposure and, 196–97
　sleep and, 21
　VEGF and, 16
　vitamin D and clots, 229
Sucralose, 83, 117
Sugar alcohols, 83, 84–85, 120
Sugar and diabetes, 82–84
Suicide, 96–99, 100
　warning signs, 97
Sumatriptan (Tosymra), 241
Sunburn, 167, 210, 242
Sundowning, 54
Sun exposure, 68, 209
　drug interactions, 167
Sunflower seeds, 119
Sunscreen, 67, 209
Superfoods, 118–19
Supplements, 226–30. *See also* specific supplements
　for bones, 227, 264
　brain health and, 44–46
　for gene repair, 296–97
　for osteoporosis, 160
　quality of, 228
　unsafe, 159–60
Support groups, 43, 97, 100, 196, 214, 267
Suprachiasmatic nucleus (SCN), 300, 303–4
Surgery
　errors, 147–48, 159
　high-intensity interval training before, 164
　rejections by surgeons, 165
Swallowing difficulties, 42, 169, 195, 208, 249, 251
Sweating, 129, 139, 206, 212, 251
Swedish massages, 231
Sweet foods, 2–3, 82–84, 112
Swimming, 246, 267, 299
　safety tips, 210
　water exercise, 130–33
Symptom diary, 143–44
Synapses, 32
Syncope, 176, 177, 181

T

Tahini, 119
Tai chi, 253, 267
Targeted cancer therapies, 62, 65, 70–71
Tea, 2, 85, 116, 222, 224, 234, 236, 313

Index

Teeth grinding, 52
Temporomandibular joint (TMJ), 52
Tendon Gliding Exercises, 10
Thermometer apps, 153
Thiopurines, 154
Thrombosis, 148, 229
Thumb C Isometric (exercise), 11
Thumb Opposition with Finger Slide, 11
Thymus gland, 72
Ticks, 210
Time, perception of, 301–3
Timed up-and-go tests, 12
Time-restricted eating, 301–2, 304
Tinnitus, 21, 50–52, 164
    CBD for, 51
Tiredness, 305
Tirzepatide, 158
To-do lists, 106
Toe pain, walking shoes for, 129
Tomatoes, canned, 118, 119
Touch (touching), 5–6, 310
Towel Stretches, 254
Toxic metals, 123–24
Transient ischemic attacks (TIAs), 48
Trans-vaccenic acid (TVA), 63
Trastuzumab (Herceptin), 70–71
Traumatic brain injuries (TBIs), 18–19, 46–47, 97
Traumatic conditioning, 103
Travel health, 209–10
Tree Pose, 262, 263
Tretinoin (Retin-A), 4
Tricyclic antidepressants, 14
Trigger point massages, 231
Triglycerides, 177–78
Trospium chloride, 43
Truffles, 126
Tulsi, 231
Turmeric, 2, 45, 116, 118, 222
TVs, and bedtime routine, 287–88, 301
Twisting Mogul, 132–33
Type 2 diabetes. *See* Diabetes

U

Ubrogepant (Ubrelvy), 241
UGT1A1, 154
Ulcerative colitis, 30, 167, 251, 313
Ulcers, 149, 233, 236, 240, 270, 272
    stomach pain and, 250
Ultra-processed foods, 69–70, 214, 222, 298
Universities, free tuition for older students, 27
Urgent-care centers, 147
Urinary tract infections (UTIs), 42, 215–17, 228
    E. coli and, 215–16
    gepotidacin for, 216–17

Urination
    painful (dysuria), 217
    UTIs and, 216

V

Vaccinations (vaccines)
    Alzheimer's disease and, 37
    COVID-19, 200
    pneumonia, 199–200, 207–8
    RSV, 200, 207
    shingles, 37, 189–91, 201–2
    skin cancer, 69
Vagal rebound, 7
Vaping, 281–82
Varicose veins, 314
Vascular endothelial growth factor (VEGF), 16
Vegetables. *See* Fruits and vegetables
Vegetarian (and vegan) diet, 1–2, 180–81, 230
Venlafaxine (Effexor), 243
Verrucae, 255
Veterinary care, 225
Vibrating capsule for constipation, 312
Vicarious learning, 103
Video calls, 102
Visceral fat. *See* Belly fat
Vision (eyesight), 6
    driving and, 27
    foods boosting, 15
Vision loss, 14–17, 19
Vitamin B, 45, 125, 207–8, 227
Vitamin C, 118, 119, 127, 207, 231, 234, 272
Vitamin D
    for bone health, 260
    diabetes risk, 80
    health benefits of, 227–30
    sun exposure, 129, 229
Vitamin D deficiencies, 36, 227, 228–30
Vitamin E, 45
    for brain health, 44, 227
Vitamin K-2, 227
Voice pitch and diabetes, 88
Volunteering, 98, 102, 239, 303
Vonoprazan, 170

W

Walking, 5, 34, 35, 76–77, 128–30
    difficulty, and fracture risk, 140
    post-stroke, 195
    steps, 136, 179
Walking-pace tests, 11–12
Walking pneumonia, 199–200
Walking shoes, 129, 253–54
"Warmlines," 99–100
Warrior II Pose, 263
Watercress, 127

Water exercise, 130–33
Water intake. *See* Hydration
Water Running, 132
Webspace Massage, 11
Wegovy, 73–74, 114–15, 121–22, 157–59, 189, 219, 241
Weight loss, 113–17
    benefits of five percent, 116
    exercise and, 130
    finding best program, 113–15
    gallstones and, 218
    genetic testing and, 114
    GLP-1 agonists, 114–15, 121–22
    for heartburn, 168
    heart disease and, 198
    for heart health, 180
    for hypertension, 186
    medications for, 114–15, 157–59, 189
    for migraines, 241
    power of mind, 292
    for prediabetes, 77
    sleep for, 116–17
    surgery and cancer, 63–64
    surgery and diabetes, 85
White blood cells, 207, 217, 224, 252, 271, 276
White matter hyperintensity (WMH), 37–38
White noise, 23, 51
Whole grains, 3, 47, 76, 78, 95, 111, 125, 180, 218, 226, 272, 311
Winter hazards, 268–70
Wood smoke, 53, 275
Workouts. *See* Exercise
Wound care centers, 271
Wounds, 270–70
Wrist Isometrics, 11
Writing pens, 9–10

X

Xylitol, 83, 85, 312
Xyloglucan, 222

Y

Yerba santa, 208
Yoga, 180
    for bone health, 261–64
    for migraines, 241
    for stress, 52
Yogurt, 2, 84, 121, 122, 123, 211, 229, 236, 312

Z

Zantac, 167–68
Zavegepant (Zavzpret), 239, 241
Zeaxanthin, 15, 17